TRAUMATIC DISSOCIATION

Neurobiology and Treatment

Edited by

ERIC VERMETTEN, M.D., PH.D.

MARTIN J. DORAHY, PH.D.

DAVID SPIEGEL, M.D.

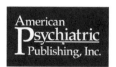

Washington, DC
London, England

Books published by American Psychiatric Publishing, Inc. (APPI), represent the views and opinions of the individual authors and do not necessarily represent the policies and opinions of APPI or the American Psychiatric Association.

To buy 25–99 copies of any APPI title, you are eligible for a 20% discount; please contact APPI Customer Service at appi@psych.org or 800-368-5777. For 100 or more copies of the same title, please e-mail us at bulksales@psych.org for a price quote.

Manufactured in the United States of America on acid-free paper
11 10 09 08 07   5 4 3 2 1
First Edition

Typeset in Adobe's Palatino and Futura.

American Psychiatric Publishing, Inc., 1000 Wilson Boulevard, Arlington, VA 22209-3901, www.appi.org

Library of Congress Cataloging-in-Publication Data
Traumatic dissociation : neurobiology and treatment / edited by Eric Vermetten, Martin J. Dorahy, David Spiegel. — 1st ed.
    p. ; cm.
    Includes bibliographical references and index.
    ISBN 978-1-58562-196-5 (pbk. : alk. paper)
    1. Dissociation (Psychology) 2. Psychic trauma. 3. Dissociative disorders. 4. Post-traumatic stress disorder. I. Vermetten, Eric, 1961– II. Dorahy, Martin J., 1971– III. Spiegel, David, 1945– IV. American Psychiatric Publishing.
    [DNLM: 1. Dissociative Disorders. 2. Dissociative Disorders—therapy. 3. Neurobiology—methods. 4. Neuropsychology—methods. 5. Stress Disorders, Post-Traumatic—complications. WM 173.6 T777 2007]

RC553.D5T735 2007
616.85′21—
dc22   2006036479

British Library Cataloguing in Publication Data
A CIP record is available from the British Library.

CONTENTS

Part 1

Conceptual Domain of Dissociation

Part II

Neurobiology of Traumaand Dissociation

Part III

Contemporary Implications for Assessment and Treatment

CONTRIBUTORS

Judith Armstrong, Ph.D.
Private Practice and Clinical Associate Professor, Department of Psychology, University of Southern California, Los Angeles, California

David M. Benedek, M.D.
Associate Professor, Department of Psychiatry and Center for the Study of Traumatic Stress, Uniformed Services University of the Health Sciences, Bethesda, Maryland

Marian J. Bakermans-Kranenburg, Ph.D.
Associate Professor, Centre for Child and Family Studies, Leiden University, The Netherlands

Robyn Bluhm, M.A.
Postdoctoral Fellow in Neuropsychiatry, Departments of Psychiatry and Philosophy, University of Western Ontario, London, Ontario, Canada

Martin Bohus, M.D., Ph.D.
Professor of Psychiatry, Psychosomatic Medicine, and Psychotherapy, University of Heidelberg, Germany; Department of Psychosomatic Medicine and Psychotherapy, Central Institute of Mental Health, Mannheim, Germany

J. Douglas Bremner, M.D.
Associate Professor of Psychiatry and Radiology, Department of Psychiatry and Radiology, Emory University School of Medicine; Emory Center for Positron Emission Tomography, Emory University Hospital; Mental Health Research, Atlanta VAMC, Atlanta, Georgia

John Briere, Ph.D.
Associate Professor of Psychiatry and Psychology, Keck School of Medicine, University of Southern California, Los Angeles, California

James A. Chu, M.D.
Chief of Hospital Clinical Services, McLean Hospital; Associate Professor of Psychiatry, Harvard Medical School, Boston, Massachusetts

Laurence Claes, Ph.D.
Professor, Department of Psychology, Catholic University of Leuven, Belgium

E. Ronald de Kloet, Ph.D.
Professor of Medical Pharmacology, Department of Medical Pharmacology, Leiden University Medical Center/Leiden Academic Center for Drug Research, Leiden University, The Netherlands

Johan A. den Boer, M.D., Ph.D.
Professor of Biological Psychiatry, Department of Psychiatry, Academic Hospital Groningen, Groningen, The Netherlands

Martin J. Dorahy, Ph.D.
Clinical Research Psychologist, The Trauma Resource Centre, North and West Belfast Health and Social Services Trust, Belfast; Research Tutor, School of Psychology, The Queen's University of Belfast, Belfast, Northern Ireland

Carol S. Fullerton, Ph.D.
Professor (Research), Department of Psychiatry; Associate Director, Center for the Study of Traumatic Stress, Uniformed Services University of the Health Sciences, Bethesda, Maryland

Dorith Harari, M.D.
Staff Psychiatrist, Altrecht Mental Health Services; University Medical Center, Utrecht, The Netherlands

Gary Hazlett, Psy.D.
Woodward-Cody Specialty Consulting, LLC.; Former selection and assessment psychologist, U.S. Army Special Operations Command, Fort Bragg, North Carolina

Rafaële J. C. Huntjens, Ph.D.
Assistant Professor, Department of Clinical and Developmental Psychology, University of Groningen, Groningen, The Netherlands

Richard P. Kluft, M.D.
Private Practice in Psychiatry and Psychoanalysis, Bala Cynwyd; Associate Clinical Professor, Department of Psychiatry, Temple University School of Medicine, Philadelphia Center for Psychoanalysis, Philadelphia, Pennsylvania

Ruth A. Lanius, M.D., Ph.D.
Harris-Woodman Chair in Psyche and Soma, Departments of Psychiatry and Neuroscience, University of Western Ontario, London, Ontario, Canada

Ulrich Lanius, Ph.D.
Psychologist, Department of Psychology, Royal Columbian Hospital, New Westminister, British Columbia, Canada

Richard J. Loewenstein, M.D.
Medical Director, Trauma Disorders Sheppard Pratt Health System; Associate Clinical Professor, Department of Psychiatry, University of Maryland School of Medicine, Baltimore, Maryland

Charles R. Marmar, M.D.
Professor in Residence and Vice Chair, Department of Psychiatry, University of California, San Francisco, California

C. Andrew Morgan III, M.D., M.A.
Departments of Psychiatry and History of Medicine, Yale University School of Medicine, New Haven and National Center for Post Traumatic Stress Disorder, VA Connecticut, West Haven, Connecticut

Ellert R. S. Nijenhuis, Ph.D.
Psychologist, Psychotherapist, and Researcher, Outpatient Department of Psychiatry of Mental Health Care Drenthe, Assen, The Netherlands

Thomas Rinne, M.D., Ph.D.
Psychiatrist and Medical Director, Pieter Baan Center, Forensic Psychiatric Observation Clinic of the Netherlands Department of Justice, Utrecht, The Netherlands

Christian Schmahl, M.D., Ph.D.
Assistant Medical Director, Department of Psychosomatic Medicine and Psychotherapy, Central Institute of Mental Health, Mannheim, Germany

Daphne Simeon, M.D.
Associate Professor of Psychiatry, Department Psychiatry, Mount Sinai
School of Medicine, New York, New York

Steven M. Southwick, M.D.
Professor of Psychiatry, Department of Psychiatry, Yale University
School of Medicine, New Haven, Connecticut; National Center for
PTSD, VA Connecticut, West Haven, Connecticut

David Spiegel, M.D.
Jack, Lulu and Sam Wilson Professor, School of Medicine; Associate
Chair, Psychiatry and Behavioral Sciences; Medical Director, Center for
Integrative Medicine, Stanford University, Stanford, California

George Steffian, Ph.D.
U.S. Navy Survival, Evasion, Resistance, and Escape Psychologist,
Brunswick NAS Maine, United States

Robert J. Ursano, M.D.
Professor of Psychiatry, Department of Psychiatry and Center for the
Study of Traumatic Stress, Uniformed Services University of the Health
Sciences, Bethesda, Maryland

Walter Vandereycken, M.D., Ph.D.
Professor of Psychiatry, Department of Psychiatry, Catholic University
of Leuven, Belgium

Onno van der Hart, Ph.D.
Professor, Psychopathology of Chronic Traumatization, Department of
Clinical Psychology, Utrecht University, Utrecht, The Netherlands

Johan Vanderlinden, Ph.D.
Academic Consultant and Psychologist, University Center St. Joseph,
Kortenberg; Department of Psychology, Catholic University of Leuven,
Belgium

Marinus J. van IJzendoorn, Ph.D.
Professor of Child and Family Studies, Centre for Child and Family
Studies, Leiden University, The Netherlands

Eric Vermetten, M.D., Ph.D.
Head of Research, Military Mental Health, Central Military Hospital,
and Associate Professor of Psychiatry at the University Medical Center
Utrecht in Utrecht, the Netherlands

DISCLOSURE OF COMPETING INTERESTS

The following contributors to this book have indicated a financial interest in or other affiliation with a commercial supporter, a manufacturer of a commercial product, a provider of a commercial service, a nongovernmental organization, and/or a government agency, as listed below:

John Briere, Ph.D.—*Product royalties:* Psychological Assessment Resources.

E. Ronald de Kloet, Ph.D.—*Scientific Advisory Board Member:* Corcept Therapeutics, Inc.

PREFACE

In this impressive volume on traumatic dissociation, Drs. Vermetten, Dorahy, and Spiegel have assembled contributions by leading authorities on theoretical models, neurobiology, and treatment. The book provides a road map to the long and complex history of the field of traumatic dissociation as well as a balanced and lively dialogue on controversies in etiology and classification. New data are reviewed on phenomenological and biological contributions that point towards a revised nosology, emphasizing psychobiologically informed phenotypes. The volume is also forward looking, setting an agenda and mapping new directions in research for understanding and treating one of the most complex and important topics in mental health.

Among the critical issues raised in this volume is the controversy regarding whether dissociation at the time of a traumatic event (including depersonalization and derealization) represents a defensive strategy whose purpose is to protect the trauma victim from overwhelming threat or a threat-driven failure of defense in which unmanageable levels of terror, horror, and helplessness interfere with integration of sensory, psychological, and biological responses. Stated differently, does peritraumatic dissociation protect against panic during a perceived threat to life or does panic overwhelm coping capacities thereby leading to altered processing of the traumatic event? This is a crucial question given recent animal and human research that sustained states of threat-driven arousal, resulting in greater fear conditioning and memory consolidation. New data emerging from studies of police officers evaluated before and after the World Trade Center attacks (Marmar et al. 2006) reveal that peritraumatic dissociation is strongly positively associated with peritraumatic panic and that both pretraumatic dissociation and peritraumatic panic independently contribute to the explanation of symptoms of posttraumatic stress disorder (PTSD) 18 months after the attacks. These findings are consistent with those of Gershuny and Thayer (1999) and Sterlini and Bryant (2002): anxious arousal associated with fear of death and fear of loss of control are central to triggering dissociative reactions and at variance with a long-held view that peritraumatic dissociation protects against immediate peritraumatic panic. Indeed, Koopman et al. (1994) found that peritraumatic dissociative symptoms not only correlated positively with anxiety but predicted the later development of PTSD. However, peritraumatic dissociation may serve to terminate runaway terror and be associated with lower levels of psychophysiological arousal with subsequent reminders.

Another important question discussed in this book regards the nature of the developing child's self-regulation of emotion. Emotion regulation is emerging as a key moderator in the relationship between perceived threat and emotional reactivity at the time of traumatic exposure and the issue is examined here from the point of view of attachment. The interesting possibility of different hypothalamic-pituitary-adrenal (HPA) axis patterns in PTSD versus chronic dissociation is also explored through the review of primate studies of maternal deprivation, which support the notion of long-term, enhanced stress reactivity to adult stressors following early maternal deprivation: early stress increases corticotropin releasing factor responses, leading to increased hippocampal glucocorticoid receptor expression, which in turn leads to greater stressor responses with subsequent exposures.

Novel directions in the study of traumatic dissociation, especially around cerebellar functioning, are reviewed. While studies using magnetic resonance spectroscopy and magnetic resonance imaging support a role for hippocampal abnormalities of a heritable or acquired nature in PTSD, cerebellar studies represent an important direction for understanding trauma-related dissociation. Intact cerebellar functions are important for procedural aspects of spatial memory whereas hippocampal functions are important for declarative spatial memory. The central role of memory in the study of traumatic dissociation is also addressed in this volume, and an important distinction is made between episodic memory retrieval driven by a sense of agency and the intrusive and unbidden emergence of trauma memories that cause PTSD patients to be retraumatized. Those who master trauma are able to dive into the sea of traumatic reminiscence while those with PTSD are drowning.

A scholarly overview of translational research issues and dissociation is undertaken, as well as an exploration of psychobiological phenotypes of trauma-related dissociation. This volume also reviews the results of fascinating new work using functional brain imaging with preliminary support for phenotypes consistent with a model of primary, secondary, and tertiary dissociation originally proposed by van der Kolk et al. (1996). The primary, secondary, and tertiary dissociation distinctions may now be reconceptualized as three different phenotypes important in the understanding of trauma-related dissociation: a highly anxious arousal pattern of responding to traumatic exposure best captured by measures of peritraumatic panic; a pattern of responding to trauma with depersonalization, derealization, altered body image, tunnel vision, and other aspects best captured by measures of peritraumatic dissociation; and a pattern of responding to early and repeated trauma inflicted by parental and other caretaking figures resulting in breaches of trust and fragmentation of ego states, best captured by measures of dissociative identity development. A structural model of traumatic dissociation is reviewed with relevance for the dissociative identity disorder phenotype.

Traumatic Dissociation: Neurobiology and Treatment concludes with an excellent and practical description of advances in the assessment and treatment of trauma-related dissociation by leading researchers and clinicians. Chief among the critical contributions are the notions that 1) PTSD-related hippocampal atrophy and associated neurocognitive impairment is reversible with selective serotonin reuptake inhibitor treatment, 2) the current diagnostic schema does not appropriately address the experiences of clinicians who treat patients with trauma-related dissociation, and 3) the treatment of traumatic dissociation should be psychotherapeutically driven and supported by pharmacotherapy where possible. This work proceeds from careful phenomenological and neurobiological studies to articulate the application of this knowledge in treatment. It provides a model for integrating dissociation into our current understanding and treatment of trauma-related disorders.

Charles R. Marmar, M.D

REFERENCES

Gershuny BS, Thayer JF: Relations among psychological trauma, dissociative phenomena, and trauma-related distress: a review and integration. Clin Psychol Rev 19:631–657, 1999
Koopman C, Classen C, Spiegel D: Predictors of posttraumatic stress symptoms among survivors of the Oakland/Berkeley, Calif., firestorm. Am J Psychiatry 151:888–894, 1994
Marmar CR, McCaslin SE, Metzler TJ, et al: Predictors of posttraumatic stress in police and other first responders. Ann N Y Acad Sci 1071:1–18, 2006
Sterlini GL, Bryant RA: Hyperarousal and dissociation: a study of novice skydivers. Behav Res Ther 40:431–437, 2002

van der Kolk, BA, van der Hart O, Marmar C: Dissociation and information processing in posttraumatic stress disorder, in Traumatic Stress. Edited by van der Kolk BA, McFarlane AC, Weisaeth L. New York, Guilford, 1996, pp 303–327

INTRODUCTION

Traumatic dissociation is that type of dissociation that occurs as a direct result of traumatic stress. Unlike dissociation evident during hypnosis, for example, this form of dissociation is a response to or by-product of exposure to trauma. Dissociation in this context can manifest as a symptom, as a process (i.e., failed integration of incoming information), or as a pattern of personality organization. Traumatic dissociation as any of these manifestations is evident in several trauma-related disorders, including acute stress disorder, posttraumatic stress disorder (PTSD), and the dissociative disorders. Although developments in theoretically and empirically based treatments of traumatic dissociation are predicated on recent developments in our understanding of the construct, a greater understanding of traumatic dissociation can also be obtained from clinical progress in treatment models and strategies. This bidirectional interaction between understanding and treatment reflects the underlying view and organization of this book.

In recent times significant steps have been taken in the understanding and treatment of traumatic dissociation. Our understanding of the disorder has been facilitated by 1) advances in neuroimaging technology; 2) developments in empirically based investigation tools, strategies, and methodologies; and 3) a willingness on behalf of mainstream researchers and theoreticians to acknowledge the importance of traumatic dissociation in psychopathology and to investigate its underpinnings. Treatment advancements have come from a greater recognition of traumatic dissociation in the clinic and a desire to effectively treat it either by developing specific treatment models or techniques or by adapting existing models to fit the latent and manifest clinical content. However, despite these advances, the construct of dissociation more broadly, and traumatic dissociation in particular, remains relatively elusive.

Consequently, the chapters in the first part of the book, "Conceptual Domain of Dissociation," explore historical, conceptual, and theoretical issues and how other domains of investigation (e.g., attachment theory, cognitive psychology) have been applied to the study of traumatic dissociation. The second part, "Neurobiology of Trauma and Dissociation," focuses specifically on how neurobiological investigations have studied and understood dissociation. The last part, "Contemporary Implications for Assessment and Treatment," explores issues pertinent for the assessment and treatment of traumatic dissociation.

Dorahy and van der Hart begin the book with an examination of the relationship between trauma and dissociation in the dissociation literature. Taking a historical perspective, they survey the literature from the commencement of the study of dissociation to contemporary times. In examining this association, they differentiate three discrete variables, one relating to trauma (exposure to traumatic stress) and two relating to dissociation (the dissociative structure or organization of the personality and dissociative phenomena). In examining the dynamic relationship between these three variables, they argue that four categories are evident in the literature. The first, dissociation per se, attributes no connection between trauma and either dissociative structure or phenomena. The second, structural dissociation, dissociative phenomena, and unacknowledged trauma, makes an association between dissociative structure and phenomena, but no link is made to the traumatic histories evident in each case profile. The third relational category between trauma, dissociative structure, and dissociative phenomena evident in the literature makes little reference to dissociative structure while explicitly linking trauma and dissociative phenomena (trauma and dissociative symptoms). The final category, trauma, dissociative structure, and dissociative symptoms, suggests that trauma exposure leads to structural divisions in the personality that, in turn, generate dissociative symptoms.

Harari and colleagues provide a review of the attachment literature in Chapter 2, with particular emphasis on the association between disorganized attachment and dissociation. After outlining the three organized types of attachment (secure, insecure-avoidant, insecure-ambivalent) as classified by the Strange Situation Procedure, they detail the more recently identified disorganized attachment style. Examining the etiological pathways to attachment disorganization, they note the importance of frightened and frightening primary caregiver behavior, but they also acknowledge the possibility of a constitutional basis for this type of attachment and provide an overview of the findings from genetic studies. In examining the link between trauma, disorganized attachment, and dissociative disorders, they point out that the available evidence indicates that the link between disorganized attachment and dissociation is mediated by trauma.

Chapter 3 presents a review of the cognitive experimental findings on attention and memory functioning in dissociative identity disorder (DID). Starting with an overview of the attentional processes and memory systems that make up human information processing, Dorahy and Huntjens present the cognitive avoidance hypothesis, which has been proffered as an explanation for psychoform amnesia. They then explore the small experimental literature on working memory and attentional functioning in DID using the larger PTSD literature as a guide. In moving along the information processing stream, they then provide a précis of the experimental literature on memory functioning within and between dissociative identities. In light of contemporary, well-designed studies they indicate that rather than objective memory retrieval deficits, the amnesia in DID may be related to dynamic processes that operate late in the memory system to keep information from being experienced as autobiographically relevant.

A review of the relationship between dissociation and PTSD is discussed by Simeon in Chapter 4. She suggests that four models can be identified to account for the association. The first model (comorbidity) views PTSD and dissociation as separate entities that may co-occur because of the nosological link to a common etiological factor (i.e., traumatic stress). The second model (shared risk factors) suggests that the link between PTSD and dissociation is through a common psychological and/or biological vulnerability (i.e., a diathesis). The third model (shared pathogenesis) posits that PTSD and dissociation have common pathogenetic mechanisms that are activated by trauma. The final model (same disorder) suggests that PTSD and dissociation are inseparable, with the current nosology unnecessarily creating artificial distinctions between them. While acknowledging that no model effectively accounts for the relationship between PTSD and dissociation, Simeon concludes that the first model, comorbidity, best captures the current data.

Vermetten and Spiegel conclude the first section with an examination of how the hypnosis literature provides a greater understanding of perceptual processing and traumatic stress. They describe hypnosis as controlled dissociation and describe dissociation as a form of self-hypnosis. The phenomenon of hypnotic influence requires a specific orientation to mind-body relations, and both hypnosis and dissociation could well be viewed as vehicles for altered control over neurophysiological and peripheral somatic functions. In search of the locus of control in the involuntary hypnotic response, they provide illustrations of studies in which persons in hypnosis are able to modulate perceptual awareness in the sensory, visual, or acoustic domains. This ability to alter perception in hypnosis can affect a sense of agency, which is disrupted as well (but with far less control) during traumatic experience. In their view, controlled dissociation using hypnosis can be a useful tool in treating the aftermath of traumatic experience, including traumatic dissociation.

Schmahl and Bohus open the second part of the book by outlining and arguing for a translational research program to better understand the correlates and mechanisms of dissociation. This program seeks to develop analogous operational definitions and multilevel indicators of dissociation in animals and humans so that experiments and findings from animal research can be translated to humans. Schmahl and Bohus highlight the importance of such a research methodology but also describe some of the difficulties in achieving it. For example, one hurdle pertains to finding an adequate experimental induction procedure (i.e., pharmacological, electrophysiological, or psychological) for dissociation. They also outline how a translational research program of dissociation could be achieved.

In Chapter 7, de Kloet and Rinne describe neuroendocrine alterations associated with stress. By reviewing the experimental literature on such changes in rodents across the life span, they note the relationship between these findings and endocrine alterations identified in PTSD and dissociative disorders. They then outline central questions drawn from the animal literature that may promote a greater understanding of the developmental effects of deprivation and trauma on PTSD.

Morgan and colleagues review a series of prospective studies on dissociation in healthy individuals in Chapter 8. Their work involved recruiting military personnel during stressful training courses and indicates that dissociative symptoms in response to extreme stress, which are often considered pathological, are common in healthy adults. However, according to these studies, "baseline" dissociation (i.e., dissociative experiences prior to acute stress) in healthy adults is related to deficits in working memory functioning and is associated with a reduced capacity for neuropeptide Y release during stress, among other biological factors.

In Chapter 9, Ursano and colleagues discuss new research findings linking cerebellar functioning to specific peritraumatic experiences. After presenting an overview of peritraumatic dissociative symptoms and their frequency, they argue that the cerebellum may be intimately connected to alterations in the sense of time and space perception, both of which are common dissociative reactions during traumatic events. They also highlight the role that the cerebellum plays in the formation of fear memories and, consequently, PTSD.

In Chapter 10, Lanius and colleagues review script-driven neuroimaging studies of PTSD and dissociative disorders. With particular reference to their own series of studies, which identify neurobiological differences between hyperarousal/flashback/reliving responses to trauma cues in PTSD and dissociative responses, they outline key brain areas and their connectivity that distinguish both responses. They suggest that results support the view of two distinct types of PTSD, one characterized by intrusions and hyperarousal and the other by dissociation. They also point out that some individuals with PTSD can experience both responses to trauma at different times. The authors argue that imaging studies that unwittingly combine these types of PTSD in one sample are likely to produce unclear, heterogeneous, neurobiological results.

Nijenhuis and den Boer open Chapter 11 with a brief summary of the structural dissociation of the personality model, arguing that this framework provides an understanding of the variable psychobiological research findings in traumatized individuals. They suggest that different dissociative parts of the personality have different neurobiological underpinnings, and they proceed to outline the functional neurobiological differences between these dissociative parts. In integrating this model with Porges's polyvagal theory, they review the neurobiological and psychophysiological literatures. They conclude that between- and within-patient variations in experimental findings are consistent with the theoretical formulations posited by structural dissociation theory that neurobiological and physiological functioning is dependent on which dissociative part of the personality is assessed.

Bremner and Vermetten open the third part of the book by briefly outlining the history and division of PTSD and the dissociative disorders in the psychiatric literature, especially in DSM. They note that although dissociation may underlie both sets of psychiatric presentations, the conceptualization of dissociative symptoms in PTSD and the dissociative disorders is different and confusing in DSM. This lack of clarity disguises the overlapping nature of the dissociative symptom complex in these disorders. In exploring this overlapping nature, the authors turn to neurobiological studies in both PTSD and the dissociative disorders. Their review includes studies of hippocampal volume along with the operation of the noradrenergic and cortisol systems. They note the association between brain areas in PTSD and dissociation and argue that the hippocampus plays a central role in dissociative symptoms. They conclude by calling for a reorganization of the diagnostic criteria for anxiety and dissociative disorders so they reflect the association between trauma, dissociation, and PTSD.

Noting the complex relationship between trauma and dissociation, Briere and Armstrong in Chapter 13 outline some of the important issues to consider when planning assessment of traumatic dissociation (e.g., problems with nonstructured clinician assessment). They then critique the primary empirically supported standardized measures of traumatic dissociation, breaking the review into three broad categories: semistructured interviews, self-report measures, and projective tests. They conclude with the important caveat that failure to detect dissociation at one assessment point in traumatized individuals may not indicate poor sensitivity on the part of the assessment tool. Rather, detection difficulties may relate to the often elusive nature of dissociation and its interaction with other dimensions of personality, the environment, and treatment.

In Chapter 14, Loewenstein outlines and discusses both the sociocognitive and trauma models of DID, noting their central characteristics. He examines the term *iatrogenesis* and its use in general medicine and psychiatry, exploring how the term relates to, but is differentiated from, terms such as *misdiagnosis*. Taking another term widely utilized in sociocognitive discussions of dissociation, *suggestibility,* he notes its many uses and reviews data indicating that one form of suggestibility may not be correlated with other forms of suggestibility. Loewenstein then examines the empirical data on the association between borderline personality disorder (BPD) and DID, countering the argument that DID is misdiagnosed BPD. The chapter concludes with a discussion of the fact that, like other psychiatric conditions, DID is influenced by interpersonal, social, and cultural factors that alone cannot explain the disorder but that are central to its presentation.

In Chapter 15, Kluft takes Tomkins's innate affect theory and its clinical application as outlined by Nathanson and explores the important contribution it can make in the understanding and treatment of DID. With particular reference to shame, Kluft examines the four scripts that have been identified in the management of shame and how these can manifest as dissociative (alter) identities in DID. Utilizing clinical material, he outlines the pervasive ways in which shame management scripts can embody alters and the importance of therapeutically dealing with these scripts and their auxiliary affects, especially before engaging in trauma processing work. He reminds the reader of the importance of mastery and competence as antidotes to shame.

In Chapter 16, Vanderlinden and colleagues examine the association between child abuse and neglect and the development of an eating disorder. They note the empirical link between childhood trauma and bulimia but also highlight the importance of other etiological factors. With particular emphasis on eating disorders with dissociative symptoms, they outline treatment principles, pointing out the central theme of loss of control in impulsivity, dissociation, and eating disorders. They note the negative experience and evaluation of the body and ways to therapeutically deal with it to reduce dissociative triggers.

Chu concludes the third part of the book with a chapter on the treatment of traumatic dissociation. After describing dominant therapeutic models and techniques used in the treatment of traumatic dissociative symptoms and the psychiatric conditions in which they are most evident, Chu explores the stage- or phase-oriented treatment of complex PTSD. After detailing treatment considerations and areas of focus in the first, foundational stage, he then explores the processing of traumatic memories and comments on the endeavors of the third stage, which attempts to consolidate treatment gains, increase active involvement in life, and further develop relational and vocational aspects of functioning. In a separate section he outlines the additional treatment considerations required for complex dissociative disorders, particularly DID.

This book was designed to provide both empirical and therapeutic insights into traumatic dissociation, drawing on the work of many of the main contributors in the field. Key issues examined include the interacting effects of traumatic experience, developmental history, neurobiological function, and specific vulnerabilities to dissociative processes that underlie the occurrence of traumatic dissociation. The maintenance of internal homeostasis in the face of traumatic input is a challenge that elicits a variety of adaptive and pathological responses. It is hoped that the research and clinical experience described in this book will provide the basis for further clinical and theoretical formulations of traumatic dissociation and will advance empirical examination of the phenomenon.

Eric Vermetten, M.D., Ph.D.
Martin J. Dorahy, Ph.D.
David Spiegel, M.D.

Part I

CONCEPTUAL DOMAIN OF DISSOCIATION

CHAPTER 1

RELATIONSHIP BETWEEN TRAUMA AND DISSOCIATION

A Historical Analysis

MARTIN J. DORAHY, PH.D.
ONNO VAN DER HART, PH.D.

The concept of psychological trauma seems to have been introduced in the literature in 1878. The German neurologist Albert Eulenburg (1878) stated that "psychic shock," the then-current concept pertaining to vehement emotions such as terror or anger in the face of overwhelming events, could better be called *psychic trauma* (van der Hart and Brown 1993). The concept of dissociation has an even longer history, with Moreau de Tours (1845), in France, being the first to use the term in a manner consistent with contemporary understanding (Crabtree 1993; van der Hart and Dorahy, in press; van der Hart and Horst 1989). Although a link between traumatic experiences and dissociation had been established in the nineteenth century (e.g., Breuer and Freud 1893/2001; P. Janet 1889, 1898), students of dissociation have differed widely in their views of this relationship. Moreover, they have also held different views on the nature of dissociation, a fact that has confounded the study of trauma and dissociation.

Various publications have focused on the history of trauma (e.g., Barrois 1988; Crocq 1999; Fischer-Homberger 1975; Herman 1992; Leys 2000; Micale and Lerner 2001; Trimble 1981; van der Kolk et al. 1996a; Young 1995). Dominant in most of these works are descriptions of the traumas of war, but they also deal with disasters and industrial trauma. In a minority of cases, and primarily in recent times, the literature on the history of trauma has dealt with child maltreatment and sexual abuse. When works in the trauma literature refer to the contributions of nineteenth-century pioneers such Jean-Martin Charcot, the young Sigmund Freud, and more particularly, Pierre Janet, they also include the notion of the division of the personality or consciousness (i.e., dissociation) as a psychological consequence of trauma. Yet the relationship between trauma and dissociation in the trauma literature remains largely unexplored. Conversely, scholars of dissociation have given considerably more attention to the association between trauma and dissociation. Historically, however, these two variables have not always been associated in the dissociation literature. In this chapter we explore the relationship between trauma and dissociation from the perspective of studies focused on dissociation. We briefly describe various, sometimes conflicting views of dissociation that have existed throughout the past two centuries. An analysis of differing views of dissociation provides the context for our attempt to systematically trace the nature of the relationship between trauma and dissociation in the history of dissociation.

VIEWS ON DISSOCIATION

Depending on how it is understood, the construct of *dissociation* describes many psychological phenomena or few. The original understanding of dissociation, one that has been reintroduced in modern times (e.g., Nijenhuis et al. 2002, 2004), relates to divisions or dissociations in the personality or consciousness (e.g., Breuer and Freud 1893/2001; P. Janet 1889; C.S. Myers 1940; F.W.H. Myers 1893).[1] From such a structural dissociative organization various negative and positive psychoform and somatoform[2] dissociative symptoms originate, such as amnesia and contractures (Holmes et al. 2005; P. Janet 1901, 1907; Kihlstrom 1992; C.S. Myers 1940; Nemiah 1991; Nijenhuis and van der Hart

---

[1]Using modern psychological terminology, *divisions* (or dissociations) of the personality (consciousness) implies the existence of two or more dissociative psychobiological systems, each with its own collection of memories, affective experiences, behavioral repertoires, and sense of self.

[2]*Psychoform dissociative symptoms* refers to symptoms experienced psychologically. *Somatoform dissociative symptoms* refer to symptoms experienced in the body or somatically.

1999; Nijenhuis et al. 2004; Steele et al., in press; van der Hart et al. 2000). This original perspective circumscribed dissociative phenomena to psychic events (usually symptoms) that resulted from a dissociative personality structure. Van der Hart and Dorahy (in press) termed this the *narrow conceptualization of dissociation* on account of the limited phenomena it seeks to explain and their *single* origin (i.e., a dissociative personality structure).[3]

In modern times the concept of dissociation has widened. Contemporary psychological and psychiatric sciences have used the term to denote alterations in conscious experience, a breakdown in integrated information processing and psychological functioning, the operation of multiple independent streams of consciousness, a dissociatively divided personality structure, and the mainly negative psychoform (as opposed to somatoform) symptoms (e.g., amnesia) that derive from a dissociative personality structure, among other things. This diffuse understanding, which presumes multiple origins for dissociative experiences, can account for many and various clinical and nonclinical psychological phenomena. Due to its conceptual breadth, van der Hart and Dorahy (in press) referred to this understanding as the *broad conceptualization of dissociation*. It has its origins in, and has been the mainstay of, contemporary models of dissociation.

The core theoretical tenet of the narrow conceptualization is that a dissociative structure gives rise to dissociative phenomena. The broad conceptualization of dissociation has focused primarily on phenomena thought to be dissociative, and recourse is not always made to its psychological origin. Therefore, in this view dissociative phenomena are not limited to the psychological experiences derived from a dissociative personality organization.

VIEWS ON THE RELATIONSHIP BETWEEN TRAUMA AND DISSOCIATION

Whether broadly understood or narrowly defined, many dissociative phenomena have a pervasive relationship with traumatic stress. The relationship between potentially traumatizing events and dissociative phenomenology has been identified through retrospective research (e.g.,

---

[3]Van der Hart and Dorahy (in press) argued that the narrow conceptualization of dissociation can be divided into two types: 1) hypnotically induced divisions of the personality or consciousness and 2) trauma-induced division of the personality or consciousness.

Boon and Draijer 1993; Chu and Dill 1990; Coons 1994; Irwin 1994; Lewis et al. 1997; Nijenhuis et al. 1998), prospective research (Ogawa et al. 1997; Putnam and Trickett 1997), clinical observation (e.g., Allison 1974; Wilbur 1985), and theoretical conjecture (e.g., P. Janet 1889). Terms such as *traumatic dissociation* or *trauma-related dissociation* have their origin in the robustness of the link between traumatic stress and various dissociative phenomena. In the broad conceptualization of dissociation, these terms also differentiate experiences that are related to trauma (e.g., the alterations in conscious experience assessed by peritraumatic dissociation measures) from those that are not (e.g., the alterations in consciousness experienced during yoga or deep meditation). In the narrow definition, *traumatic dissociation* or *trauma-related dissociation* differentiates trauma-induced divisions of the personality (e.g., dissociative identity disorder [DID]) from non-trauma-induced divisions of the personality (e.g., deep hypnosis).

Historically, the attributes of trauma have been nonspecifically associated with dissociation. However, since the rejuvenation of interest in dissociation in the 1970s, which crystallized in 1980 with the recognition of dissociative disorders in DSM-III (American Psychiatric Association 1980) and several core clinical papers on multiple personality disorder, greater attention has been given to the relationship between the characteristics and timing of trauma and specific dissociative manifestations.

We propose that, from the inception of the study of dissociation until contemporary time, the nature of the relationship between trauma and dissociation can be divided into four discrete categories. This classification is based on the overt connection made between three factors: exposure to traumatic stress, the structure or organization of the personality, and dissociative phenomena. The first category, dissociation per se, attributes no relationship between trauma and either dissociative phenomena or the structural organization of the psyche from which these phenomena originate (i.e., no relationship between trauma and the broad or narrow conceptualizations of dissociation). Attention is given purely to the nature of dissociation. The second category, structural dissociation, dissociative phenomena, and unacknowledged trauma, pertains to literature in which dissociative phenomena are viewed as deriving from a division (dissociation) of the personality (i.e., narrow conceptualization of dissociation), but no link is made to the traumatic experience evident in the case history. The third category, trauma and dissociative symptoms, demonstrates a connection between trauma and dissociative phenomena but makes little or no reference to a dissociative personality structure (i.e., no relationship between trauma and the narrow conceptualization of dissociation). The fourth category, trauma, structural dissociation, and dissociative symptoms, posits that traumatic stress leads to a division or dissociation of consciousness or the personality that in turn gives rise to dissociative phenomena (primarily dissociative symptoms). This category links trauma with the narrow conceptualization of dissociation.

In the latter three categories, dissociation can be referred to as trauma-related or traumatic. However, this is not strictly the case in the first category, in which some dissociative experiences (e.g., posthypnotic amnesia) may be unrelated to trauma. These four relational dynamics between trauma, dissociative organization, and dissociative phenomena are explored in turn in this chapter. The literature pertaining to each category is generally presented in chronological order.

Dissociation Per Se

Dissociation in the nineteenth century pertained not only to hysteria but also to a wealth of more or less related phenomena: somnambulism, artificial somnambulism, spiritist séances, talking tables, possession, and even dreams (Crabtree 1993, 2003; van der Hart 1997). According to the various authors that studied these phenomena, they were all explained by divisions in the personality wherein, unknown to the primary part of the personality, a secondary part of the personality would be responsible for the behavior. Trauma was not implicated in these phenomena (e.g., Gale 1900), nor were the phenomena always seen as pathological (e.g., Gurney's 1888 studies of hypnotic and posthypnotic suggestions). Despite the fact that the broad conceptualization of dissociation encapsulates much of the narrow conceptualization, this category would fall into the narrow conceptualization. This is primarily because of the emphasis on psychic organization being the basis of dissociative phenomena in this category, which is distinct from the phenomenological emphasis in the broad conceptualization. The study of dissociation per se characterized the birth of the study of dissociation.

Following Mesmer's discovery of "animal magnetism," one of his students, the Marquis de Puységur (1751–1825), found that the "convulsive crisis" central to Mesmer's original induction was not necessary for inducing a lucid state.[4] He also noted that in one of his first patients, Victor Race, a distinct change in his character occurred during the "passive crisis," and amnesia for what occurred in the lucid state accompanied a return to normal waking functioning (Crabtree 1993; Forrest 1999). As-

---

[4] In the lucid state Puységur found he could talk with the patient, answer questions, explain the origins of the illness, and suggest a remedy.

tounded by the alteration in his patient's personality between the lucid and waking states, as well as the amnesia that demarcated them, Puységur and several of his colleagues (e.g., Deleuze 1819) hypothesized that those capable of this phenomenon manifested a structural division or dissociation of consciousness or the personality that gave rise to two different states of being. These observations marked the commencement of the study of dissociation (Crabtree 1993; van der Hart and Dorahy, in press). The induced structural division of the personality (i.e., dissociation in the narrow sense) and the amnesia that highlighted it were initially referred to as *somnambulism* and subsequently as *artificial somnambulism*. The magnetizers soon found that this state could best be induced in patients with hysteria (van der Hart 1997). However, it was not until the late 1800s that theorists and clinicians began to observe the link between divisions of the personality (i.e., dissociation), hysteria, and trauma. Neither the birth of the study of dissociation nor of its relationship to hysteria, which soon followed, shared any association with exposure to traumatic stress.

Examples of noninduced, spontaneous dissociation were also given in the early nineteenth century. Dwight (1818) presented three cases in which he identified a dissociative personality structure and resultant amnesia (i.e., dissociative symptom). He noted that the dissociative personality exemplified "the human mind in a diseased state" (p. 431), where there was a rational and a delirious part of the personality. Dwight's case vignettes demonstrated that amnesia was an expected phenomenological feature in people who have "two souls, each occasionally dormant, and occasionally active, and utterly ignorant of what the other was doing" (p. 433).

Tascher (1855), in his work on mediums and other phenomena characterized by divisions in consciousness, proposed that thoughts could be separated into discrete streams that represent distinct parts of the personality and have their own self-identity. Writing mediums may exhibit a second part of the personality that is "inflamed, passionate, and unrestrained" and momentarily blot out the normal part of the personality, or the medium may exhibit "two simultaneous currents of thought, one which constitutes the ordinary person, the other which develops outside of it" (p. 23). On the other hand, with somnambulism "we are now in the presence of the second personality only, the other being annihilated in sleep" (p. 44).

Some members of the Society for Psychical Research (SPR), a British group that studied the varying clinical and nonclinical manifestations of dissociation (Alvarado 2002), fully supported the existence of a dissociated or secondary personality that operated behind, and was concealed from, the primary personality or consciousness. This secondary consciousness—called by various names, including *duplex consciousness*—was a permanent and ongoing facet of the human psychological apparatus that could be induced or evoked spontaneously. Venman (1889) professed

> I would suggest that it may *not* really be a "supervening" or special "state" or "condition" at all, but a "*constant*" one, always existing though ordinarily unmanifesting, and that its seemingly peculiar supersensuous powers of perception, and capacities of acquiring knowledge otherwise than through ordinary sensory channels, are constantly in action, though veiled from observation by the influence of the ordinary (normal or primary) consciousness. (p. 76, italics in original)

Some SPR members who advocated a natural structural dissociation of the personality into two parts vehemently argued against the possibility of "multiplex" personality, or consciousness being divided into more than two parts (e.g., Barkworth 1889). Trauma was unrelated to a dissociative psychic organization. In addition, many SPR members did not associate dissociative structure with pathology (Alvarado 2002), which was the dominant view of dissociation held in France at that time.

F.W.H. Myers, a founding member of the SPR, extensively and influentially studied divisions of the personality and its various manifestations (Alvarado 2002; Crabtree 2003). He incorporated into his domain of exploration human experiences that were deemed "normal, pathological and extraordinary" (Crabtree 2003, p. 60). His theoretical concept of subliminal consciousness posited the existence of separate and relatively independent streams of consciousness that operated outside awareness. He used this concept to draw together diverse human phenomena, from sensory and motor automatism (e.g., posthypnotic hallucinatory suggestions; automatic writing) evident in the nonclinical population to "diseases of the hypnotic stratum" that "for convenience's sake we may continue to give...the meaningless name 'hysteria'" (F.W.H. Myers 1893, p. 5). The focus for Myers was the expression of divisions of consciousness in their many guises. Issues related to the origins of the divisions (e.g., trauma) were of less interest.

Neurological accounts were proffered to explain dissociation per se in the nineteenth-century literature. For example, Bruce (1895) forwarded a hemispheric lateralization explanation of H.P., a 47-year-old Welshman who alternated with apparent amnesia between two distinct phases. Bruce referred to these different personality states as the English stage and the Welsh stage on account of the dominant language used during the activation of each phase. Bruce argued that H.P. "appeared to have two separate and distinct states of consciousness, and in whom the right and left brain alternately exert a preponderating influence over the motor functions" (p. 54). The left hemisphere, according to Bruce, was dominant and regulated mental and behavioral activities during the English phase, in which H.P. was right-handed and somewhat hypomanic. During his Welsh phases H.P. was left-handed, spoke Welsh or some "unintelligible" language, and had a presentation of dementia. Bruce also identified different heart rate tracings between the two different states of consciousness. He concluded by noting that

> the cerebral hemispheres are capable of individual mental action, and that the mentally active cerebrum has a preponderating influence over the control of the motor functions, the patient living two separate existences during the two stages through which he passes; the mental impressions received during each of these separate existences being recorded in one cerebral hemisphere only. (p. 64)

At the time, this neurobiological theory was a rather popular explanation for divisions in the personality, but it later met with strong opposition, as is summarized by P. Janet (1929):

> A first explanation has been spread everywhere. Today it is ridiculous; it is the explanation by the two brains. The anatomists have always a disposition toward giving a material and physical form to the phenomena that they observe in their subjects. They are only satisfied when they localize the troubles they observe in a part of the nervous system. Well, here they have two persons. People have two cerebral hemispheres. Eh, good, it's very simple: one personality will be in one hemisphere; the other one will be in the other hemisphere. This hypothesis...doesn't have, I believe, great value. In any case, it is without any real anatomical value. What one does know very well is that the suppression of one half of the brain determines motor troubles and sensory troubles of a particular kind. A cerebral hemorrhage which destroys one hemisphere leads to hemiplegias of a very special form: it leads to hemianopsias, of ways of seeing from one side and not from both sides. In one word, there are very specific physiological symptoms with the suppression of one brain and the existence of one single brain. Well, never, in these observations of double personalities, does one find real hemiplegias or real hemianopsias. We thus don't have any really physiological symptom that corresponds with the suppression of a hemisphere. (pp. 501–502)

The two-hemispheres explanation of dual personality becomes even more awkward in cases of multiple personality.

In contemporary times Hilgard (1977) used laboratory-based studies of hypnosis to investigate the nature of dissociation per se in non-clinical, nontraumatized participants. In hypnotic procedures that initially started with the induction of analgesia (Hilgard 1974), Hilgard observed a striking division in consciousness in highly hypnotizable participants. When asked to report the level of pain they experienced, the hypnotic self accepted the analgesic suggestion and reported experiencing no pain. However, outside the awareness of this stream of consciousness another stream, accessed through "automatic" procedures such as writing or ideomotor responding, communicated that the painful stimulus was being experienced. Seemingly in those individuals who demonstrated these phenomena, consciousness was divided or dissociated so that at least two streams of consciousness were operating independently and in parallel to process two different types of information, one concordant with the hypnotic suggestion and one concordant with phenomenal experience (Hilgard 1977). This is not dissimilar to the studies of artificial somnambulism that marked the birth of the study of dissociation; Hilgard observed not only the division of consciousness but also the operation of one stream outside the awareness of another (i.e., one stream had amnesia for the other's experience and behavior).

In summary, perhaps unsurprisingly, the study of dissociation was initiated by the investigation of its nature. The Marquis de Puységur and other magnetizers noted the structural division in consciousness or the personality and the accompanying amnesia that characterized dissociation. Later investigators of dissociation per se moved from the study of artificial somnambulism to the study of other phenomena believed to derive from divisions of consciousness, including hysteria. Finally, Hilgard brought the investigation of dissociation per se full circle by using the more contemporary variant of artificial somnambulism—hypnosis—as a study tool. In his multiple streams of consciousness model, Hilgard also offered a contemporary, nonclinical understanding of the structural divisions of the personality that Puységur and many authors who followed him advocated as clinical manifestations of dissociation. In the study of dissociation per se correlates of the construct, such as trauma, were generally outside the interest of investigators; the focus was on the dissociative structure of the psyche and the phenomena it led to.

Structural Dissociation, Dissociative Phenomena, and Unacknowledged Trauma

Many initial clinical reports of dissociation are characterized by a failure to recognize the existence and importance of traumatic antecedents. Several retrospective studies of classic DID and possession cases have demonstrated the unacknowledged existence of trauma in the patient's history or the failure to recognize its etiological significance. The original authors of these case studies understood dissociation as divisions in the personality and some identified trauma, especially in childhood, in the patient's history. However, no connection was made between trauma and divisions of the personality (i.e., dissociation). Strictly speaking, this would be encompassed by the narrow conceptualization of dissociation because it emphasizes a dissociative organization, which is not the primary concern of the phenomenologically oriented broad conceptualization of dissociation.

The sixteenth-century case of Jeanne Fery possibly represents the earliest example of unacknowledged trauma in a dissociative presentation. Although the case was initially presented as a example of possession (van der Hart et al. 1996), Bourneville (1886) observed in his republication of the case that Jeanne Fery demonstrated a most perfect case of "doubling of the personality"(*dédoublement de la personnalité*)—that is the nineteenth-century French diagnostic category of DID. He compared Fery with the famous nineteenth-century cases of Félida X and Louis Vivet (van der Hart et al. 1996). Although there were clear indications of early physical and verbal abuse and, possibly, of childhood sexual abuse, Bourneville did not relate the disorder to childhood traumatization.

Mary Reynolds, one of the first American presentations of DID,[5] represents an example in which records of her life and times demonstrated significant childhood trauma, especially extrafamilial, but no mention was made of this trauma history in the initial clinical accounts of her dissociation (e.g., E. T. Carlson 1984; Greaves 1980; S. L. Mitchell 1816; S. W. Mitchell 1888). In a reanalysis of Mary Reynolds's history that outlines several key traumatic events in her childhood, Goodwin (1987) offered a posttraumatic interpretation of the etiology of Mary's DID. Goodwin argued that the development of divisions in Mary's personality allowed her to "erase from her mind the first 8 years of her life and thereby all feelings of loss and fear connected to the family's life in Birmingham [England] and their experience there of riots and discrimination" (p. 97).

In presenting an analysis of Antoine Despine's 1840 work on multiple personality disorder and his child index-case of Estelle, Fine (1988) noted that Despine never recognized the etiology of multiple personality nor the importance of trauma. Fine (1988) suggested that Estelle experienced a number of life events in childhood that may have precipitated the development of DID, including her own near death and the

---

[5] Benjamin Rush had written of two cases of DID before Mary Reynolds, one being the famous 1791 case from Springfield, Massachusetts (E.T. Carlson 1981; Crabtree 1993). Both cases were characterized by alterations in identities, each of which had their own discrete memories and were amnesic for the other.

death of her father. Despine had not associated these factors with Estelle's dissociative presentation. He had treated many DID patients before Estelle and therefore recognized a dissociative personality organization, although he was never able to make sense of it: "Despine was unable to advance a satisfactory theory to explain the phenomena that he documented" (Fine 1988, p. 38).

The childhood trauma history of Louis Vivet was acknowledged but not linked to his dissociative presentation. Vivet is the most famous nineteenth-century male case of DID, and his presentation first attracted the name "multiple personality." The loss of time, amnesia, and many somatic symptoms experienced by Vivet were explained as divisions in his personality (Faure et al. 1997). In addition, many of the various physicians who treated Vivet noted the childhood maternal neglect and physical abuse in his case history, but they made no direct link from these experiences to his presenting symptoms. Much was made of his ordeal with a viper at age 14 (e.g., Bourru and Burot 1888; Camuset 1882; F. W. H. Myers 1887), but little attention was given to his childhood history (Faure et al. 1997).

The importance of Louis Vivet in this current text goes beyond the missing link between trauma and dissociative divisions of the personality evident in his case. Like Bruce's (1895) case of H.P., Vivet was also the subject for one of the early, tentative attempts to provide a neurobiological explanation of dissociation. In presenting many examples of what he called multiplex personality, F. W. H. Myers (1887) provided a brief synopsis of Vivet in which he cautiously, "and with many reserves and technicalities perforce omitted" (p. 499), offered some neurobiological insights. Paraphrasing the explanation given by the French physicians who at different times treated Vivet (e.g., Camuset, Bourru, Burot, Voisin), Myers stated, "A sudden shock [e.g., the viper attack]…has effected in this boy a profounder severance between the functions of the right and left hemispheres of the brain than has perhaps ever been observed before" (p. 499). Myers went on to describe three of Vivet's dissociative identities using the functions of each hemisphere and hemispheric lateralization or equilibrium. He argued,

> [I]nhibit his left brain (and right side) and he becomes,…not only left handed but *sinister*; he manifests himself through nervous arrangements which have reached a lower degree of evolution. And he can represent in memory those periods only when his personality had assumed the same attitude…. Inhibit the right brain, and the higher qualities of character remain, like the power of speech, intact. There is self control;…there is a sense of duty…. But nonetheless he is only half himself. Besides the hemiplegia, which is a matter of course, memory is truncated too, and he

can summon up only such fragments of the past as chance to have been linked with this one abnormal state, leaving unrecalled not only the period of sinister inward ascendency [sic], but the normal period of childhood…. And now if by some art we can restore the equipoise of the two hemispheres again… [h]e is, if I may say, born again; he becomes as a little child; he is set back in memory, character, knowledge, power, to the days before this trouble came upon him. (pp. 499–500)

Although they offered what was then a cogent neurological account of dissociative divisions of the personality, as discussed earlier in the hemispheric lateralization theory offered by Bruce (1895), such explanations were too crude to account for the psychological data.

The classic case studies of DID from the nineteenth century were prominent in moving the exploration of dissociation beyond the induced divisions in the personality created by artificial somnambulism that dominated the eighteenth-century study of dissociation. These later case studies demonstrated dissociation in a spontaneous and clinical form. Yet despite the trauma histories evident in several of these presentations, including Bourneville's (1886) reanalysis of the Jeanne Fery case, trauma was not entertained as an etiological factor in the division of the personality that was the central characterological feature of these cases. It would not be until Pierre Janet and several of his late-nineteenth-century contemporaries developed sophisticated theoretical models of dissociation that trauma would gain its etiological significance.

Trauma and Dissociative Symptoms/Phenomena

Modern views on dissociation generally agree that the term refers to the compartmentalization (e.g., Kluft 1993; Putnam 1989; van der Kolk et al. 1996b) or structured separation of mental processes (e.g., perceptions, conation, emotions, memories, and identity) that are ordinarily integrated in and accessible to conscious awareness (Spiegel 2003; Spiegel and Cardeña 1991). This belief is consistent with a structural view of dissociation as divisions of the personality. However, in the contemporary non-DID study of dissociation, very little—if any—attention is given to the dissociative organization of the psyche, even though it forms the basis of several definitions of dissociation. Rather, the primary emphasis in the modern study of dissociation is on dissociative phenomenology (van der Hart and Dorahy, in press). The study of trauma and dissociative symptoms thus falls under the broad conceptualization of dissociation.

The Expansion of Dissociative Phenomenology

The initial understanding of dissociation, as well as contemporary understandings that have remained true to the original conceptualization, limits dissociative phenomena to those experiences that derive from a dissociative personality structure. Since the 1980s, and perhaps with its impetus in the rise of interest in altered states of consciousness in the late 1960s (e.g., Ludwig 1966; Tart 1969), phenomena described under the heading of dissociation have considerably broadened to include experiences that are not directly related to divisions in the personality (or consciousness). Thus, a dissociative personality structure plays a smaller role in the conceptualization of dissociation in modern times, and the structure of the psyche no longer determines the nature of dissociative phenomena in the mainstream study of dissociation.

Under the expanded definition of *dissociation* as a breakdown or disruption in integrated functioning, these experiences may include flights into the imaginary world (e.g., daydreams), alterations in consciousness (e.g., trance states), alterations in perception (e.g., derealization), the operation of multiple and more or less independent streams of consciousness (e.g., inadvertently changing gears while engrossed in a conversation), as well as the phenomena that derive from divisions in the personality[6] (e.g., amnesia).

Subsuming such a broad range of phenomena under the label of *dissociation* has serious consequences for the validity of the construct. As one of the authors of the Dissociative Experiences Scale (DES; Bernstein and Putnam 1986) concluded, "Total DES scores sometimes have different meanings for subjects from different populations.... DES scores for nonclinical groups tend to reflect experiences of absorption and imaginative involvement, whereas DES scores across a wide spectrum of psychiatric disorders reflect a wide range of dissociative experiences" (E. B. Carlson 1994, pp. 44–45). Contemporary work has given considerably less attention to the *psychological origins* of dissociative phenomena than to the phenomena themselves. The study of trauma and dissociative phenomenology has tended to be conducted in the absence of attention to, or acknowledgment of, dissociative structure.

Trauma and Dissociative Phenomenology

Research using questionnaires has typified the study of trauma and dissociative phenomenology. Trait measures of dissociation began to develop in the 1980s following the increase of interest in dissociative phenomena.

---

[6] The contemporary study of dissociative phenomena in clinical cases of dissociation (i.e., divisions in the personality) has tended to focus on psychoform expressions, to the relative neglect of somatoform dissociative symptoms.

Scales such as the DES (Bernstein and Putnam 1986), the Dissociation Questionnaire (DIS-Q; Vanderlinden et al. 1993) and the Somatoform Dissociation Questionnaire (SDQ-20; Nijenhuis et al. 1996) tap dissociative phenomena such as amnesia and anesthesia believed to originate from a dissociative personality. However, with the exception of the SDQ-20, these scales also tap experiences related to alterations in consciousness (e.g., trance states), the activation of multiple streams of consciousness (e.g., highway hypnosis), absorption phenomena, and alterations in perceptual experience (e.g., derealization). Many studies have shown a positive relationship between trauma and trait dissociation (Chu and Dill 1990; Irwin 1994). The emphasis in these studies has been on the relationship between traumatic stress and dissociative experience (i.e., phenomena). Links have rarely been made to how these experiences came about (i.e., their underlying psychological origin). This may be largely due to the fact that dissociative phenomena in modern psychological and psychiatric science have been associated with several different origins (i.e., the broad conceptualization) rather than a single origin (i.e., dissociative personality structure; the narrow conceptualization). In addition, the trend in contemporary psychiatric thought has been toward psychological phenomenology (e.g., symptoms) rather than psychic organization. As E.B. Carlson (1994) noted in discussing the development of the DES,

> The definition of dissociation incorporated into the DES was intentionally broad. The authors attempted to include as wide a range of items as possible in the DES and tried to avoid including items that also measured some other distinct construct (such as modulation of affect). Consequently, the authors included many different kinds of *experiences* that had been previously *associated* with dissociation. There are items inquiring about amnestic experiences, gaps in awareness, depersonalization, derealization, absorption, and imaginative involvement. (p. 42, italics added)

Like trait measures of dissociation, state and peritraumatic questionnaires assess a vast range of experiences that come from multiple origins. These measures have consistently found a positive relationship between traumatic experience and the phenomena indicated on state and peritraumatic surveys of dissociation (Marmar et al. 1997). There is also some indication that peritraumatic dissociative phenomena are related to the development of posttraumatic stress disorder (PTSD; e.g., Birmes et al. 2001; Koopman et al. 1994; Shalev et al. 1996; Weiss et al. 1995). However, the direct nature of this association is uncertain (Marshall and Schnell 2002; Spiegel 2003), and studies have rarely linked the phenomena with the dissociative structure that some have argued characterizes

PTSD (e.g., Chu 1998; Nijenhuis et al. 2004; Spiegel and Cardeña 1991; van der Hart et al. 1998, 2006).

The empirical relationship between traumatic stress and dissociative phenomenology has been underpinned by theoretical frameworks that attempt to explain this association. One dominant framework posits that dissociation acts as a psychological defense against the integration of overwhelming, highly aversive psychosomatic stimuli (e.g., Vaillant 1992). From this perspective, peritraumatic dissociative experiences occur in the face of trauma and impede the successful creation of an integrated psychobiological representation of that event. According to the broad view of dissociation, dissociative experiences after the trauma may mirror the peritraumatic dissociative experience (e.g., depersonalization) or may be the result of the breakdown of integrated processing (e.g., amnesia, retraction of the field of consciousness).

A brief note is required here regarding the term *retraction of the field of consciousness* and its two distinct meanings: 1) It is often understood as the narrowing of the perceptual field that is common in the face of trauma. Senses sharpen and become selectively focused on the traumatizing object or situation. These perceptual alterations represent phenomenal experiences. According to Janet's original definition of dissociation, these experiences may accompany dissociation (divisions of the personality). However, retraction from a phenomenal perspective is not an example of dissociation (contrary to what the broad conceptualization of dissociation may advocate) nor a by-product of it. 2) Retraction of the field of consciousness also has a structural meaning and refers to the dissociative psychological consequences of traumatic stress and the fact that once the personality is divided, conscious awareness is no longer able to access the full range of experiences that have been encoded (e.g., P. Janet 1889; F.W.H. Myers 1887). Retraction in this sense is most grandly highlighted in DID, in which dissociative identities often experience extreme retractions so that only small portions of the person's overall experience are available to conscious awareness. From the narrow conceptualization of dissociation, both of these meanings hold that retraction of the field of consciousness is related to dissociation but not analogous with it.

Moving back to the relationship between trauma and dissociative phenomena, the more traumatic stressors experienced and the earlier their occurrence, the more dissociation will become the automatic (involuntary) means of responding to them. The theoretical association between trauma and the broad view of dissociation may be construed as follows: Traumatic stress leads to defensive peritraumatic dissociative experiences, which lead to a greater frequency and perhaps type of trait dissociative episodes. One of many critical issues in this understanding is whether peritraumatic phenomena, such as depersonalization and narrowing of the perceptual field, actually represent defensive dissociative strategies in and of themselves, or whether the defensive properties of dissociation are secondary to the brain's inability to successfully integrate the numerous sensory, psychological, and biological elements of a highly stressful event. The latter would be in keeping with a Janetian understanding of dissociation, which is discussed in the next section.

The near-exclusive focus on phenomenology, which characterizes the broad conceptualization of dissociation and epitomizes most dissociation questionnaires, has dominated the study of dissociation since at least 1980 when DSM-III offered a phenomenological account of dissociative disorders (although it should be noted that somatoform dissociative disorders were not included). The emphasis on phenomenology has had a major positive impact on the empirical and clinical study of dissociation. Yet the broad conceptualization does not provide a clear and explicit psychological understanding of what gives rise to dissociative phenomena. In addition, there has been little attention given to what becomes of the unintegrated psychological remnants of a traumatic experience (except in the study of DID). The failure since the 1980s to seriously address the growing conceptual cloudiness in the meaning of dissociation is perhaps not surprising given the enthusiasm and many significant insights that the study of dissociative phenomenology has produced. However, the fuzzy concept characteristic of the modern study of trauma-related dissociation makes it distinct from the late nineteenth and early to mid-twentieth century studies of dissociation.

The contemporary association between trauma and dissociative phenomenology in the absence of dissociative structure is not without historical precedent. For example, Voisin (1883), in his chapter on madness caused by the siege of Paris (1870–1871), argued that a person in complete mental health could become mad when confronted with certain extremely demanding circumstances. He noted the development of this madness in those exposed to bombardments during the siege and the subsequent violence between the warring commune and government forces. In ignoring dissociative structure and emphasizing the association between trauma and dissociative phenomena, he presented an example of a healthy 17-year-old girl who witnessed the decapitation of her mother when a sudden bombardment took place as they walked in the Rue de Grenelle. Among the girl's acute responses were syncope and shaking. Later that same day she had an "hystero-epileptic attack" followed by others on consecutive days. In between these attacks she was either in a stupor or was laughing for hours. Voisin pointed out that, "[e]stranged of everything that took place around her, and having become paraplegic, she had lost completely the memory of the catastrophe which had brought about such a state" (p. 188).

Although this example demonstrates a case of pre-1900s writing in which dissociation was limited to specific phenomena, Voisin's focus on the symptoms of his patient represented a departure from the focus on structure favored by his contemporaries. Attention given to dissociative phenomena in the absence of links to dissociative personality structure is more a contemporary feature than one handed down from the forefathers of dissociation study. Investigators of dissociation up until the renaissance of interest in the topic in the early 1980s were generally cognizant of the structural basis of dissociative phenomena.

Trauma, Structural Dissociation, and Dissociative Symptoms

The contemporary posttraumatic model of DID, the study of war neuroses in World Wars I and II (which is also known by other names, including *shell shock,* and became known as PTSD in DSM-III), and many psychiatric studies of hysteria, especially in France from the 1880s, share a similar view on the association between trauma and dissociation. In all cases, traumatic events such as child abuse, combat exposure, or the generically named *traumatic shock* used by the early investigators of hysteria led to divisions or dissociative separations in consciousness or the personality. From these divisions arose specific symptoms that were described as dissociative. The category of trauma, structural dissociation, and dissociative symptoms is the defining position of the narrow conceptualization of dissociation, but it can also be subsumed under the broad understanding due to its conceptual breadth.

The Study of Hysteria From the Late Nineteenth Century

France in the late nineteenth century was the international hub for the clinical study of dissociation. Theorists and clinicians such as Binet (1890, 1892/1896), J. Janet (1888), Charcot (1887), Azam (1876), and Gilles de la Tourette (1887) tackled the subject of divisions in the personality and the resultant clinical symptoms. However, Pierre Janet was one of the first to systematically study the association between traumatic or psychic shock, structural divisions of the personality, and resultant dissociative phenomena (P. Janet 1889, 1898, 1911, 1919). His theoretical contribution eclipsed his contemporaries, and like many of the French insights of that time, Janet's observations remain pertinent to the study of trauma and dissociation today (Ellenberger 1970; Nijenhuis et al. 2004; van der Hart et al. 2006). Janet observed that patients diagnosed with hysteria had "an

illness of the personal synthesis" (P. Janet 1907, p. 332)—that is, insufficient capacity for psychological integration that manifested in the development and existence of dissociative parts of the personality. Thus he
defined *hysteria* as "a form of mental depression characterized by the retraction of the field of consciousness and a tendency to the dissociation
and emancipation of the systems of ideas and functions that constitute
personality" (P. Janet 1907, p. 322). Each of these systems was characterized by its own rudimentary or more developed sense of self.

Janet (1889, 1909, 1911) acknowledged a role for constitutional vulnerability, such as physical ill health and exhaustion, in illnesses of personal synthesis. Yet he regarded the vehement emotions inherent in
traumatic experiences as being the primary cause of this integrative failure. Traumas, according to Janet (1909), "produce their disintegrative effects in proportion to their intensity, duration, and repetition" (p. 1556).
Janet (1889, 1907) roughly distinguished dissociative parts of the personality—that is, "habitual" parts—that had to accomplish the tasks of daily
life, parts that kept the traumatic memories, and parts that fulfilled a
kind of observing role. Whereas amnesia often existed between other
parts, "observing" parts of the personality often remained aware of the
other parts' experiences. Dissociative parts of the personality could be
present side by side (i.e., co-conscious) and/or alternate with each other.

According to Janet (1901, 1907, 1911), this dissociation of the personality manifested in mental stigmata and mental accidents (i.e., negative
and positive dissociative symptoms). The negative symptoms included
losses of memory (amnesia), sensation (anesthesia), and motor control
(e.g., paralysis). The positive symptoms involved acute, usually transient intrusions, such as additional sensations (e.g., pain), movements
(e.g., tics), and perceptions, up to an apparently complete reexperiencing
of reactivated traumatic memories. In general, many of these positive
symptoms were viewed by Janet as directly connected with traumatic
memories. Unfortunately, his view that dissociative symptoms could
also pertain to movements and sensations is one that was somewhat lost
in the second half of the twentieth century (e.g., DSM's division between
dissociation and somatoform/conversion experiences). However, dissociative symptoms of movement and sensation recently have become
once again the focus of attention (Kihlstrom 1992; Nemiah 1991; Nijenhuis 1999; Nijenhuis and van der Hart 1999; van der Hart et al. 2000).

Acknowledging their indebtedness to Pierre Janet, his brother Jules,
and Alfred Binet, Breuer and Freud (1893/2001) clearly argued in their
thesis on the mechanisms of hysteria that exposure to traumatic stress
leads to dissociative divisions in the personality, which subsequently
gives rise to hysterical (dissociative) symptoms. They first pointed out

that a dissociative personality organization is central in hysteria: "The splitting of consciousness which is so striking in the well-known classical cases under the form of 'double conscience' is present to a rudimentary degree in every hysteria…a tendency to such a dissociation, and with it the emergence of abnormal states of consciousness [dissociative personality structure]…is the basic phenomena of this neurosis" (p. 12). Breuer and Freud (1893/2001) then implicated trauma in the etiology of a dissociative personality structure: "Severe trauma (such as occurs in a traumatic neurosis)…can bring about a splitting-off of groups of ideas even in people who are in other respects unaffected [i.e., those who were not what Breuer and Freud termed *dispositional hysterics*]; and this would be the mechanism of *psychically acquired* hysteria" (pp. 12–13, italics in original).

According to Breuer and Freud, symptoms are experienced either when the hypnoid, traumatic, or second consciousness remains relatively unassociated with the "normal consciousness" (e.g., amnesia) or when the second consciousness (that holding the traumatic memories) intrudes on the normal consciousness (e.g., contractures, flashback, or intrusive thoughts). Freud (1896/1953) subsequently postulated that the dissociated traumatic memories invariably pertained to childhood sexual abuse, a view strongly criticized by Pierre Janet (1919) and one that Freud soon moved away from (e.g., Freud 1906/1953).

The European study of dissociation generated significant interest in North America in the late nineteenth and early twentieth centuries. This interest initially came courtesy of William James and his 1896 lecture series on dissociative structure and phenomena (see Taylor 1983) as well as subsequent work by other leading New England scholars such as Boris Sidis (1902; Sidis and Goodhart 1904) and Morton Prince (1906a).

Prince was initially influenced by the groundbreaking French observations and theories on hysteria in the late 1800s. However, he soon become quite critical of their understanding of dissociation (e.g., Prince 1906b) and began to develop his own model of psychic functioning (Hales 1975). Crucially, however, he never turned his back on French wisdom and retained dissociation as a central tenet for understanding the human personality. Although not clearly explicated (Hales 1975), Prince's theory was essentially a structural one in which systems of ideas, emotions, behaviors, and so on become associated and disassociated based on environmental and psychic experience as well as factors such as suggestion and trauma. In the face of trauma (although Prince [1909], identified other possible factors), sophisticated sets of associations that represent the overwhelming experience could develop (i.e., the personality could become divided). For Prince, a division in consciousness resulted from the failed integration of "trauma" complexes, and this dissociation led to symptoms such as anesthesia and amnesia (Prince 1906b).

Several post–World War I clinical theorists clearly acknowledged the link between trauma, dissociative personality structure, and dissociative phenomena (e.g., McDougall 1926; T.W. Mitchell 1922). Charles Myers provided a lucid account of the dynamics between dissociative structure and phenomena following trauma. Of an acutely traumatized soldier in a state of stupor, Myers (1940) wrote the following:

> At this stage, the normal personality is in abeyance. Even if it is capable of receiving impressions, it shows no signs of responding to them. The recent emotional (i.e., traumatic) experiences of the individual have the upper hand and determine his conduct: the normal has been replaced by what we call the "emotional" personality. Gradually or suddenly an "apparently normal" personality usually returns—normal save for the lack of all memory of events directly connected with the shock, normal save for the manifestation of other ("somatic") hysterical disorders indicative of mental dissociation. Now and again there occur alterations of the "emotional" and the "apparently normal" personalities, the return of the former being often heralded by severe headache, dizziness or by a hysteric convulsion. On its return, the "apparently normal" personality may recall, as in a dream, the distressing experiences revived during the temporary intrusion of the "emotional" personality. The "emotional" personality may also return during sleep, the "functional" disorders of mutism, paralysis, contracture, etc., being then usually in abeyance. On waking, however, the "apparently normal" personality may have no recollection of the dream state and will at once resume his mutism, paralysis, etc. (p. 66–67)

The link between trauma, dissociative structure, and dissociative phenomena that characterized nineteenth-century thinking on hysteria and early twentieth-century theorizing about PTSD is clearly evident in the contemporary understanding of DID.[7] (DID is examined in several chapters in this book, and thus it is not examined in detail here.) In short, childhood trauma is believed to evoke dissociative divisions in the personality (Kluft 1996; Putnam 1989; Ross 1989). Assisted by the fluidity of the personality in childhood and its lack of integrated functioning, trauma-

---

[7] In recent times, Spiegel and colleagues (e.g, Butler et al. 1996; Spiegel et al. 1988), among a small number of others, have extended the link between trauma, dissociative structure, and dissociative phenomena beyond DID to incorporate other conditions with a dissociative underpinning (e.g., PTSD, conversion disorder). For example, Butler et al. (1996) proposed a diathesis-stress model of dissociative symptoms and structure in which hypnotizability is the biologically derived psychological diathesis between traumatic stress and dissociation.

related divisions of the personality become more stable psychological structures as the personality solidifies in late childhood (Putnam 1997). The different dissociative identities are believed to house different psychological and behavioral experiences. Dissociative identities are also believed to differ in their neurobiological and physiological operation, an issue that is addressed in subsequent chapters. Dissociative symptoms in DID are directly related to the dissociative personality structure. Consequently, symptoms of loss (i.e., negative symptoms such as amnesia) are accounted for by discrete divisions between identities, whereas symptoms of intrusion (i.e., positive symptoms such as flashbacks and identity alterations) relate to the incursion of one dissociative identity on another.

The connection between trauma, dissociative structure, and dissociative phenomena (symptoms) advocated in the DID literature reflects the nineteenth-century French understanding of trauma-induced hysteria. A distinguishing facet of the contemporary literature, however, is that greater attention is given to understanding the type, chronicity, age at onset, and psychological meaning of traumatic events. These specifications were rarely examined in detail by Prince, Janet, James, and other early investigators, who presumably lumped the different aspects of trauma together under labels such as "traumatic shock."

CONCLUSION

From the historical literature we have identified four differing relationships between trauma and dissociation. In the first, dissociation per se, trauma was not a feature of the intrinsic link between dissociative personality organization and dissociative phenomena. The second category, structural dissociation, dissociative phenomena, and unacknowledged trauma, related more exclusively to early clinical cases of dissociation. Like the first category, no association was made between trauma and dissociation (i.e., structure or phenomena). The case records of these historically well-known dissociative patients suggested considerable childhood trauma, yet this trauma was given no etiological significance in the dissociative personality structure evident in each case. The third category (trauma and dissociative symptoms) connected dissociative phenomena with a trauma history, but no association was made to the organization of the personality or the underlying origin of the dissociative phenomena. The more contemporary literature on non-DID dissociation has largely operated out of this category. The direct association from trauma to dissociative symptoms has had a positive impact on the expansion of dissociation research, but a failure to acknowledge structure has led to some phenomena being largely ignored (i.e., negative somatoform dissociative phenomena). Finally, the fourth type of relationship between trauma and dissociation (trauma, structural dissociation, and dissociative symptoms) theoretically proposes a link between trauma exposure, a dissociative personality organization, and dissociative phenomena. This viewpoint dominated the early clinical history of dissociation, but despite not being lost in the DID literature it has been rather obscured from modern mainstream accounts of dissociation. Dissociation described in the latter three views, whether the focus is on phenomenology, structure, or both, would be classified as traumatic or trauma-related dissociation. However, dissociation described in the first category could not be so classified.

REFERENCES

Allison RB: A guide to parents: how to raise your daughter to have multiple personalities. Fam Ther 1:83–88, 1974

Alvarado CS: Dissociation in Britain during the late nineteenth century: the Society for Psychical Research, 1882–1900. J Trauma Dissociation 3:9–33, 2002

American Psychiatric Association: Diagnostic and Statistical Manual of Mental Disorders, 3rd Edition. Washington, DC, American Psychiatric Association, 1980

Azam E: Amnésie périodique ou dédoublement de la vie. Ann Med Psychol (Paris) 16:5–35, 1876

Barkworth T: Duplex versus multiplex personality. Journal of the Society for Psychical Research 4:58–60, 1889

Barrois C: Les Névroses Traumatiques. Paris, Dunod, 1988

Bernstein EM, Putnam FW: Development, reliability, and validity of a dissociation scale. J Nerv Ment Dis 174:727–735, 1986

Binet A: On Double Consciousness: Experimental Psychological Studies. Chicago, IL, Open Court, 1890

Binet A: Les Altérations de la Personnalité (1892). New York, D. Appleton and Company, 1896

Birmes P, Carreras D, Charlet J-P, et al: Peritraumatic dissociation and posttraumatic stress disorder in victims of violent assault. J Nerv Ment Dis 189:796–798, 2001

Boon S, Draijer N: Multiple personality disorder in the Netherlands: a clinical investigation of 71 patients. Am J Psychiatry 150:489–494, 1993

Bourneville D (ed): La Possession de Jeanne Fery, Religieuse Professe du Couvent des Soeurs Noires de la Ville de Mons (1584). Paris, Progrès Médical/ A. Delahaye et Lecrosnier, 1886

Bourru H, Burot P: Les Variations de la Personnalité. Paris, J.B. Baillière, 1888

Breuer J, Freud S: On the psychical mechanism of hysterical phenomena (1893), in The Standard Edition of the Complete Psychological Works of Sigmund Freud, Vol 2. Translated and edited by Strachey J, Strachey A. London, Hogarth Press, 2001

Bruce LC: Notes of a case of dual brain action. Brain 18:54–65, 1895

Butler LD, Duran RE, Jasiukaitis P, et al: Hypnotizability and traumatic experience: a diathesis-stress model of dissociative symptomatology. Am J Psychiatry 153:42–63, 1996

Camuset L: Un cas de dédoublement de la personnalité; période amnésique d'une année chez un jeune homme. Ann Med Psychol (Paris) 40:75–86, 1882

Carlson EB: Studying the interaction between physical and psychological states with the Dissociative Experiences Scale, in Dissociation: Culture, Mind, and Body. Edited by Spiegel D. Washington, DC, American Psychiatric Press, 1994, pp 41–58

Carlson ET: The history of multiple personality in the United States, I: the beginnings. Am J Psychiatry 138:666–668, 1981

Carlson ET: The history of multiple personality in the United States: Mary Reynolds and her subsequent reputation. Bull Hist Med 58:72–82, 1984

Charcot J.-M: Leçons sur les Maladies du Système Nerveux Faites à la Salpêtrière. Paris, Progrès Médical/A. Delahaye et Lecrosnier, 1887

Chu JA: Rebuilding Shattered Lives: The Responsible Treatment of Complex Posttraumatic Stress and Dissociative Disorders. New York, John Wiley, 1998

Chu JA, Dill DL: Dissociative symptoms in relation to childhood physical and sexual abuse. Am J Psychiatry 147:887–892, 1990

Coons PM: Confirmation of childhood abuse in child and adolescent cases of multiple personality disorder and dissociative disorder not otherwise specified. J Nerv Ment Dis 182:461–464, 1994

Crabtree A: From Mesmer to Freud: Magnetic Sleep and the Roots of Psychological Healing. New Haven, CT, Yale University Press, 1993

Crabtree A: "Automatism" and the emergence of dynamic psychiatry. J Hist Behav Sci 39:51–70, 2003

Crocq L: Les Traumatismes Psychiques de Guerre. Paris, Odile Jacob, 1999

Deleuze JPF: Histoire Critique du Magnétisme Animal, Vol 1, 2nd Edition. Paris, Mame, 1819

Dwight BW: Facts illustrative of the powers and operations of the human mind in a diseased state. Am J Sci 1:431–433, 1818

Ellenberger HF: The Discovery of the Unconscious. New York, Basic Books, 1970

Eulenburg A: Lehrbuch der Nervenkrankheiten. Berlin, August Hirschwald, 1878

Faure H, Kersten J, Koopman D, et al: The 19th century DID case of Louis Vivet: new findings and re-evaluation. Dissociation 10:104–113, 1997

Fine CG: The work of Antoine Despine: the first scientific report on the diagnosis and treatment of a child with multiple personality disorder. Am J Clin Hypn 31:33–39, 1988

Fischer-Homberger E: Die Traumatische Neurose: Vom Somatischen zum Sozialen Leiden. Bern, Switzerland, Hans Huber, 1975

Forrest D: The Evolution of Hypnotism. Forfar, Scotland, Black Ace Books, 1999

Freud S: The etiology of hysteria (1896), in The Standard Edition of the Complete Psychological Works of Sigmund Freud, Vol 1. Translated and edited by Strachey J. London, Hogarth, 1953, pp 189–221

Freud S: My views on the part played by sexuality in the etiology of the neuroses (1906), in The Standard Edition of the Complete Psychological Works of Sigmund Freud, Vol 7. Translated and edited by Strachey J. London, Hogarth, 1953, pp 269–279

Gale H: A case of alleged loss of personal identity. Proceedings of the Society for Psychical Research 15:90–95, 1900

Gilles de la Tourette G: L'Hypnotisme et les États Analogues au Point de Vue Médico-Légal. Paris, Librairie Plon, 1887

Goodwin J: Mary Reynolds: a post-traumatic reinterpretation of a classic case of multiple personality disorder. Hillside J Clin Psychiatry 9:89–99, 1987

Greaves GB: Multiple personality: 165 years after Mary Reynolds. J Nerv Ment Dis 168:577–596, 1980

Gurney E: Recent experiments in hypnotism. Proceedings of the Society for Psychical Research 5:3–17, 1888

Hales NG: Morton Prince. Psychotherapy and Multiple Personality: Selected Essays. Cambridge, MA, Harvard University Press, 1975

Herman JL: Trauma and Recovery. New York, Basic Books, 1992

Hilgard ER: Toward a neo-dissociation theory: multiple cognitive controls in human functioning. Perspect Biol Med 17:301–316, 1974

Hilgard ER: Divided Consciousness: Multiple Controls in Human Thought and Action. New York, Wiley, 1977

Holmes EA, Brown RJ, Mansell W, et al: Are there two qualitatively distinct forms of dissociation? A review and some clinical implications. Clin Psychol Rev 25:1–23, 2005

Irwin HJ: Proneness to dissociation and traumatic childhood events. J Nerv Ment Dis 182:456–460, 1994

Janet J: L'hystérie et l'hypnotisme d'après la théorie de la double personnalité. Revue Scientifique 1:616–623, 1888

Janet P: L'Automatisme Psychologique: Essai de Psychologie Expérimentale Sur les Formes Inférieures de l'Activité Humaine. Paris, Félix Alcan, 1889

Janet P: Névroses et Idées Fixes. Paris, Félix Alcan, 1898

Janet P: The Mental State of Hystericals. New York, Putnam's Sons, 1901

Janet P: The Major Symptoms of Hysteria. New York, Macmillan, 1907

Janet P: Problèmes psychologiques de l'émotion. Revue de Neurologie 17:1551–1687, 1909

Janet P: L'État Mental des Hystériques, 2nd Edition. Paris, Félix Alcan, 1911

Janet P: Les Médications Psychologiques. Paris, Félix Alcan, 1919

Janet P: L'Évolution Psychologique de la Personnalité. Paris, A. Chahine, 1929

Kihlstrom JF: Dissociative and conversion disorders, in Cognitive Science and Clinical Disorders. Edited by Stein DJ, Young JE. San Diego, CA, Academic Press, 1992, pp 248–270

Kluft RP: Multiple personality disorder, in Dissociative Disorders: A Clinical Review. Edited by Spiegel D. Lutherville, MD, Sidran Press, 1993, pp 17–44

Kluft RP: Dissociative identity disorder, in Handbook of Dissociation: Theoretical, Empirical, and Clinical Perspectives. Edited by Michelson LK, Ray WJ. New York, Plenum, 1996, pp 337–366

Koopman C, Classen C, Spiegel D: Predictors of posttraumatic stress symptoms among survivors of the Oakland/Berkeley, Calif., firestorm. Am J Psychiatry 151:888–894, 1994

Lewis DO, Yeager CA, Swica Y, et al: Objective documentation of child abuse and dissociation in 12 murderers with dissociative identity disorder. Am J Psychiatry 154:1703–1710, 1997

Leys R: Trauma: A Genealogy. Chicago, IL, University of Chicago Press, 2000

Ludwig AM: Altered states of consciousness. Arch Gen Psychiatry 15:225–234, 1966

Marmar CR, Weiss DS, Metzler T: The Peritraumatic Dissociative Experiences Questionnaire, in Assessing Psychological Trauma and PTSD. Edited by Wilson JP, Keane TM. New York, Guilford, 1997, pp 412–428

Marshall GN, Schell TL: Reappraising the link between peritraumatic dissociation and PTSD symptom severity: evidence from a longitudinal study of community violence survivors. J Abnorm Psychol 111:626–636, 2002

McDougall W: An Outline of Abnormal Psychology. London, Methuen and Co., 1926

Micale MS, Lerner P: Traumatic Pasts: History, Psychiatry, and Trauma in the Modern Age, 1870–1930. Cambridge, MA, Cambridge University Press, 2001

Mitchell SL: A double consciousness, or a duality of persons in the same individual. Medical Repository 3:185–186, 1816

Mitchell SW: Mary Reynolds: a case of double consciousness. Transactions of the College of Physicians of Philadelphia 10:366–389, 1888

Mitchell TW: Medical Psychology and Psychical Research. London, Methuen and Co., 1922

Moreau de Tours JJ: Du Hachisch et de l'Aliénation Mentale: Études Psychologiques. Paris, Fortin, Masson et Cie, 1845

Myers CS: Shell Shock in France 1914–1918. Cambridge, MA, Cambridge University Press, 1940

Myers FWH: Multiplex personality. Proceedings of the Society for Psychical Research 4:496–514, 1887

Myers FWH: The subliminal consciousness: the mechanism of hysteria. Proceedings of the Society for Psychical Research 9: 2–25, 1893

Nemiah JC: Dissociation, conversion, and somatization, in Review of Psychiatry, Vol. 10. Edited by Tasman A, Goldfinger SM. Washington, DC, American Psychiatric Press, 1991, pp 248–260

Nijenhuis ERS: Somatoform Dissociation: Phenomena, Measurement, and Theoretical Issues. Assen, The Netherlands, Van Gorcum, 1999

Nijenhuis ERS, van der Hart O: Somatoform dissociative phenomena: a Janetian perspective, in Splintered Reflections: Images of the Body in Trauma. Edited by Goodwin JM, Attias R. New York, Basic Books, 1999, pp 89–127

Nijenhuis ERS, Spinhoven P, Van Dyck R, et al: The development and psycho-metric characteristics of the somatoform dissociation questionnaire (SDQ-20). J Nerv Ment Dis 184:688–694, 1996

Nijenhuis ERS, Spinhoven P, Vanderlinden J, et al: Somatoform dissociative symptoms as related to animal defensive reactions to predatory threat and injury. J Abnorm Psychol 107:63–73, 1998

Nijenhuis ERS, van der Hart O, Steele K: The emerging psychobiology of trauma-related dissociation and dissociative disorders, in Biological Psychiatry. Edited by D'Haenen H, den Boer JA, Willner P. Chicester, England, Wiley, 2002, pp 1079–1098

Nijenhuis ERS, van der Hart O, Steele K: Trauma-related structural dissociation of the personality. Trauma Information Pages Web site, January 2004. Available online at http://www.trauma-pages.com/a/nijenhuis-2004.php. Accessed August 17, 2006

Ogawa JR, Sroufe LA, Weinfield NS, et al: Development and the fragmented self: longitudinal study of dissociative symptomatology in a nonclinical sample. Dev Psychopathol 9:855–879, 1997

Prince M: The Dissociation of a Personality. New York, Longmans, Green, 1906a

Prince M: Hysteria from the point of view of dissociated personality. J Abnorm Psychol 1:170–187, 1906b

Prince M: The psychological principles and field of psychotherapy. J Abnorm Psychol 4:72–98, 1909

Putnam FW: Diagnosis and Treatment of Multiple Personality Disorder. New York, Guilford, 1989

Putnam FW: Dissociation in Children and Adolescents: A Developmental Perspective. New York, Guilford, 1997

Putnam FW, Trickett P: The psychobiological effects of sexual abuse: a longitudinal study. Ann NY Acad Sci 821:150–159, 1997

Ross CA: Multiple Personality Disorder: Diagnosis, Clinical Features, and Treatment. New York, Wiley, 1989

Shalev AY, Peri T, Canetti L, et al: Predictors of PTSD in injured trauma survivors: a prospective study. Am J Psychiatry 153:219–225, 1996

Sidis B: Psychopathological Researches: Studies in Mental Dissociation. New York, G.E. Stechert, 1902

Sidis B, Goodhart SP: Multiple Personality: An Experimental Investigation Into the Nature of Human Individuality. New York, D. Appleton and Company, 1904

Spiegel D: Hypnosis and traumatic dissociation: therapeutic opportunities. J Trauma Dissociation 4:73–90, 2003

Spiegel D, Cardeña E: Disintegrated experience: the dissociative disorders revisited. J Abnorm Psychol 100:366–378, 1991

Spiegel D, Hunt T, Dondershine HE: Dissociation and hypnotizability in post-traumatic stress disorder. Am J Psychiatry 145:301–305, 1988

Steele K, Dorahy M, van der Hart O, et al: Dissociation versus alterations in consciousness: related but different concepts, in Dissociation and the Dissociative Disorders: DSM-V and Beyond. Edited by Dell P, O'Neil JA. New York, Routledge, in press

Tart CT (ed): Altered States of Consciousness. New York, Anchor Books, 1969

Tascher P: Seconde Lettre de Gros-Jean à Son Évêque au Sujet des Tables Parlantes, des Possessions, des Sibylles, du Magnétisme et Autres Diableries. Paris, Ledoyen, 1855

Taylor E: William James On Exceptional Mental States: The 1896 Lowell Lectures. Amherst, MA, The University of Massachusetts Press, 1983

Trimble MR: Post-Traumatic Neurosis: From Railway Spine to the Whiplash. Chichester, England, Wiley, 1981

Vaillant GE: The historical origins of Sigmund Freud's concept of the mechanisms of defense, in Ego Mechanisms of Defense: A Guide for Clinicians and Researchers. Edited by Vaillant GE. Washington, DC, American Psychiatric Press, 1992, pp 3–28

van der Hart O: Dissociation: past developments. Keynote address presented at the 14th International Congress of Hypnosis, San Diego, CA, June 1997

van der Hart O, Brown P: Concept of psychological trauma. Am J Psychiatry 147:1691, 1993

van der Hart O, Dorahy MJ: Dissociation: history of a concept, in Dissociation and the Dissociative Disorders: DSM-V and Beyond. Edited by Dell P, O'Neil JA. New York, Routledge, in press

van der Hart O, Horst R: The dissociation theory of Pierre Janet. J Trauma Stress 2:397–412, 1989

van der Hart O, Lierens R, Goodwin J: Jeanne Fery: a sixteenth-century case of dissociative identity disorder. J Psychohist 24:18–35, 1996

van der Hart O, van der Kolk BA, Boon S: Treatment of dissociative disorders, in Trauma, Memory, and Dissociation. Edited by Bremner JD, Marmar CR. Washington, DC, American Psychiatric Press, 1998, pp 253–283

van der Hart O, Van Dijke A, Van Son M, et al: Somatoform dissociation in traumatized World War I combat soldiers: a neglected clinical heritage. J Trauma Dissociation 1:33–66, 2000

van der Hart O, Nijenhuis E, Steele K: The Haunted Self: Structural Dissociation and the Treatment of Chronic Traumatization. New York, Norton, 2006

van der Kolk BA, McFarlane AC, van der Hart O: History of trauma in psychiatry, in Traumatic Stress. Edited by van der Kolk BA, McFarlane AC, Weisaeth L. New York, Guilford, 1996a, pp 47–74

van der Kolk BA, van der Hart O, Marmar CR: Dissociation and information processing in posttraumatic stress disorder, in Traumatic Stress. Edited by van der Kolk BA, McFarlane AC, Weisaeth L. New York, Guilford, 1996b, pp 303–327

Vanderlinden J, Van Dyck R, Vandereycken W, et al: The Dissociation Question-naire (DIS-Q): development and characteristics of a new self-report ques-tionnaire. Clin Psychol Psychother 1:1–7, 1993

Venman H: The probably continuous activity of what is known as our secondary consciousness. Journal of Society for Psychical Research 4:76–77, 1889

Voisin A: Leçons Cliniques sur les Maladies Mentales et sur les Maladies Nerveuses. Paris, J.B. Bailliere et Fils, 1883

Weiss DS, Marmar CR, Metzler TJ: Predicting symptomatic distress in emer-gency service workers. J Consult Clin Psychol 63:361–368, 1995

Wilbur CB: The effects of childhood abuse on the psyche, in Childhood Ante-cedents of Multiple Personality Disorder. Edited by Kluft RP. Washington, DC, American Psychiatric Press, 1985, pp 21–35

Young: A: The Harmony of Illusions: Inventing Post-Traumatic Stress Disorder. Princeton, NJ, Princeton University Press, 1995

C H A P T E R 2

ATTACHMENT, DISORGANIZATION, AND DISSOCIATION

DORITH HARARI, M.D.
MARIAN J. BAKERMANS-KRANENBURG, PH.D.
MARINUS J. VAN IJZENDOORN, PH.D.

Since the 1970s, attachment theory has developed into one of the most influential and productive lines of research in developmental, social, and clinical psychology. The strength of attachment theory lies in the combination of a strong empirical foundation and a theoretical integration of approaches from various scientific disciplines, combining insights from ethology, evolutionary biology, cognitive science, and developmental and analytical psychology.

Attachment theory deals with the way children and adults handle fear and with the organization and transformation of reactions to fear into attachment representations in the course of emotional and cognitive development. Secure attachment has been associated with adequate psychological functioning, whereas insecure attachments have been associated with a variety of psychopathological conditions (Dozier et al. 1999).

The insecure style of disorganized/disoriented attachment has been linked both conceptually and empirically to the occurrence of dissociative phenomena (Carlson 1998; Main and Morgan 1996; Ogawa et al. 1997; van IJzendoorn et al. 1999). Moreover, some researchers have conceptualized disorganization of attachment as a condition prototypical of the development of dissociative disorders (Liotti 1999a, 1999b). Although other developmental pathways leading to dissociation are possible, and although dissociation is not an inevitable outcome of disorganization, there is some evidence for disorganization of attachment as a risk factor for the development of dissociation.

This chapter begins with a short overview of attachment theory and the organized types of secure and insecure attachment. Next, disorganization of attachment is discussed in terms of observable behavior in children and adults and of the phenotypical resemblance of this behavior to dissociative phenomena. Concomitants and sequelae of attachment disorganization, along with its determinants, are reviewed, followed by an hypothesized model of cognitive processes associated with disorganized attachment. The model implies a causal relation between disorganized attachment and later dissociative disorders. Finally, clinical implications for the prevention of disorganized attachment and for the treatment of dissociative disorders are discussed.

OVERVIEW OF ATTACHMENT THEORY

A central notion in attachment theory is that infants' reactions to anxiety and fear consist of a repertoire of innate behaviors aimed at increasing proximity to a central caregiver—the attachment figure. In the course of the first year of life, these behaviors crystallize within the context of the infant's relationship with the caregiver into organized strategies for dealing with stressful situations and negative emotions, particularly fear. Thus, infants with a *secure* attachment exhibit attachment behavior when distressed and are readily comforted by the parent, whom they can use efficiently as a secure base from which to explore their world (Weinfield et al. 1999).

Infants demonstrating *insecure-avoidant* attachment tend to have consistently experienced parental rejection of negative emotions. When distressed, they minimize attachment behavior and shift their attention away from the parent, thereby avoiding the additional stress of rejection. Infants classified as *insecure-ambivalent* supposedly experience their parents as unpredictably responsive and maximize or heighten their display of attachment behavior in an attempt to ensure their parents' response. They remain passively or angrily focused on the parent, even in the absence of fearful stimuli (Weinfield et al. 1999).

These behavioral strategies are considered to correspond to internal working models, which contain both an image of the self and of the attachment figure and reflect the infant's relational experiences with his or her primary caregiver (usually a parent). Internal working models, termed *attachment representations,* are essential in the infant's self-regulation of emotion and in his or her cognitive functioning around attachment-related issues. Attachment representations influence the meaning assigned to attachment-related experiences as well as their conscious accessibility (Bretherton and Munholland 1999).

Attachment representations in nonclinical samples appear to be consistently distributed across cultures, with roughly two-thirds of cases securely attached (van IJzendoorn and Sagi 1999). In infants, the gold standard for assessing attachment quality is the Ainsworth Strange Situation Procedure (SSP; Ainsworth et al. 1978; Hesse 1999), which consists of a series of separation and reunion episodes in a laboratory setting. In adolescents and adults, attachment representation is assessed with the Adult Attachment Interview (AAI; C. George, N. Kaplan, M. Main: "Adult Attachment Interview," unpublished manuscript, University of California at Berkeley, 1985; Hesse 1999; M. Main, R. Goldwyn, "Adult Attachment Scoring and Classification System," unpublished manuscript, University of California at Berkeley, 1984). This semistructured interview evaluates the subject's way of recounting and reflecting on salient attachment experiences. In the adult's verbal responses, preoccupation with attachment issues, avoidance, and clear acknowledgment of painful emotions correspond with child ambivalent, avoidant, and secure attachment behaviors in stressful situations (Hesse 1999). Parental AAI score has been found to strongly predict the quality of the parent–infant attachment relationship as measured by the SSP and to also predict parental responsiveness to infant attachment signals (van IJzendoorn 1995). In varying clinical and forensic adult samples, insecure attachments are strongly overrepresented (van IJzendoorn and Bakermans-Kranenburg 1996).

DISORGANIZED ATTACHMENT: OBSERVABLE BEHAVIOR

Whereas secure, insecure-avoidant, and insecure-ambivalent attachments can be considered *organized* strategies that are adaptive to the child's (sometimes suboptimal) environment, in nonclinical populations approximately 15%–20% (van IJzendoorn et al. 1999) of the attachment relationships appear to be characterized by the absence or breakdown of an otherwise organized strategy, hence defined as *disorganized* (Main and Solomon 1990). The classification of *disorganized attachment* represents the fourth identified attachment style.

Disorganized attachment behaviors are considered to mirror the infant's acute dilemma in the face of stressful circumstances, namely in the presence of a frightening parent. This is evident, for example, after a brief separation in the SSP; the child's dilemma is that he or she cannot

resolve the stress and anxiety created by the parent being simultaneously the source of fear and the only possible protective figure. In the
face of this paradoxical situation, in which the child experiences "fright
without solution" (Hesse and Main 2000), the infant's organized attachment strategy is expected to fall apart, at least momentarily (Main and
Hesse 1990). Indices of disorganized attachment behavior as expressed
in the SSP reflect this dilemma: sequential or simultaneous displays of
contradictory behavior, such as distress and avoidance; undirected or
misdirected movements and expressions; stereotypical and anomalous
movements or postures; freezing or stilling behaviors; expressions of
fear or apprehension regarding the parent; and clear indices of confusion in the presence of the parent (Main and Solomon 1990). In the SSP,
contradictory behavior may be observed when the infant shows indiffer-
ence upon reunion after excessive distress during separation. *Misdirected behavior* may consist of seeking proximity to the stranger instead of
to the parent upon reunion. *Stereotypical behaviors* include the repeated
pulling of hair with a dazed expression in a context in which the child is
clearly stressed and the parent is available. *Freezing* refers to occasions
when the child stops moving for several moments as though in a trance
and dissociated from regular thought processes (Main and Morgan
1996). It appears to be associated with the child's inability to choose between seeking proximity and avoiding the parent. *Apprehension* means
showing fear of the parent immediately after a brief separation, such as
by a hand-to-mouth movement. *Disorientation* may occur when—after
the entrance of the parent—the child suddenly becomes clumsy and
falls down without visible cause or reason. Disorganized behavior in the
SSP may be very brief, and episodes of less than 30 seconds may suffice
for placement in the category of disorganized attachment.

In adults, the unresolved category of the AAI is akin to the disorganized attachment type in the SSP. An adult is categorized as unresolved if
his or her narrative exhibits disorganization when he or she is attempting
to discuss traumatic experiences, such as loss or abuse. Disorganization
may be the result of lapses in the monitoring of reasoning or discourse
(M. Main, R. Goldwyn, "Adult Attachment Scoring and Classification
System," unpublished manuscript, University of California at Berkeley,
1984). Examples of lapses in the monitoring of reasoning are statements
that are logically incompatible with one another or with common understanding of time and causality. For example, a subject may state in the interview that he or she has never experienced the death of a close relative
but in the same interview state that his or her mother died last year. As a
second example, a person may speak about someone deceased as though
that person were still alive; for example, a patient whose mother had

been dead for several years stated, "my mother always gets angry with the wrong person." Lapses in the monitoring of discourse include prolonged silences and inability to finish sentences as well as changes in discourse register, moving to eulogistic speech or to extreme attention for detail. Finally, reported lapses in monitoring of behavior, such as being unable to work for a long period after a loss, are considered an index of disorganization but are rarely sufficient reason for placement in the unresolved category (M. Main, R. Goldwyn, "Adult Attachment Scoring and Classification System," unpublished manuscript, University of California at Berkeley, 1984; Main and Morgan 1996).

Like disorganization in infant attachment behavior, lapses in the monitoring of reasoning or discourse may be very brief and subtle, amounting to only a few sentences in an otherwise coherent transcript. Disorganization in a parental AAI has been consistently found to predict disorganized attachment in the infant (van IJzendoorn et al. 1999).

PHENOTYPICAL RESEMBLANCE OF DISORGANIZED ATTACHMENT IN DISSOCIATIVE STATES

Main (1996) pointed out the phenotypical resemblance between some forms of disorganized infant attachment behavior, lapses in monitoring in AAI transcripts, and dissociative states. In disorganized infants, freezing, trance-like states, and sudden intrusion of incompatible behavior or aggressive actions in an otherwise nonaggressive context (e.g., accompanied by smiling) bear a strong resemblance to dissociative states as diagnosed in adults. In unresolved AAI transcripts, prolonged silences can be considered trance-like states in which the subject is no longer aware of the interview context. When a trauma is discussed, a sudden and temporary change of discourse into a different, visual-sensory detailed style of speech reflects intrusion of traumatic memory into consciousness, interfering with normal monitoring of discourse. The same applies for breakdown of discourse into incoherent speech. A lack of integration and dissociation of traumatic memory from conscious functioning can be seen when incompatible beliefs coexist; for example, a belief that a person is dead and at the same time a belief that the person is not dead, or a belief that one witnessed a traumatic event and at the same time a belief that one was not present at this event.

Thus, disruption in the usually integrated functions of consciousness, memory, identity, or perception of the environment, which is the central feature of the dissociative disorders, can be observed in instances of attachment disorganization both in children in the SSP and in adults in the AAI.

CONCOMITANTS AND SEQUELAE OF DISORGANIZED ATTACHMENT

Several studies have shown that disorganized attachment in infancy is predictive of problematic stress management as indicated by increased cortisol excretion and heart rate variability in stressful settings (Hertsgaard et al. 1995; Spangler and Grossman 1993, 1999; Willemsen-Swinkels et al. 2000) and an elevated risk of externalizing behavior problems (e.g., Carlson 1998; Hubbs-Tait et al. 1994; Lyons-Ruth et al. 1997). It is unclear why disorganized children would be especially liable to develop externalizing problem behaviors instead of other developmental problems, such as internalizing problems. One possible explanation may be that externalizing behavior, more specifically reactive aggression, is committed in dissociative states of mind. Attachment disorganization, as is discussed later in this chapter, is considered a major vulnerability factor for dissociative states and thus possibly for reactive aggression as well. A somewhat different conceptualization is advanced by Liotti (1999a), who speculated that in order to avoid painful and confusing attachment experiences, disorganized children may deactivate their attachment motivational system by routinely activating other biological motivational systems, such as sexual or antagonistic systems, the latter resulting in aggressive, antagonistic behavior.

Three studies identified in a comprehensive meta-analysis that examined 80 studies of attachment disorganization (van IJzendoorn et al. 1999) documented significant effects of disorganized attachment on infants' physical stress reactions. Spangler and Grossman (1993) found increased cortisol after the SSP in both insecure-avoidant and disorganized infants. Hertsgaard et al. (1995) found elevated cortisol following the SSP in disorganized but not insecure-avoidant infants. Willemsen-Swinkels et al. (2000) found that disorganized attachment was associated with an increase in heart rate during parting from the caregiver and a decrease in heart rate during reunion in children with pervasive developmental disorder, developmental language disorder, and those developing normally. Disorganized attachment has been found to be associated with hyperreactive neurophysiological responses to stressors in descriptive, nonexperimental studies. Attachment theory suggests that this hyperreactivity is one of the consequences of disorganized attachment and does not constitute a causal determinant. The corollary of *organized* attachment relationships as regulators of negative emotions is the idea of *disorganized* attachments leading to dysregulation of negative emotions, evidenced by a hyperreactive hypothalamic-pituitary-adrenal axis and larger heart rate variability in response to major stresses (van IJzendoorn and Bakermans-Kranenburg 2002).

DETERMINANTS OF DISORGANIZED ATTACHMENT

Determinants of disorganized attachment have been found in specific family phenomena, other environmental factors, genetic factors, and forms of parenting, specifically frightening parental behavior. Associations between specific family phenomena and later infant disorganization have been established in several studies (for an overview, see Lyons-Ruth and Jacobvitz 1999; van IJzendoorn et al. 1999). In samples of maltreated children, most infants appear to be classified as disorganized (Carlson et al. 1989; Cicchetti and Barnett 1991). Also, parental unresolved loss or exposure to trauma, as assessed in the AAI, appears to be significantly associated with infant disorganized attachment (see van IJzendoorn 1995). Furthermore, marital discord (Owen and Cox 1997) and parental depression (in particular bipolar mood disorder, e.g., Teti et al. 1995) have been suggested as precursors for disorganization. Adopted children are also at risk of attachment disorganization, particularly when they live in disturbing, depriving, or otherwise adverse circumstances before being placed for adoption (Marcovitch et al. 1997; Rutter 1998; Vorria et al. 2003).

From these findings, Main and Hesse (1990) derived their hypothesis of disorganized attachment as "fright without solution" (Main 1996). They suggested that parental unresolved loss or trauma would lead to involuntary expressions of fright and unexpected and threatening dissociative behaviors in the presence of their children. These children would then experience their parents as both the most important source of security and at the same time a source of overwhelming fear. The unpredictable transitions of their attachment figures into a different state of mind and subsequent frightening behaviors would cause a momentary breakdown of the children's otherwise organized attachment pattern (see Figure 2–1).

One of the implications of the Main and Hesse (1990) hypothesis is the prediction of a link between frightening or frightened parental behavior and disorganized attachment, which has been tested and demonstrated in four recent studies (Abrams 2000; Lyons-Ruth et al. 1999; Schuengel et al. 1999; True et al. 2001). In the study by Schuengel et al. (1999), 85 nonclinical middle-class mothers who had experienced an important loss were assessed for unresolved status in the AAI and for parental behavior during two home visits that lasted 2 hours each. Infants were seen in the SSP with their mothers. The Main and Hesse model was found to only apply to mothers with currently insecure attachment representations. Both in secure and insecure mothers, frightening behavior predicted infant disorganization. However, secure mothers with unre-

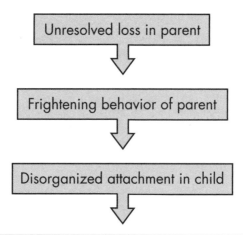

FIGURE 2–1. Parental unresolved loss leading to disorganized attachment in child.

solved loss displayed less frightening behavior than insecure mothers. Thus, whereas unresolved loss in insecure mothers predicted frightening behavior and ultimately disorganized attachment of their infants, in secure mothers unresolved loss did not predict frightening behavior to the extent that would lead to disorganized attachment in their infants. Security of attachment appears to be a protective factor in the relationship between parental unresolved loss, subsequent frightening behavior, and infant attachment disorganization (see Figure 2–2).

Postulating a model of unbalanced relationships predicting attachment disorganization, Lyons-Ruth et al. (1999) described two relational patterns in which the parent either coercively opposes and counters the attachment initiatives of the child through negative and intrusive behavior or withdraws from the interaction by being (extremely) unresponsive to the needs of the child. Solomon and George (1999) hypothesized that a profound lack of response, or "a failure to terminate" the child's attachment system, may lead to infant disorganization. In a meta-analysis on the studies using assessments of frightening, frightened, or extremely insensitive (neglectful or intrusive) parental behaviors, it was concluded that such anomalous parenting is rather strongly associated with attachment disorganization (Madigan et al., unpublished data).

Genetics of Disorganized Attachment

The studies just mentioned all focused on anomalous parenting behavior as a precursor of disorganized attachment. However, constitutional factors in the child may contribute to the emergence of disorganized attachment. In

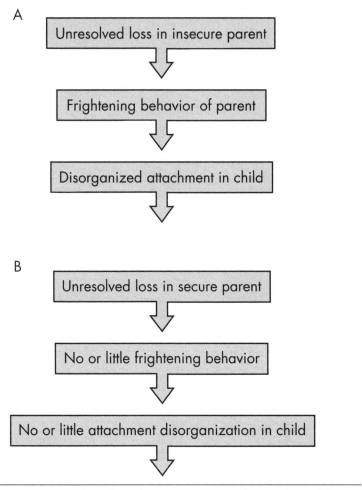

FIGURE 2-2. Parental attachment security as a protective factor in the possible development of attachment disorganization.

the first meta-analysis of disorganized attachment, it was documented that attachment disorganization did not appear to be associated with gender or temperament (van IJzendoorn et al. 1999), but child characteristics might nevertheless be important. For example, children with medical or physical problems (e.g., neurological abnormalities, Down syndrome) are supposed to be at risk for elevated rates of attachment disorganization (Rutgers et al. 2004), although this may be as a consequence of measurement problems (van IJzendoorn et al. 1999). Furthermore, Spangler et al. (1996) found that attachment disorganization was best predicted by newborn behavioral organization in terms of less optimal orienting ability and regulation.

In the first molecular genetic study, Lakatos et al. (2000) found an association between the dopamine D4 receptor (DRD4) gene polymorphism and attachment disorganization. In previous studies the DRD4 gene polymorphism had shown associations with pathological impulsive behavior and substance abuse in adults and attention-deficit/hyperactivity disorder in children. The dopaminergic system is engaged in attentional, motivational, and reward mechanisms (Robbins and Everitt 1999). A second study with the same group of infants showed that the association between disorganized attachment and the 7-repeat DRD4 allele was enhanced in the presence of a specific allele in the promoter region of the DRD4 gene. In the presence of both the exon III 48-bp 7-repeat allele and the –521 C/T or T/T allele in the upstream regulatory region of the DRD4 gene, the odds ratio for disorganized attachment was suggested to increase tenfold (Lakatos et al. 2002). These studies point to a genetic explanation for the development of attachment disorganization in normal, low-risk populations.

However, in a recent behavioral genetic study on monozygotic and dizygotic twins, the role of genetic factors in disorganized attachment was found to be negligible (Bokhorst et al. 2003). Because Lakatos et al. (2000, 2002) themselves pointed to the need for independent replication of their provocative findings, and in the past several examples of irreplicable molecular genetic findings have been detected, Bakermans-Kranenburg and van IJzendoorn (2004) replicated Lakatos et al.'s studies as an extension of a behavioral genetic study. The role of the DRD4 7-repeat allele and the –521 C/T promoter gene in disorganized attachment was not confirmed. Although the replication sample was larger (132 infants compared with 90 infants) and contained more children with C/T or T/T alleles, which enhanced the probability of finding the *DRD4* and C/T interaction, the association was not found. However, because of the modest percentage of disorganized children in nonclinical samples, lack of power might still explain the absence of genetic effects. Replication in a much larger sample is needed to address more accurately the issue of a genetic bias for disorganized attachment.

The issue of a genetic basis for disorganized attachments is important in view of the possible genetic determination of dissociation found in some behavior-genetic studies. If both disorganized attachment and dissociation were largely genetically determined, we would find potentially spurious associations between disorganization and dissociation through their common genetic basis. Becker-Blease et al. (2004) examined genetic and environmental sources of variance in dissociative behaviors in an adoption sample and in a twin sample. In the adoption sample, 86 pairs of adopted siblings were compared with 102 pairs of full siblings followed from ages 9 to 12 years. In the twin sample, 218 pairs of identical twins were compared with 173 pairs of same-sex fraternal twins ranging from 8 to 16 years of age. A measure of nonpathological dissociation derived from the Child Behavior Checklist was used. Results showed moderate to substantial amounts of genetic and nonshared (e.g., witnessing a serious car accident) environmental variance and negligible shared (e.g., neglect of all children by an alcoholic and depressed parent) environmental variance. These findings are consistent with an earlier study that found that genetic and environmental factors each made a contribution to nonpathological dissociation in adolescents and adults (Jang et al. 1998). In contrast, using the taxometric subscale of the Dissociative Experiences Scale (DES-T) in an adolescent twin sample, Waller and Ross (1997) found no genetic variance and both a large shared and nonshared environment component. Because the DES-T measures pathological dissociation, a possible explanation for these diverging findings may be that genetics play a larger role in normative dissociative behaviors, whereas environmental factors play a larger role in the etiology of dissociative disorders.

Interplay Between Neurobiological and Environmental Risks

Overall, the available empirical evidence to date appears to support variability in parenting rather than genetic factors as the most important contributor to the presence or absence of disorganized attachment. A modest genetic effect would not be incompatible with an environmental explanation of disorganized attachment: Some children may be especially susceptible to developing this type of attachment, whereas other children might be genetically protected against some of the negative consequences of similar parenting. Such differential susceptibility moderated by the DRD4 gene was found in a study by van IJzendoorn and Bakermans-Kranenberg (2006), where maternal unresolved loss or trauma was associated with infant disorganization only in the presence of the DRD4 polymorphism. This hypothesis is consistent with the evolutionary theory of differential susceptibility, which suggests that children with high temperamental reactivity may be more susceptible to childrearing influences in the socio-emotional domain than other children (Belsky 1997). An alternative or complementary explanation pertains to the possibility of a gene–environment interaction, the interplay between "nature" and "nurture" deriving from genetic effects on liability to risk exposure and susceptibility to environmental risks (e.g., Bennet et al. 2002; Caspi et al. 2002, 2003). So far, the associations between disorganized attachment and the two gene polymorphisms have been studied without reference to environmental risk. As demonstrated by Suomi (1999) in primates and by

Caspi et al. (2002, 2003) in humans, an individual's response to environmental influences may be moderated by his or her genetic makeup (gene–environment interaction) or by neurological status (e.g., high levels of monoamine oxidase A expression). In Bokhorst et al.'s (2003) twin study mentioned earlier, only unique environmental or error components could explain the variance in disorganized versus organized attachment, but it has been noted that a failure to include the gene–environment interaction is liable to lead to an overestimate of the genetic component (Rutter et al. 2001) as well as the nonshared environmental effects (Eaves et al. 2003).

RESEMBLANCE IN RISK FACTORS FOR THE DEVELOPMENT OF DISORGANIZED ATTACHMENT AND DISSOCIATIVE DISORDERS

In clinical samples, child physical and sexual abuse has been found to correlate with prevalence and severity of dissociative symptoms (Chu and Dill 1990; Draijer and Langeland 1999). Moreover, in a meta-analysis of the DES in clinical and nonclinical studies, van IJzendoorn and Schuengel (1996) found a rather strong association between dissociation and childhood physical and sexual abuse experiences. Associations with familial loss in a nonclinical sample (Irwin 1994) and with emotional abuse in clinical samples (Simeon et al. 2001, 2003) have also been documented. Focusing explicitly on caregiving experiences that may be common to disorganized attachment and dissociative disorders, Pasquini et al. (2002) found in a clinical case-control study that early traumatic experiences and maternal major losses within 2 years of the patient's birth were the greatest risk factors for the development of dissociative disorders. A similarly designed study with borderline personality disorder patients, a condition associated with dissociative phenomena (American Psychiatric Association 1994), established also that early traumatic experiences and maternal major loss within 2 years of the patient's birth were risk factors for borderline personality (Liotti and Pasquini 2000).

Thus, abuse and early familial loss have been associated with both attachment disorganization and dissociative disorders. Different mechanisms have been hypothesized underlying these associations. In terms of disorganized attachment, abuse is considered to lead to attachment disorganization through fright without solution and the collapse of attentional and behavioral strategies (Hesse and Main 2000). Familial loss is considered to contribute to the development of disorganized attachment through parental unresolved status leading to parental frightening behavior in interactions with the child, and again to fright without solution and the collapse of attentional and behavioral strategies (Lyons-Ruth and Jacobvitz 1999; Schuengel et al. 1999). In the relationship between dissociation and abuse or early trauma, attachment disorganization itself has been suggested as part of the causal mechanism, as is discussed in the next section.

A THEORETICAL MODEL OF ATTACHMENT DISORGANIZATION IN THE DEVELOPMENT OF DISSOCIATIVE DISORDERS

A theoretical model linking attachment disorganization and later dissociative disorders has been advanced by Liotti (1999a, 1999b), who proposed that disorganization in infancy increases a child's vulnerability to altered states of consciousness and dissociative disorders. According to this model, an unresolved caregiver who exhibits frightened and frightening behavior in interactions with the child leads the child to experience rapid shifts in perception of the self and other. With each shift, a different model of the self (as perpetrator of fright, as victim of fright, as rescuer, or as loved child) and of the other (as victim, as perpetrator, as rescued victim, and as caregiver) is operative. These rapidly shifting models effectively represent the young child's unpredictable relational environment and cannot be integrated. They continue to exist as multiple internal working models of self and other in attachment relationships. In a situation of acute distress, the multiple internal models not only hinder the search for help and comfort but also increase the experience of fear and lead to a paradoxical loop of ever-increasing fear: when approaching the parent, the child expects to be further frightened or to be frightening. Moreover, Liotti proposed that in this situation of overwhelming contradictory affects the child might cope by entering a minor dissociative state and that repeated minor dissociative states will result in a vulnerability to dissociative reactions to trauma. This latter statement is consistent with the concept of use-dependent development of the brain, advanced by Perry et al. (1995), which suggests that repeated dissociative experiences in the young child influence neural development and result in a sensitized neurobiology and a vulnerability to altered states.

Liotti proposed that disorganized attachment in itself does not lead to the development of dissociative disorders. In an attempt to override the psychological confusion, children with disorganized attachment may in the first years of life develop a strategy for handling fear and distress, often in the form of a role-inverting, controlling approach to the parent (Hesse and Main 2000), that fits in with one of the child's multiple contradictory internal working models. However, when a traumatic experience is superimposed on a disorganized attachment, this adopted

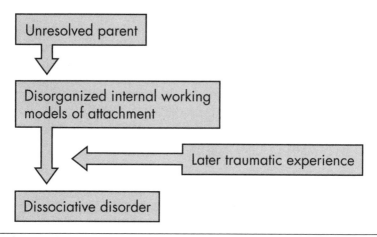

FIGURE 2–3.   Traumatic experience superimposed on attachment disorganization may lead to development of a dissociative disorder.

strategy may not suffice, and in the emerging disorganization dissociative disorders may develop (see Figure 2–3).

Trauma superimposed on an organized attachment representation is more likely to become integrated and resolved over time. Children and adults with an organized attachment representation are less likely to become overwhelmed in potentially traumatic circumstances, because their reactions to fear are integrated into an organized strategy. The fear and helplessness that are part of a traumatic experience are not increased by fear resulting from disintegration. In traumatic circumstances, these children and adults are less likely to enter a dissociative state, a phenomenon that would hinder integration and resolution.

Thus this model offers a possible explanation for the finding that not all attachment disorganization or traumatic experiences result in dissociative disorders. If no trauma is superimposed on attachment disorganization, or when trauma is experienced by persons with firmly established organized attachment strategies, the risk of dissociation is lowered. The model also explains why, in the limited findings currently available, dissociation strongly correlates with attachment disorganization, because attachment disorganization entails a strong vulnerability to develop dissociative disorder as a reaction to superimposed trauma.

This theoretical model is supported by various findings. First, there is a phenomenological resemblance between some disorganized attachment behaviors and dissociation, as discussed earlier in this chapter. Second, the contradictory tendencies the child experiences toward a frightening parent have been compared with the confusion technique used in certain forms of hypnotic induction (Liotti 1992, 1995). Moreover, propensities toward absorption have been related to unresolved status in the AAI (Hesse and van IJzendoorn 1999) and to parental loss of close family members (Hesse and van IJzendoorn 1998). This latter argument, however, presupposes a relation between hypnotizability and dissociative disorders for which no evidence was found in the meta-analysis conducted by van IJzendoorn and Schuengel (1996).

A third group of studies supportive of Liotti's model are those by Pasquini and colleagues (Liotti and Pasquini 2000; Pasquini et al. 2002), in which maternal early trauma and maternal loss around the birth of the child were predictive of dissociative disorders and borderline personality disorder in that child's adulthood. Finally, two further studies are supportive of Liotti's connection between attachment disorganization, early trauma, and dissociative disorders or phenomena later in life. In a cross-sectional study of 133 clinical adolescents (i.e., adolescents receiving different types of clinical treatment), West et al. (2001) found a relationship between unresolved and unclassifiable AAI status and dissociative symptomatology as assessed using a subscale of the Youth Self Report behavior checklist. Carlson (1998), in a longitudinal study of 128 socially deprived participants, found the combination of attachment disorganization in infancy and trauma was correlated ($r = 0.36$) with dissociative tendencies at ages 17.5 and 19 years and with greater risk for psychopathology in adolescence. In this study disorganization was measured with the SSP and dissociation was rated not only with a self-report questionnaire but also with teacher-rated episodes of elevated dissociation (Egeland and Susman-Stillman 1996).

CLINICAL IMPLICATIONS OF ATTACHMENT RESEARCH

Implications of attachment research are relevant in the areas of prevention of attachment disorganization and treatment of dissociative disorders. In the area of prevention, Schuengel et al.'s (1999) finding of maternal security as a protective factor suggests that maternal insecurity should be addressed first to minimize the occurrence of frightening behavior and ensuing disorganization (Byng-Hall 1999). Most attachment-based intervention studies have not aimed exclusively at prevention of attachment disorganization, but in 15 studies ($N=842$) disorganization was included as an outcome measure. A recent meta-analysis of these studies by Bakermans-Kranenburg et al. (2005) showed that sensitivity-focused interventions that aim at increasing the mother's sensitivity to her infant's needs and signals were most effective in preventing infant attachment disorganization. An example of such sensitivity-focused interventions is direct personal feedback or personal video feedback on the mother's interaction with her infant. The authors speculated that sensitivity-focused interventions may qualitatively affect certain forms of insensitive behavior that are linked to attachment disorganization but are not (yet) measurable—for example, parental intrusiveness and interfering or other disruptive behavior. Alternatively, they suggested that these interventions may have successfully affected the mothers' attentional processes, promoting the focusing of attention on the child. As a consequence of stronger focusing on the child, mothers would experience in the presence of the child both fewer intrusions of traumatic experiences and less frightening/frightened behaviors (Juffer et al. 2004).

Interventions aiming at parental sensitivity and attachment security in general, without addressing attachment disorganization, have recently been reviewed (Bakermans-Kranenburg et al. 2005). From a meta-analysis of 70 studies ($N=7{,}636$), the authors concluded that the sensitivity-focused type of interventions that were the most effective in reducing attachment disorganization were also most effective in enhancing attachment security, which supports the notion of a causal role of sensitivity in shaping attachment and the effectiveness of rather brief but behaviorally focused approaches.

In the area of therapy of dissociative disorders, attachment theory has inspired the study of transference. Liotti (1995) described five different internal working models of the attachment relationship that typically in rapid alternation shape the dissociative patient's experience in therapy. These internal working models are the child as victim; the child as persecutor (the cause of the parent's fear); the child as victim of impending danger from which he or she is rescued by the parent; the child as rescuer of a helpless and frightened parent; and the child and parent together as victims of external danger. The understanding of these different internal working models may be of therapeutic importance and is a means to increase the therapist's and the patient's insight into their interactions. Moreover, Liotti stated that in order to escape the painful and confusing experience of disorganized attachment, many disorganized patients deactivate their attachment system by routinely activating other biological behavioral systems, such as the sexual, the antagonistic, or the caregiving system. This may be the basis for the erotizing, chronic aggressive, or compulsory caring behavior often seen in early traumatized patients. A number of other theorists have been inspired by attachment research in conceptualizing the dynamics and specific phenomena in the treatment of dissociative disorders (Barach 1991; Blizard 2003; Steele et al. 2001).

Fonagy (1998) developed a treatment approach aimed at fostering patients' metacognitive skills. This approach is inspired by the assumption that children of abusive or frightened caregivers face an intolerable view of themselves as reflected by their caregiver and may have suspended their ability to reflect on their own and others' representational worlds. Because they are unable to see the actions of others, as well as their own actions, as resulting from intentional states, these children and later adults disavow self-agency and ownership of their actions. In Fonagy's approach, the aim of therapy is not insight but recovery of reflective functioning by ongoing clarification of moment-to-moment changes in the patient's mental state. Successful therapy is considered a maturational process in which mentalizing capacity is restored.

Because therapies promoting security of attachment in parents indirectly lower the risk of dissociation in their children (by reducing attachment disorganization), it is worthwhile to consider the influence of both client and clinician attachment in the context of corrective emotional experience. Bernier and Dozier (1994, 2002) found that case managers who were more secure were better able to respond to the underlying neediness of clients, whether these clients were using dismissing or preoccupied strategies. (An example of a *preoccupied strategy* is presenting oneself as very vulnerable, thus eliciting caretaking in others. An example of a *dismissing strategy* is presenting oneself as strong and self-reliant, thus eliciting very little caretaking behavior in others). Analyzing the phenomenon of corrective emotional experience, Bernier and Dozier stated that the most effective combinations are probably those of somewhat dismissing therapists with preoccupied clients and somewhat preoccupied therapists with dismissing clients. The counterbalancing of the client's attachment bias to dismissiveness or preoccupation appeared to provide the best fit between therapist and client (Bernier and Dozier 2002). It is hypothesized that the therapist's natural style helps him or her to resist the pull to react to the client in a complementary way. Thus the client's often rigid strategies are not reinforced, and an opportunity is created for changing and adapting strategies.

Another important therapeutic approach aimed at enhancing security of attachment is family and couple therapy. Byng-Hall (1995) introduced the concept of a *secure family base*, defined as a family that provides a reliable network of attachment relationships, which enables all family members of whatever age to feel sufficiently secure to explore relationships with each other and with others outside the family. The concept involves shared responsibility among family members who collaborate in order to assure care of any member in need of it. For young children this implies the expectation of reliable handover and continuity of care. A family functioning as a secure base promotes security of attachment in all members, particularly children. Byng-Hall (1995, 1999) described how a family therapist can provide a temporary secure base for the family during therapy and improve security in the family as a whole. In order to provide a secure therapeutic base for the family, the therapist has to prove him- or herself to be available and has to fulfill two important functions of an attachment figure: to be alert to potential danger by addressing core anxieties and conflicts, and to facilitate exploration. By helping family members to explore ways of improving the security of the family base, the therapist also helps them to explore and solve their own problems during and after therapy.

CONCLUSION

Attachment disorganization constitutes a major vulnerability in children to react to traumatic experiences with psychopathology, most notably dissociative disorders. Attachment disorganization may be related to genetic factors that are still being studied and, very probably, to early parenting experiences. These parenting experiences include not only frightening, abusive behavior, which has long been recognized as an important determinant of dissociation, but also frightened behavior in parents with unresolved loss or their own trauma history. Because attachment disorganization is both empirically and conceptually linked to dissociation, attachment theory has inspired several conceptual approaches to the prevention and treatment of dissociative disorders and disorganized attachment. In summary, attachment theory provides a new perspective on the etiology, prevention, and treatment of dissociative disorders, emphasizing the early relational basis of increased vulnerability to dissociate in the aftermath of traumatic experiences.

REFERENCES

Abrams KY: Pathways to disorganization: a study concerning varying types of parental frightened and frightening behaviors as related to infant disorganized attachment. Doctoral dissertation, University of California at Berkeley, Berkeley, California, 2000
Ainsworth MDS, Blehar MC, Waters E, et al: Patterns of Attachment: A Psychological Study of the Strange Situation. Hillsdale, NJ, Erlbaum, 1978
American Psychiatric Association: Diagnostic and Statistical Manual of Mental Disorders, 4th Edition. Washington, DC, American Psychiatric Association, 1994
Bakermans-Kranenburg MJ, van IJzendoorn M: No association of the dopamine D4 receptor (DRD4) and -521C/T promoter polymorphisms with infant attachment disorganization. Attach Hum Dev 6:211–218, 2004

Bakermans-Kranenburg MJ, van IJzendoorn M, Juffer F: Disorganized infant attachment and preventive interventions: a review and meta-analysis. Infant Ment Health J 26:191–216, 2005

Barach PM: Multiple personality disorder as an attachment disorder. Dissociation 4:117–123, 1991

Becker-Blease KA, Deater-Deckard K, Eley T, et al: A genetic analysis of individual difference in dissociative behaviors in childhood and adolescence. J Child Psychol Psychiatry 45:522–532, 2004

Belsky J: Theory testing, effect-size evaluation and differential susceptibility to rearing influence: the case of mothering and attachment. Child Dev 68:598–600, 1997

Bennet AJ, Lesch KP, Heils A, et al: Early experience and serotonin transporting gene variation interact to influence primate CNS function. Mol Psychiatry 7:118–122, 2002

Bernier A, Dozier M: Clinicians as caregivers: role of attachment organization in treatment. J Consult Clin Psychol 62:793–800, 1994

Bernier A, Dozier M: The client-counselor match and the corrective emotional experience: evidence from interpersonal and attachment research. Psychotherapy 39:32–43, 2002

Blizard RA: Disorganized attachment, development of dissociated self states, and a relational approach to treatment. J Trauma Dissociation 4:27–50, 2003

Bokhorst CL, Bakermans-Kranenburg MJ, Fearon P, et al: The importance of shared environment in mother-infant attachment security: a behavioral genetic study. Child Dev 74:1769–1782, 2003

Bretherton I, Munholland KA: Internal working models in attachment relationships, in Handbook of Attachment: Theory, Research, and Clinical Applications. Edited by Cassidy J, Shaver PR. New York, Guilford, 1999, pp 89–111

Byng-Hall J: Rewriting Family Scripts: Improvisation and Systems Change. New York, Guilford, 1995

Byng-Hall J: Family and couple therapy: toward greater security, in Handbook of Attachment: Theory, Research, and Clinical Applications. Edited by Cassidy J, Shaver PR. New York, Guilford, 1999, pp 625–648

Carlson EA: A prospective longitudinal study of attachment disorganization/disorientation. Child Dev 69:1107–1128, 1998

Carlson EA, Cicchetti D, Barnett D, et al: Disorganized/disoriented attachment relationships in maltreated infants. Devel Psychol 25:525–531, 1989

Caspi A, McClay J, Moffit T E, et al: Role of genotype in the cycle of violence in maltreated children. Science 297:852–854, 2002

Caspi A, Sugden K, Moffit TE, et al: Influence of life stress on depression: moderation by a polymorphism in the 5-HTT gene. Lancet 361:865–872, 2003

Chu JA, Dill DL: Dissociative symptoms in relation to childhood physical and sexual abuse. Am J Psychiatry 147:887–892, 1990

Cicchetti D, Barnett D: Attachment organization in maltreated preschoolers. Special issue: attachment and developmental psychopathology. Dev Psychopathol 3:397–411, 1991

Dozier M, Stovall KC, Albus KE: Attachment and psychopathology in adult-hood. in Handbook of Attachment: Theory, Research, and Clinical Applications. Edited by Cassidy J, Shaver PR. New York, Guilford, 1999, pp 497–519

Draijer N, Langeland W: Childhood trauma and perceived parental dysfunction in the etiology of dissociative symptoms in psychiatric inpatients. Am J Psychiatry 156:379–385, 1999

Eaves L, Silberg JL, Erkanli A: Resolving multiple epigenetic pathways to adolescent depression. J Child Psychol Psychiatry 44:1006–1014, 2003

Egeland B, Susman-Stillman A: Dissociation as a mediator of child abuse across generations. Child Abuse Negl 20:1123–1132, 1996

Fonagy P: An attachment theory approach to the treatment of the difficult patient. Bull Menninger Clin 62:147–169, 1998

Hertsgaard L, Gunnar M, Erickson MF, et al: Adrenocortical responses to the strange situation in infants with disorganized/disoriented attachment relationships. Child Dev 66:1100–1106, 1995

Hesse E: The adult attachment interview: historical and current perspectives, in Handbook of Attachment: Theory, Research, and Clinical Applications. Edited by Cassidy J, Shaver PR. New York, Guilford, 1999, pp 395–343

Hesse E, Main M: Disorganized infant, child, and adult attachment: collapse in behavioral and attentional strategies. J Am Psychoanal Assoc 48:1097–1127, 2000

Hesse E, van IJzendoorn M: Parental loss of close family members and propensities toward absorption in the offspring. Dev Sci 1:299–305, 1998

Hesse E, van IJzendoorn M: Propensities toward absorption are related to lapses in the monitoring of reasoning or discourse during the Adult Attachment Interview: a preliminary investigation. Attach Hum Dev 1:67–91, 1999

Hubbs-Tait L, Osofsky DJ, Hahn JM, et al: Predicting behavior problems and social competence in children of adolescent mothers. Family Relations: Interdisciplinary Journal of Applied Family Studies 43:439–446, 1994

Irwin HJ: Proneness to dissociation and traumatic childhood events. J Nerv Ment Dis 182:456–460, 1994

Jang KL, Paris J, Zweig-Frank H, et al: Twin study of dissociative experience. J Nerv Ment Dis 186:345–351, 1998

Juffer F, Bakermans-Kranenburg MJ, van IJzendoorn M: The importance of parenting in the development of disorganized attachment: evidence from a preventive intervention study in adoptive families. J Child Psychol Psychiatry 45:1–13, 2004

Lakatos K, Toth I, Nemoda Z, et al: Dopamine D4 receptor (DRD4) gene polymorphism is associated with attachment disorganization in infants. Mol Psychiatry 5:633–637, 2000

Lakatos K, Nemoda Z, Toth I, et al: Further evidence for the role of the dopamine D4 receptor (DRD4) gene in attachment disorganization: interaction of the exon III 48-bp repeat and the 521 C/T promoter polymorphisms. Mol Psychiatry 7:27–31, 2002

Liotti G: Disorganized/disoriented attachment in the etiology of the dissociative disorders. Dissociation 4:196–204, 1992

Liotti G: Disorganized/disoriented attachment in the psychotherapy of the dissociative disorders, in Attachment Theory: Social, Developmental and Clinical Perspectives. Edited by Goldberg SA, Muir R, Kerr I. Hillsdale, NY, Analytic Press, 1995, pp 343–364

Liotti G: Organization of attachment as a model for understanding dissociative psychopathology, in Attachment Disorganization. Edited by Solomon J, George C. New York, Guilford, 1999a, pp 291–317

Liotti G: Understanding the dissociative processes: the contribution of attachment theory. Psychoanal Inq 19:757–783, 1999b

Liotti G, Pasquini P: Predictive factors for borderline personality disorder: patients' early traumatic experiences and losses suffered by the attachment figure. Acta Psychiatr Scand 102:282–289, 2000

Lyons-Ruth K, Jacobvitz D: Attachment disorganization: unresolved loss, relational violence and lapses in behavioral and attentional strategies, in Handbook of Attachment: Theory, Research, and Clinical Applications. Edited by Cassidy J, Shaver PR. New York, Guilford, 1999, pp 520–554

Lyons-Ruth K, Easterbrooks MA, Cibelli CD: Infant attachment strategies, infant mental lag, and maternal depressive symptoms: predictors of internalizing and externalizing problems at age 7. Dev Psychol 33:377–396, 1997

Lyons-Ruth K, Bronfman E, Parsons E: Maternal frightened, frightening or atypical behavior and disorganized infant attachment patterns. Monogr Soc Res Child Dev 64:67–96, 1999

Madigan S, Bakermans-Kranenburg MJ, van IJzendoorn MH, et al: Unresolved states of mind, anomalous parental behavior, and disorganized attachment: a review and meta-analysis of a transmission gap. Attach Hum Dev 8:89–111, 2006

Main M: Introduction to the special section on attachment and psychopathology, 2: overview of the field of attachment. J Consult Clin Psychol 64:237–243, 1996

Main M, Hesse E: Parents' unresolved traumatic experiences are related to infant disorganized attachment status: is frightened and/or frightening parental behavior the linking mechanism?, in Attachment in the Preschool Years: Theory, Research, and Intervention. Edited by Greenberg MT, Cicchetti D, Cummings EM. Chicago, IL, University of Chicago Press, 1990, pp 161–118

Main M, Morgan H: Disorganization and disorientation in infant strange situation behavior: phenotypic resemblance to dissociative states, in Handbook of Dissociation: Theoretical, Empirical, and Clinical Perspectives. Edited by Michelson LK, Ray WJ. New York, Plenum, 1996, pp 107–138

Main M, Solomon J: Procedures for identifying infants as disorganized/disoriented during the Ainsworth strange situation, in Attachment in the Preschool Years: Theory, Research, and Intervention. Edited by Greenberg MT, Cicchetti D, Cummings EM. Chicago, IL, University of Chicago Press, 1990, pp 121–182

Marcovitch S, Goldberg SA, Gold A, et al: Determinants of behavioral problems in Romanian children adopted in Ontario. Int J Behav Dev 20:17–31, 1997

Ogawa JR, Sroufe LA, Weinfield NS, et al: Development and the fragmented self: longitudinal study of dissociative symptomatology in a nonclinical sample. Dev Psychopathol 9:855–879, 1997

Owen MT, Cox MJ: Marital conflict and the development of infant parent attachment relationships. J Fam Psychol 11:152–164, 1997

Pasquini P, Liotti G, Mazzoti E, et al: Risk factors in the early family life of patients suffering from dissociative disorders. Acta Psychiatr Scand 105:110–116, 2002

Perry BD, Pollard RA, Blakley TL, et al: Childhood trauma, the neurobiology of adaptation, and "use-dependent" development of the brain: how "states" become "traits." Infant Ment Health J 16:271–291, 1995

Robbins TW, Everitt BJ: Motivation and reward, in Fundamental Neuroscience. Edited by Zigmond MJ, Bloom FE, Landis SC, et al. San Diego, CA, Academic Press, 1999, pp 1246–1260

Rutgers AH, Bakermans-Kranenburg MJ, van IJzendoorn M, et al: Autism and attachment: a meta-analytic review. J Child Psychol Psychiatry 25:1123–1134, 2004

Rutter M: Some research considerations on intergenerational continuities and discontinuities: comment on the special section. Hum Dev 34:1269–1273, 1998

Rutter M, Pickles A, Murray R, et al: Testing hypotheses on specific environmental causal effects on behavior. Psychol Bull 127:291–324, 2001

Schuengel C, Bakermans-Kranenburg MJ, van IJzendoorn M: Frightening maternal behavior linking unresolved loss and disorganized infant attachment. J Consult Clin Psychol 67:54–63, 1999

Simeon D, Guralnik O, Schmeidler J, et al: The role of childhood interpersonal trauma in depersonalization disorder. Am J Psychiatry 158:1027–1033, 2001

Simeon D, Nelson D, Elias R, et al: Relationship of personality to dissociation and childhood trauma in borderline personality disorder. CNS Spectr 8:755–762, 2003

Solomon J, George C: Attachment and caregiving: the caregiving behavioral system, in Handbook of Attachment: Theory, Research, and Clinical Applications. Edited by Cassidy J, Shaver PR. New York, Guilford, 1999, pp 649–670

Spangler G, Grossman K: Biobehavioral organization in securely and insecurely attached infants. Child Dev 64:1439–1450, 1993

Spangler G, Grossman K: Individual and physiological correlates of attachment disorganization in infancy, in Handbook of Attachment: Theory, Research, and Clinical Applications. Edited by Cassidy J, Shaver PR. New York, Guilford, 1999, pp 95–126

Spangler G, Fremmer-Bombik E, Grossman K: Social and individual determinants of infant attachment security and disorganization. Infant Ment Health J 17:127–139, 1996

Steele K, van der Hart O, Nijenhuis ERS: Dependency in the treatment of complex posttraumatic stress disorder and dissociative disorders. J Trauma Dissociation 2:79–116, 2001

Suomi SJ: Attachment in rhesus monkeys, in Handbook of Attachment: Theory, Research, and Clinical Applications. Edited by Cassidy J, Shaver PR. New York, Guilford, 1999, pp 181–197

Teti DM, Messinger DS, Gelfand DM, et al: Maternal depression and the quality of early attachment: an examination of infants, preschoolers, and their mothers. Dev Psychol 31:364–376, 1995

True M, Pisani L, Oumar F: Infant-mother attachment among the Dogon of Mali. Child Dev 72:1451–1466, 2001

van IJzendoorn M: Adult attachment representations, parental responsiveness, and infant attachment: a meta-analysis on the predictive validity of the adult attachment interview. Psychol Bull 117:387–403, 1995

van IJzendoorn M, Bakermans-Kranenburg MJ: Attachment representations in mothers, fathers, adolescents, and clinical groups: a meta-analytic search for normative data. J Consult Clin Psychol 64:8–21, 1996

van IJzendoorn M, Bakermans-Kranenburg MJ: Disorganized attachment and the dysregulation of negative emotions, in Emotional Regulation and Developmental Health: Infancy and Early Childhood. Edited by Zuckerman BS, Lieberman AF, Fox NA. New Brunswick, NJ , Johnson & Johnson Pediatric Institute, 2002, pp 159–180

van IJzendoorn MH, Bakermans-Kranenburg MJ: DRD4 7-repeat polymorphism moderates the association between maternal unresolved loss or trauma and infant disorganization. Attach Hum Dev 8:291–307, 2006

van IJzendoorn MH, Sagi A: Cross-cultural patterns of attachment: universal and contextual dimensions, in Handbook of Attachment: Theory, Research, and Clinical Applications. Edited by Cassidy J, Shaver PR. New York, Guilford, 1999, pp 713–734

van IJzendoorn MH, Schuengel C: The measurement of dissociation in normal and clinical populations: meta-analytic validation of the Dissociative Experiences Scale (DES). Clin Psychol Rev 16:365–382, 1996

van IJzendoorn M, Schuengel C, Bakermans-Kranenburg MJ: Disorganized attachment in early childhood: meta-analysis of precursors, concomitants, and sequelae. Dev Psychopathol 11:225–249, 1999

Vorria P, Papaligoura Z, Dunn J, et al: Early experiences and attachment relationships of Greek infants raised in residential group care. J Child Psychol Psychiatry 44:1208–1220, 2003

Waller NG, Ross CA: The prevalence and biometric structure of pathological dissociation in the general population: taxometric and behavior genetic findings. J Abnorm Psychol 106:499–510, 1997

Weinfield NS, Sroufe LA, Egeland B, et al: The nature of individual differences in infant-caregiver attachment, in Handbook of Attachment: Theory, Research, and Clinical Applications. Edited by Cassidy J, Shaver PR. New York, Guilford, 1999, pp 68–88

West M, Adam K, Spreng S, et al: Attachment disorganization and dissociative symptoms in clinically treated adolescents. Can J Psychiatry 46:627–631, 2001

Willemsen-Swinkels SHN, Bakermans-Kranenburg MJ, Buitelaar JK, et al: Insecure and disorganized attachment in children with a pervasive developmental disorder: relationship with social interaction and heart rate. J Child Psychol Psychiatry 41:759–767, 2000

C H A P T E R   3

MEMORY AND ATTENTIONAL PROCESSES IN DISSOCIATIVE IDENTITY DISORDER

A Review of the Empirical Literature

MARTIN J. DORAHY, PH.D.
RAFAËLE J. C. HUNTJENS, PH.D.

Clinical reports and empirical findings suggest that the human memory system is particularly sensitive to highly threatening information (Butler and Spiegel 1997; Spiegel et al. 1993). Victims of trauma often report continuous intrusions of traumatic memories they would rather forget or the inability to recall trauma-related memories they should remember. Dissociative identity disorder (DID) is considered a trauma-induced psychiatric condition characterized by psychogenic disruptions to memory functioning (American Psychiatric Association 2000). As well as more generic memory and awareness problems (e.g., blank spells, periods of missing time, coming to in unfamiliar places, being unaware of reported actions), individuals with DID frequently experience the inability to recall trauma-related information from their auto-

We would like to thank Onno van der Hart, Ph.D, Anne DePrince, Ph.D, and Marcel van den Hout, Ph.D, for their thoughtful comments on earlier versions of this chapter.

graphical history (Boon and Draijer 1993; Coons et al. 1988; Putnam et al. 1986; Ross et al. 1989, 1990). Arguably this information is "stored" in other dissociative identities, and a failure to retrieve the traumatic material is attributed to the lack of awareness of material contained in those identities (i.e., interidentity amnesia; see Dorahy 2001).

Experimental research on memory functioning in DID is beginning to offer insights into the conceptual and clinical understanding of the condition. Although the experimental study of memory functioning in DID can be traced back to at least 1908,[1] the purpose of this chapter is to review more recent cognitive experimental studies. Many recent studies of memory functioning in DID have moved beyond single-case designs and have attempted to utilize various control strategies to assist in the interpretation of experimental findings. Where appropriate, research conducted on posttraumatic stress disorder (PTSD), another disorder characterized by traumatic dissociation, and studies of dissociation in the nonclinical general population are drawn upon to highlight overlapping and divergent findings. First, to guide the examination of memory functioning in DID, some central concepts in cognitive memory and attention theory are discussed. Subsequently, studies examining attentional and working memory processes in DID are examined, followed by research investigating long-term memory functioning.

A COGNITIVE SYNOPSIS OF HUMAN MEMORY

Tulving (2000), among others (e.g., Schacter and Tulving 1994), has elucidated the systems, processes, expressions, and kinds of awareness underpinning the cognitive science of human memory. Figure 3–1 shows a schematic representation of this framework. The human memory system can be broadly divided into *procedural* or behavioral memory and *cognitive* memory. The procedural memory system is involved in the acquisition of behavioral skills. Cognitive memory is made up of three discrete long-term memory systems: *episodic memory*, which refers to the system mediating the contextually rich material of the individual's personal history (e.g., specific time and place memories from childhood); *semantic memory*, which is involved in the use of general information and knowledge of the world; and *perceptual representation*, which operates to allow the recognition of perceptual objects.

---

[1] Prince and Peterson (1908) examined the transfer of cued associations between dissociative identities.

The retrieval of information stored in memory systems can be explicit or implicit. *Explicit* or *implicit* retrieval refers to the degree of awareness, during retrieval, of the relationship between retrieved information and prior experience (i.e., encoding) of that information. Broadly speaking, if an individual is consciously aware on retrieval that they have previously encoded that information, the retrieved material is said to be an *explicit* memory. *Implicit* memory, in Tulving's (2000) words, refers to the "retrieval of stored information in the *absence* of the awareness that the current behavior and experience have been influenced by a particular earlier happening" (p. 730, italics in original).

Besides the distinction between the explicit and implicit expressions of memory, Tulving (1985, 2002) proposed a further division related to the individual's state of consciousness during retrieval, namely the distinction between anoetic, noetic, and autonoetic consciousness. *Anoetic* consciousness refers to memory retrieval without conscious awareness (i.e., implicit). *Noetic* consciousness relates to when the individual knows he or she experienced the retrieved memory but has no self-awareness of the experience. Self-awareness of having personally experienced the retrieved memory characterizes *autonoetic* consciousness—that is, autonoetic consciousness makes a retrieved event feel personal.

One or the other of the qualitatively different states of noetic and autonoetic awareness accompany the identification of test items in recognition tasks. Recognition tasks require participants to acknowledge whether they have been exposed to presented stimuli in a previous learning trial. An affirmative response to a stimulus piece characterized by noetic awareness evokes a subjective feeling of familiarity, or *knowing* the stimulus piece has been seen before, without conscious recollection of contextual details (e.g., *when* the stimulus was encoded). An affirmative response to a stimulus piece characterized by autonoetic awareness, or *remembering* seeing the stimulus piece, involves conscious recollection of aspects of the original encounter with the particular item (Conway and Dewhurst 1995; Gardiner and Java 1993; Knowlton and Squire 1995; Postma 1999).

Before new stimuli are encoded in the long-term memory system, a whole range of processes are activated.[2] Contemporary models view information processing as a combination of bottom-up analysis with massive, top-down influences. Information processing at its earliest stage involves preattentive analysis of the stimuli perceived by the senses. According to Cowan (1988, 1997), physical characteristics and some se-

---

[2] These processes are part of the short-term memory and cognitive control processes and operations referred to as *working memory.* Although not depicted explicitly in Figure 3–1, working memory is part of the cognitive memory system in Tulving's model.

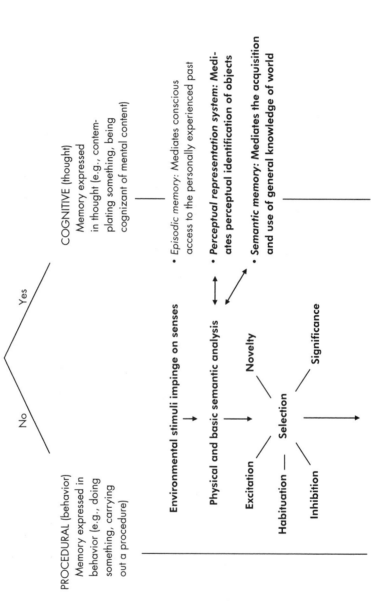

Memory systems

Can one hold in mind the PRODUCT of the act of memory?

No — PROCEDURAL (behavior) Memory expressed in behavior (e.g., doing something, carrying out a procedure)

Yes — COGNITIVE (thought) Memory expressed in thought (e.g., contemplating something, being cognizant of mental content)

- *Episodic memory:* Mediates conscious access to the personally experienced past
- **Perceptual representation system: Mediates perceptual identification of objects**
- **Semantic memory: Mediates the acquisition and use of general knowledge of world**

Environmental stimuli impinge on senses → Physical and basic semantic analysis → Selection →

Novelty

Significance

Excitation

Habituation

Inhibition

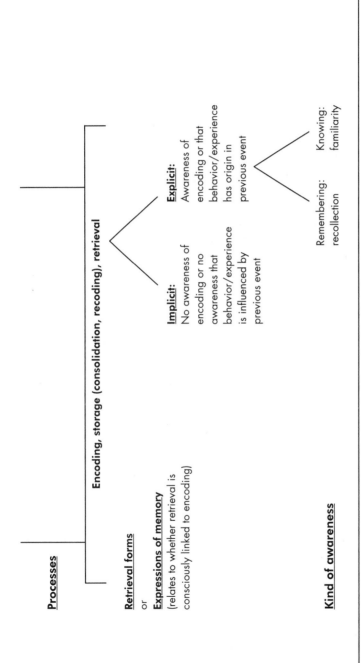

Processes

Encoding, storage (consolidation, recoding), retrieval

Retrieval forms
or
Expressions of memory
(relates to whether retrieval is
consciously linked to encoding)

Implicit:
No awareness of
encoding or no
awareness that
behavior/experience
is influenced by
previous event

Explicit:
Awareness of
encoding or that
behavior/experience
has origin in
previous event

Kind of awareness

Remembering:
recollection

Knowing:
familiarity

FIGURE 3–1. The information processing stream (in bold) has been overlaid on Tulving's model of memory.

mantic (i.e., meaning) features of incoming stimuli are analyzed (i.e., bottom-up processing) and compared with information from long-term memory (top-down processing) before attentional resources are allocated.[3] Preattentive analysis that deems stimuli unchanged from previous experience gives the stimuli a quality of familiarity. These stimuli become habituated to and can be processed automatically, without requiring conscious attention. Alternatively, preattentive analysis that deems stimuli novel or important to the individual attracts attentional resources to the stimuli. Preattentive processing therefore provides the possibility for very early detection of significant (e.g., emotional) stimuli. Selection of information for attentional processing is assisted by excitatory and inhibitory mechanisms. Excitatory processes allow selected information to receive further analysis while inhibitory processes simultaneously restrain the competitive impact of nonselected information (Tipper et al. 1989). The information processing stream (in bold) has been overlaid on Tulving's model of memory in Figure 3–1.

With the tenets of human memory now laid out, we give brief attention to the cognitive avoidance hypothesis for amnesia in DID in order to lay the theoretical foundations for the empirical literature review.

THE COGNITIVE AVOIDANCE HYPOTHESIS

Most studies of amnesia start from the so-called cognitive avoidance hypothesis—that is, the premise that DID patients have the ability to selectively avoid internally generated or externally presented trauma-related information (Cloitre 1992; Elzinga et al. 2000). Whether the avoidance of trauma-related information is an intentional or automatic process is a matter of disagreement, as is the question regarding at which stage of information processing avoidance of traumatic material is accomplished. Avoidance of traumatic stimuli may be related to the allocation of attentional resources away from information that is deemed threatening at the initial stage of information processing. Alternatively, avoidance of traumatic stimuli may occur at a slightly later stage, during the encoding and consolidation of events in memory. Then again, trauma-stimuli avoidance may operate even later, during retrieval from memory. It also may be possible that memory failure in DID is relatively independent of some

---

[3] Because preattentive processing occurs before conscious awareness and episodic memory is by definition conscious, this memory system is not believed to be active in preattentive processing.

form of avoidance and reflects, for example, extreme shifts in state between dissociative identities. The encoding specificity hypothesis in normal human memory, which accounts for state-dependent memory findings, suggests that retrieval will be impeded if the conditions between encoding and later retrieval (e.g., context, mood) differ considerably (Tulving and Thomson 1973). It is likely that the encoding of trauma memories differs significantly in many contextual and psychological ways from later retrieval, especially if the dissociative identity that attempts to retrieve the information differs in its emotional and cognitive composition from the dissociative identity that encoded the information.

Studying the complete information processing and memory retrieval stream in DID will allow a greater understanding of the origin of symptoms of memory, such as amnesia. For example, amnesia in DID may be related to deficits in the operations of memory processes such as encoding, storage, and retrieval. Yet amnesia could also occur in the presence of effectively operating memory processes. This may happen if preattentive or attentive processes impede (e.g., due to avoidance) information from reaching memory processes. Alternatively, processes may operate in the presence of effective memory retrieval that direct attention away from, or influence the interpretation of, certain retrieved information, thereby creating the experience of amnesia. In moving from theory to empirical research, we first discuss studies of attention and working memory that assess the initial stages of information processing.

STUDIES OF ATTENTION AND WORKING MEMORY

In experimental psychology, the most widely used task to study attention is the Stroop task (Stroop 1935). This task examines the effects of distracting semantic information (i.e., interference effects) early in the information processing stream. Participants are required to ignore semantic information (e.g., the *meaning* of a color word, such as "blue") and respond to perceptual (physical) information (in this case, the *actual ink color* of the words, e.g., green). Studies of psychopathology often use the "emotional" Stroop task (see Williams et al. 1996), in which color words are replaced with specific and nonspecific emotional words. Research, particularly in anxiety disorders, has consistently found that patients selectively attend to stimuli consistent with core psychological fear structures (i.e., schemas; Mathews and MacLeod 1985). This "attentional bias" appears to be limited to fear schema–specific information rather than general threat information (e.g., Foa et al. 1991; Watts et al. 1986). Although classed as an anxiety disorder, PTSD, like DID, is characterized by traumatic dissociation (see Chapter 4, "Relationships Between Dissociation and Posttraumatic Stress Disorder," and Chapter 11, "Psychobiology of Traumatization and Trauma-Related Structural Dissociation of the Personality," for review). Therefore, the more-developed empirical understanding of attentional functioning in PTSD may offer insight into information processing in DID, especially regarding whether threatening material is being shunted beyond attentional processes and onto memory processes (e.g., memory encoding).

Studies of PTSD samples have consistently displayed a response bias (i.e., slower responding) to stimuli consistent with the trauma-related etiology of the condition. For example, rape victims with PTSD display slower color naming to rape-related words than general threat words (Foa et al. 1991), whereas combat veterans with PTSD demonstrate greater interference when exposed to combat-related words (McNally et al. 1990). The attentional bias evident in these two groups is also present in motor vehicle accident survivors with PTSD when presented with accident-related stimuli (Bryant and Harvey 1995). Given the physical and basic semantic processing that takes place before the allocation of attention, much of the information processing that may lead to threat-specific biases in attention probably occurs automatically (i.e., without willful intention). Consistent with this idea, PTSD studies have found attentional bias to schema-specific threat stimuli at the subliminal (i.e., preattentive) processing stage (e.g., Bryant et al. 1996).

To date, little dedicated attention has been given to interference effects and the (early) processing of threat stimuli in DID. One study, using a word naming task, reported slower responses to non-schema-specific negative words than neutral words in a DID sample tested in an anxiety-provoking context (Dorahy et al. 2005). However, by its nature, this over-simplified task provided no insight as to the locus of interference (i.e., whether interference occurred at an early, automatic stage of processing or later when more controlled, strategic processes were employed). There was also no attempt to control for the type of dissociative identity assessed, and an initial study of this issue has highlighted the possibility of different response patterns to threat stimuli between trauma-fixated and trauma-avoidant dissociative identities (Hermans et al. 2006). Finally, this bias in naming negative words was not replicated in another sample of DID participants using the same task (Dorahy et al. 2006). Thus it remains possible but as yet untested that, as in PTSD samples, attentional bias in DID is related to fear-specific rather than generic negative information and the bias is generated at an early, automatic stage of processing.

Whereas interference effects in PTSD may primarily occur as a result of the semantic processing that takes place before the allocation of attention and the activation of excitatory and inhibitory mechanisms to information streams, weakened inhibitory mechanisms may also contribute to slower response time for threat stimuli (Fox 1994). If not effectively inhibited, the semantic meaning of a threat word will receive excitatory processing and further analysis. Consequently, deficits in inhibitory functioning may have important implications for intrusion-related symptoms in PTSD and DID.

Amir et al. (2002) found deficits in the inhibition of threat-related meaning in a PTSD sample compared with a traumatized group without PTSD. This deficit in inhibiting the threat meaning of words was not evident in the very early stage of information processing. Rather, individuals with PTSD demonstrated inhibitory difficulties when they had marginally longer to process the negative connotation of the word (i.e., at a slightly later stage of processing). Inhibitory ability appears to be weakened in PTSD following the identification of a threat-related meaning, which is achieved through greater semantic processing. In individuals without PTSD this semantic "judgment" of threat attributed to the stimulus is inhibited if such an appraisal is irrelevant to the task being performed. In individuals with PTSD irrelevant threat judgments are not effectively inhibited. Therefore instead of being suppressed these semantic threat appraisals receive further activation and processing.

Wood et al. (2001) found only equivocal support for reduced inhibition of threat versus nonthreat stimuli in sample of high nonclinical anxiety, including a group that experienced a violent assault. However, their results, along with supporting data from the Amir et al. (2002) PTSD study, suggest that patients with an anxiety disorder may experience general deficits in the ability to inhibit irrelevant mental information (e.g., competing physical details or semantic meaning), rather than deficits specifically related to threat stimuli. Concordant findings were reported in an initial study of inhibitory functioning in DID (Dorahy et al. 2002). However, more sensitive assessment of the operation of cognitive inhibitory mechanisms in DID, using the so-called Flanker task (B.A. Eriksen and Eriksen 1974; see C.W. Eriksen 1995 for overview), revealed a more complex pattern of functioning. The cognitive inhibitory processes of selective attention covaried in DID with the level of task anxiety (i.e., state rather than trait) experienced.

When DID participants were assessed using neutral word stimuli in the initial study (Dorahy et al. 2002), they displayed evidence of ineffective cognitive inhibition. On debriefing after the study, several DID participants reported finding the study stressful because they did not know if the next presentation of "neutral" stimuli would contain a word that was idiosyncratically stressful for them. Using more unequivocally neutral stimuli (i.e., single-digit numbers), two subsequent studies demonstrated effective cognitive inhibitory functioning in DID (Dorahy et al.

2004a, 2004b). To examine whether inhibition was a function of state anxiety, Dorahy et al. (2005) used the Flanker task with single-digit number stimuli and assessed DID, depressed, and control participants in a neutral and negative context. The emotional context was manipulated via task instructions (e.g., "emotionally negative words will be presented") and word stimuli (e.g., neutral or negative) presented between trials designed to assess inhibition. The DID sample displayed efficient cognitive inhibition in the neutral context but no evidence of inhibition when tested in the negative context. The depressed sample failed to display inhibition in both contexts, whereas the control sample displayed cognitive inhibition in the neutral and negative environments. In controlling for the effects of anxiety, a further study (Dorahy et al. 2006) replicated the DID findings across contexts and found that a generalized anxiety disorder sample displayed the opposite results (i.e., effective inhibition in the negative but not neutral contexts). Extrapolating from these findings it could be tentatively suggested that reduced inhibition in DID during moments of increased anxiety may be the cognitive precursor for experiencing intrusive (i.e., positive) psychoform and somatoform dissociative symptoms. With inhibitory processes not effectively withholding distracting associations, the dissociative individual is more vulnerable to dissociative symptoms.

Although weakened inhibition in anxiety-provoking situations may increase vulnerability to dissociative episodes in DID, Dorahy et al. (2006) argued that reduced inhibition in situations of heightened anxious arousal may be an adaptive response. Weakened inhibitory processes provide the cognitive architecture for faster defensive orientation to environmental threat stimuli outside the immediate focus of attention (i.e., on the periphery of focal attention). The reduced inhibition evident in DID provides the possibility of greater initial processing of peripheral stimuli before attention is focused. Theoretically, the early detection of a potential threat stimulus in the environment afforded by weakened inhibition would allow faster activation of defensive responses in DID. However, the slower reactions to threat stimuli found in one DID study (Dorahy et al. 2005), and alluded to by attentional bias findings in PTSD, suggest slower responses to environmental threat once detected. Thus although reduced inhibition may facilitate initial processing and detection of potentially threatening stimuli, the conversion from cognition (i.e., identification) to behavioral response (e.g., defensive action) that occurs later in processing may be impeded in DID. This model awaits sensitive and controlled empirical assessment.

STUDIES OF LONG-TERM MEMORY

Memory Functioning Within Individual Dissociative Identities

Schacter et al. (1989) asked a female DID participant to briefly describe and date specific life episodes cued from different types of word triggers such as "object" (e.g., window, game) and "affect" (e.g., happy, hurt). Compared with a control group, the DID patient displayed substantial recall preference for events occurring later in her life, especially when given affective cues. No memories were recalled before the age of 10 in either this task or a task in which she was asked to recall therapeutically relevant childhood events (e.g., "earliest memory of your father" and "earliest unhappy memory").

Bryant (1995) had the fortuitous opportunity to assess a participant on two separate occasions (28 months apart), once before the participant was diagnosed with DID and once after her diagnosis. Bryant used a procedure similar to that used by Schacter's group (Schacter et al. 1989), and his results before diagnosis were not unlike those reported by that group (Bryant's patient did recall more childhood memories, but still far fewer than control subjects). On the second assessment (after diagnosis), the patient could retrieve no events from childhood and relied on a child identity to retrieve those memories. The postdiagnosis result suggests that childhood memories were accessible only through other identities.

The studies by Schacter et al. (1989) and Bryant (1995) support the existence of amnesia for autobiographical events in DID outlined by criterion C in DSM-IV-TR (i.e., the "inability to recall important personal information that is too extensive to be explained by ordinary forgetfulness" [American Psychiatric Association 2000, p. 529]). In both studies, however, the single-case method was used in combination with a self-report measure, which limits generalization given a possible resistance to volunteer memories (e.g., because they are painful) or the possibility of learned socio-cognitive responses (i.e., participants have learned to respond in a manner consistent with DID).

In an attempt to more systematically study amnesia within individual dissociative identities, Elzinga et al. (2000, 2003) used a so-called directed, or intentional, forgetting paradigm. Subjects were shown a word list, and an instruction to either *forget* or *remember* followed the presentation of each word. In the literature, two possible explanations have been suggested for the directed forgetting effect: encoding bias of to-be-remembered words and retrieval inhibition of to-be-forgotten words. Procedures that present the instruction to remember or forget immediately following the presentation of *each* word stimulus (i.e., item method) are thought to generate a directed forgetting effect by relying on a favorable bias toward the encoding of to-be-remembered words (MacLeod 1989). The directed forgetting effect in procedures that present the remember or forget instruction after the presentation of a *block* of word stimuli (i.e., list method) is believed to rely on retrieval inhibition of to-be-forgotten words (Wilhelm et al. 1996).

In using the item method, directed forgetting effects in the Elzinga et al. (2000, 2003) studies would implicate differential encoding of to-be-remembered word stimuli. To further focus attention on differential encoding, Elzinga et al. (2000, 2003) told participants that they would only be tested on to-be-remembered words. However, at test time, participants were asked to complete word stems (test of implicit memory retrieval) to either to-be-remembered or to-be-forgotten words. Words with a sexual connotation (e.g., petting, orgy, pregnant), threat words (e.g., danger, trembling, nauseous), and neutral words were used as stimuli. Clinical dissociators (e.g., patients with DID in the 2003 study) showed a striking absence of directed forgetting when tested in the same identity. They even showed an enhanced recall of the to-be-forgotten sex words compared with the to-be-remembered sex words and other words, resembling the famous "white bear" effect (Wegner 1989), which demonstrated that greater conscious effort to forget a stimulus often results in greater intrusions from that stimulus. The failure of the clinical dissociator groups to show directed forgetting effects suggests that, rather than withholding encoding resources from to-be-forgotten stimuli, substantial encoding was taking place. This was particularly the case for words with a sexual connotation. Even compared with threat stimuli, words with a sexual connotation are likely to be more consistent with core pathological fear schemas in clinical dissociators, given that many report childhood histories of sexual abuse (e.g., Middleton and Butler 1998; Putnam et al. 1986; Ross et al. 1989).

The failure of Elzinga's group to demonstrate directed forgetting effects in clinical dissociators and the enhanced recall of word stimuli with a sexual connotation is in line with predictions from the attentional bias literature, which shows greater processing of information related to trauma schemas (e.g., Foa et al. 1991). In support, De Ruiter et al. (2003) have shown that dissociation-prone, nonclinical individuals display enhanced (not reduced) attention to threat stimuli. These authors have argued that enhanced attention given to negative stimuli by high dissociators is independent of anxiety. They maintain that dissociation as an individual differences variable makes a significant and independent contribution to attentional functioning. Consequently, it seems likely that to-be-forgotten words with a sexual connotation in Elzinga et al.'s

(2003) DID participants would have received greater rather than lesser processing that would wash out the directed forgetting effect. Presuming problems were not evident at retrieval, greater processing of schema-specific stimuli during encoding would produce greater recall of words with a sexual connotation.

Nonclinical findings contrary to the notion of increased attention to threat stimuli in high dissociators (i.e., nonclinical participants with high dissociation scores) administered the directed forgetting task were reported by DePrince and Freyd (2001, 2004). They have consistently found more effective cognitive functioning in high dissociators (compared with low dissociators) during divided attention (rather than selective attention) tasks (e.g., DePrince and Freyd 1999). In a directed forgetting task using neutral and threat stimuli, DePrince and Freyd (2004) found reduced recall of to-be-remembered threat stimuli and reduced recognition of to-be-forgotten threat stimuli in high dissociators under divided attention conditions. They concluded that a selective avoidance of threat stimuli during preattentive processing most parsimoniously accounted for their findings. Thus instead of being attracted to threat stimuli, attentional resources in high nonclinical dissociators avoided them. Future work in DID will need to determine whether attentional resources are drawn toward or directed away from threat stimuli in different dissociative identity types (e.g., trauma-fixated vs. trauma-avoidant).

Memory Functioning Between Dissociative Identities

The studies by Schacter et al. (1989), Bryant (1995), and Elzinga et al. (2000, 2003) examined memory functioning within individual dissociative identities. However, most experimental studies have tested patients in more than one dissociative identity, thereby evaluating the more specific dissociative ability to compartmentalize (trauma-related) information in separate dissociative identities. This line of research follows numerous clinical observations of DID patients displaying differences across dissociative identities in remembered autobiographical history (episodic memory), knowledge base such as languages spoken (semantic memory), and even behavioral skills such as driving a car or riding a bicycle (procedural memory). Essentially, DID is thought to involve a division between dissociative identities that remain fully aware and fixated on their trauma history and identities that avoid trauma-reminding cues and lack a full awareness of their history of trauma (e.g., due to partial or total amnesia of trauma memories or noetic awareness of traumatic events [It happened, but not to me]) (Nijenhuis and van der Hart 1999; Nijenhuis et al. 2004; van der Hart et al. 2006).

In experimental research, interidentity amnesia is assessed by testing one identity (identity A) that has learned a set of stimuli and another identity (identity B) that self-reports amnesia for the learning trial on retrieval ability for the learned information. In earlier studies of interidentity amnesia (Dick-Barnes et al. 1987; Eich et al. 1997b; Ludwig et al. 1972; Nissen et al. 1988; Peters et al. 1998; Silberman et al. 1985) that were performed with neutral stimulus material, it was usually found that DID patients demonstrated amnesia on explicit memory retrieval tasks where learned stimuli were open to identity-specific interpretations of material. However, evidence of information transfer on more implicit memory retrieval tasks was often found (Eich et al. 1997b; Nissen et al. 1988). Most of the more recent studies on interidentity amnesia have found evidence of intact interidentity memory functioning both on implicit and explicit memory retrieval tasks (Allen and Movius 2000; Eich et al. 1997a; Elzinga et al. 2003; Huntjens et al. 2002, 2003, 2005, 2006). Like previous work, the majority of these studies have used neutral stimulus material, but they have employed much more sophisticated methodological designs and larger patient samples. In addition, some recent studies have included trauma-related stimulus material (e.g., Elzinga et al. 2003; Huntjens et al. submitted) and have assessed both age- and education-matched control subjects as well as participants instructed to simulate DID.

In one study, explicit memory retrieval was tested in a so-called interference paradigm (Huntjens et al. submitted). First, participants were asked to learn a list of words designated as wordlist A that contained trauma-related, positive, and neutral words. Subjects were then tested for free recall. Subsequently, and following a switch to an amnesic identity, they learned a list of different words (i.e., wordlist B) that resembled wordlist A and again were tested for free recall. Results indicated no evidence of interidentity amnesia: DID participants recalled words from wordlist A in their amnesic identity (i.e., the identity learning wordlist B). After a 2-hour interval, the amnesic identity was given a surprise recognition test in which they were shown all of the words from *both* lists intermixed with "distractor" (i.e., new) words and asked to indicate which words were old and which were new. Participants recognized trauma-related (as well as neutral and positive) wordlist A words in their amnesic dissociative identity. Interestingly, they were inclined to assign recognized wordlist A (learned in a different dissociative identity) and wordlist B (learned in the same dissociative identity) words to wordlist B, the test identity's own list.

Evidence of transfer across amnesic barriers in DID has also been found for conditioned emotional information. Huntjens et al. (2005) administered to DID participants an evaluative conditioning procedure in which previously neutral words gained a positive or negative connotation. In a subsequent affective priming procedure, participants displayed transfer of this newly acquired emotional valence in amnesic identities (i.e., transfer of emotional material between identities).

Recent studies of interidentity information transfer have examined the kind of awareness experienced during stimulus recognition (Huntjens et al. 2003, submitted). Participants were asked whether recognized words generated a feeling of *remembering* (i.e., autonoetic awareness) or *knowing* (i.e., noetic awareness). Clinical indications suggest that recognition of events learned by the same identity should be characterized more by a remember kind of awareness, whereas recognition of events learned by another identity should evoke primarily knowing responses (Cardeña 2000; Steele et al. 2004). Although test stimuli and conditions only indirectly reflect real-life experience, there was no significant confirmation of differences in kind of awareness for information learned in the identity assessed versus information learned in another identity.

Although acknowledging important, and possibly meaningful, differences between laboratory-based tasks and real-life autobiographical events, the most striking finding in recent experimental studies of compartmentalization is an absence of objective evidence for interidentity amnesia. This absence of objective amnesia has been noted when DID participants subjectively reported complete amnesia in the "test" identity for material and instructions given to the "learn" identity. These findings do not support the cognitive avoidance hypothesis, which posits that DID patients have some special ability to avoid trauma-related material, either within and/or between different dissociative identities. In fact, the hypothesis is even challenged by the results of enhanced recall of words with a threatening or sexual connotation in the studies by Elzinga et al. (2000, 2003), suggesting dissociative patients may actually have a reduced ability to forget trauma-related material.

Huntjens (2003) argued that the discrepancy between subjective reports of amnesia without objective evidence of memory impairment is consistent with the view that DID entails a subjective, rather than objective, psychological organization. As such, different memories (as well as emotions and behaviors) are conceived as being compartmentalized in different dissociative identities. In support of this view, a recent study in a nonclinical population found evidence for subjective but not objective memory fragmentation in high dissociators compared with low dissociators (Kindt and Van den Hout 2003). Rather than an impairment in memory encoding and/or retrieval, the problem may be DID patients' appraisal of memories as either ego-dystonic or ego-syntonic after correct retrieval. Their preconscious or conscious appraisal of their memories being compartmentalized in separate identities may lead to the non-use of correctly retrieved material that is believed to "belong" to other identities. Failed identification of material from other identities may be especially evident for information incongruent or conflictual with the psychological makeup of the identity attempting to retrieve the material. This suggests, for example, that one identity's ability to drive a motor vehicle and another identity's inability to do so may have less to do with procedural memory compartmentalization for the required behaviors and more to do with the identity's "job" or role in the system (i.e., the learned behavioral repertoire of an identity).

Despite needing further elaboration and development, this explanation for amnesia is not altogether dissimilar from Brenner's (2001) psychoanalytic model of DID. Brenner postulated that the defense mechanism underlying the subjective experience of separateness between alter identities is a form of denial in which identities are perceived as "it's not me" selves through the use of *negation*, which refers to the ability to "disown intolerable behavior and mental content" (p. 88). Amnesia between identities is therefore created not by consciously and unconsciously avoiding the mental content of other identities but by negating it, or defensively attributing the mental content of other identities to something *other* than the autobiographical experience.

CONCLUSION

Most studies of information processing in DID start from the premise that DID patients are capable of either automatically or willfully avoiding information that, because of its traumatic nature, is too painful to confront. However, from recent experimental studies of information processing in DID, a different picture is beginning to emerge. In contrast to the hypothesis of cognitive avoidance, the processing of trauma stimuli seems to result in an increased activation of trauma-related material, whether through enhanced attention to traumatic stimuli resulting from deficits in inhibitory functioning or through enhanced memory for words with a threatening or sexual connotation. In addition, well-controlled studies of compartmentalization and information transfer across amnesic identities appear to indicate normal functioning of memory encoding and retrieval mechanisms.

To explain patient reports of the inability to process and retrieve traumatic information, an alternate viewpoint—and one admittedly not based on studies utilizing personally threatening or traumatic stimuli—holds that individuals with DID can effectively retrieve traumatic or amnesic information, but this information is deemed ego-alien or ego-dystonic. Therefore, the retrieved information is not perceived as belonging to the person's autobiographical experience and is consequently discarded. Thus, appraisal processes operating very late (i.e., following retrieval) in the memory stream account for subjective amnesia. Models of amnesia between identities in DID will develop with further empirical and theoretical work and the overcoming of several limitations in current experimental research. The most significant of these limitations is difficulties generalizing from laboratory studies to real life. Although some recent studies included stimulus material specifically related to sexual and physical abuse, the use of single words does not reflect the contextual, meaningful, multifaceted, and highly emotional episodes of abuse reported by patients. Moreover, greater control is required of the type of dissociative identities (e.g., trauma-fixated, trauma-avoidant) assessed in studies of attention and memory functioning in DID. Memory research in DID is beginning to provide valuable empirical data on the nature of amnesia within and between dissociative identities. However, greater efforts need to be made to objectively assess retrieval deficits for personally experienced traumatic events, given the reported prevalence of this phenomenon in the DID clinical literature.

REFERENCES

Allen JJB, Movius HL: The objective assessment of amnesia in dissociative identity disorder using event-related potentials. Int J Psychophysiol 38:21–41, 2000

American Psychiatric Association: Diagnostic and Statistical Manual of Mental Disorders, 4th Edition, Text Revision. Washington, DC, American Psychiatric Association, 2000

Amir N, Coles ME, Foa EB: Automatic and strategic activation and inhibition of threat-relevant information in posttraumatic stress disorder. Cognit Ther Res 26:645–655, 2002

Boon S, Draijer N: Multiple personality disorder in The Netherlands: a clinical investigation of 71 patients. Am J Psychiatry 150:489–494, 1993

Brenner I: Dissociation of Trauma: Theory, Phenomenology, and Technique. Madison, CT, International Universities Press, 2001

Bryant RA: Autobiographical memory across personalities in dissociative identity disorder: a case report. J Abnorm Psychol 104:625–631, 1995

Bryant RA, Harvey AG: Processing threatening information in posttraumatic stress disorder. J Abnorm Psychol 104:537–554, 1995

Bryant RA, Harvey AG, Rapee RM: Preconscious processing of threat in post-traumatic stress disorder. Cognit Ther Res 20:613–623, 1996

Butler LD, Spiegel D: Trauma and memory, in American Psychiatric Press Review of Psychiatry, Vol 16. Edited by Dickstein LJ, Riba MB, Oldham JM. Washington, DC, American Psychiatric Press, 1997, pp 13–53

Cardeña E: Dissociative disorders, in Encyclopedia of Psychology. Edited by Kazdin AE. New York, Oxford University Press, 2000, pp 55–59

Cloitre M: Avoidance of emotional processing: a cognitive perspective, in Cognitive Science and Clinical Disorders. Edited by Stein DJ, Young JE. San Diego, CA, Academic Press, 1992, pp 19–41

Conway MA, Dewhurst SA: Remembering, familiarity, and source monitoring. Q J Exp Psychol A 48:125–140, 1995

Coons PM, Bowman ES, Milstein V: Multiple personality disorder: a clinical investigation of 50 cases. J Nerv Ment Dis 176:519–527, 1988

Cowan N: Evolving conceptions of memory storage, selective attention and their mutual constraints within the human information processing system. Psychol Bull 104:163–191, 1988

Cowan N: Attention and Memory: An Integrated Framework. Oxford, England, Oxford University Press, 1997

DePrince AP, Freyd JJ: Dissociation, attention and memory. Psychol Sci 10:449–452, 1999

DePrince AP, Freyd JJ: Memory and dissociative tendencies: the role of attentional context and word meaning. J Trauma Dissociation 2:67–82, 2001

DePrince AP, Freyd JJ: Forgetting trauma stimuli. Psychol Sci 15:488–492, 2004

De Ruiter MB, Phaf RH, Veltman DJ, et al: Attention as a characteristic of nonclinical dissociation: an event-related potential study. Neuroimage 19:376–390, 2003

Dick-Barnes M, Nelson RO, Aine CJ: Behavioral measures of multiple personality: the case of Margaret. J Behav Ther Exp Psychiatry 18:229–239, 1987

Dorahy MJ: Dissociative identity disorder and memory dysfunction: the current state of experimental research, and its future directions. Clin Psychol Rev 21:771–795, 2001

Dorahy MJ, Irwin HJ, Middleton W: Cognitive inhibition in dissociative identity disorder (DID): developing an understanding of working memory function in DID. J Traum Dissociation 3:111–132, 2002

Dorahy MJ, Irwin HJ, Middleton W: Assessing markers of working memory function in dissociative identity disorder using neutral stimuli: a comparison with clinical and general population samples. Aust NZ J Psychiatry 38:47–55, 2004a

Dorahy MJ, Middleton W, Irwin HJ: Investigating cognitive inhibition in dissociative identity disorder compared to depression, posttraumatic stress disorder and psychosis. J Trauma Dissociation 5:93–110, 2004b

Dorahy MJ, Middleton W, Irwin HJ: The effect of emotional context on cognitive inhibition and attentional processing in dissociative identity disorder. Behav Res Ther 43:555–568, 2005

Dorahy MJ, McCusker CG, Loewenstein RJ, et al: Cognitive inhibition and interference in dissociative identity disorder: the effects of threat on specific executive functions. Behav Res Ther 44:749–764, 2006

Eich E, Macaulay D, Loewenstein RJ, et al: Implicit memory, interpersonality amnesia, and dissociative identity disorder: comparing patients with simulators, in Recollections of Trauma: Scientific Research and Clinical Practice. Edited by Read JD, Lindsay DS. New York, Plenum, 1997a, pp 469–474

Eich E, Macauley D, Loewenstein RJ, et al: Memory, amnesia, and dissociative identity disorder. Psychol Sci 8:417–422, 1997b

Elzinga BM, De Beurs E, Sergeant JA, et al: Dissociative style and directed forgetting. Cognit Ther Res 24:279–295, 2000

Elzinga BM, Phaf RH, Ardon AM, et al: Directed forgetting between, but not within, dissociative personality states. J Abnorm Psychol 112:237–243, 2003

Eriksen BA, Eriksen CW: Effects of noise letters upon the identification of a target letter in a search task. Percept Psychophys 16:143–149, 1974

Eriksen CW: The Flanker task and response competition: a useful tool for investigating a variety of cognitive problems. Vis Cogn 2:101–118, 1995

Foa EB, Feske U, Murdock TB, et al: Processing of threat-related information in rape victims. J Abnorm Psychol 100:156–162, 1991

Fox E: Attentional bias in anxiety: a deficit inhibition hypothesis. Cogn Emot 8:165–195, 1994

Gardiner JM, Java RI: Recognition memory and awareness: an experimental approach. European Journal of Cognitive Psychology 5:337–346, 1993

Hermans EJ, Nijenhuis ERS, Van Honk J, et al: Identity state-dependent attentional bias for facial threat in dissociative identity disorder. Psychiatry Res 141:233–236, 2006

Huntjens RJC: Apparent amnesia: interidentity memory functioning in dissociative identity disorder. Doctoral thesis, Utrecht University, Utrecht, The Netherlands, 2003

Huntjens RJC, Postma A, Hamaker EL, et al: Perceptual and conceptual priming in patients with dissociative identity disorder. Mem Cognit 30:1033–1043, 2002

Huntjens RJC, Postma A, Peters ML, et al: Interidentity amnesia for neutral, episodic information in dissociative identity disorder. J Abnorm Psychol 112:290–297, 2003

Huntjens RJC, Postma A, Peters M, et al: Transfer of newly acquired stimulus valence between identities in dissociative identity disorder. Behav Res Ther 43:243–255, 2005

Huntjens RJC, Postma A, Peters M, et al: Memory transfer for emotionally valenced words between identities in dissociative identity disorder. Behav Res Ther, Aug 21 (Epub ahead of print), 2006.

Kindt M, Van den Hout M: Dissociation and memory fragmentation: experimental effects on meta-memory but not on actual memory performance. Behav Res Ther 41:167–178, 2003

Knowlton BJ, Squire LR: Remembering and knowing: two different expressions of declarative memory. J Exp Psychol 21:699–710, 1995

Ludwig AM, Brandsma JM, Wilbur CB, et al: The objective study of a multiple personality. Arch Gen Psychiatry 26:298–310, 1972

MacLeod CM: Directed forgetting affects both direct and indirect tests of memory. J Exp Psychol 15:13–21, 1989

Mathews A, MacLeod C: Selective processing of threat cues in anxiety states. Behav Res Ther 23:563–569, 1985

McNally RJ, Kaspi SP, Reimann BC, et al: Selective processing of threat cues in posttraumatic stress disorder. J Abnorm Psychol 99:398–402, 1990

Middleton W, Butler J: Dissociative identity disorder: an Australian series. Aust NZ J Psychiatry 32:794–804, 1998

Nijenhuis ERS, van der Hart O: Forgetting and reexperiencing trauma: from anesthesia to pain, in Splintered Reflections: Images of the Body in Trauma. Edited by Goodwin J, Attias R. New York, Basic Books, 1999, pp 39–65

Nijenhuis ERS, van der Hart O, Steele K: Trauma-related structural dissociation of the personality. Trauma Information Pages Web site, January 2004. Available online at http://www.trauma-pages.com/a/nijenhuis-2004.php. Accessed August 18, 2006

Nissen MJ, Ross JL, Willingham DB, et al: Memory and awareness in a patient with multiple personality disorder. Brain Cogn 8:117–134, 1988

Peters ML, Uyterlinde SA, Consemulder J, et al: Apparent amnesia on experimental memory tests in dissociative identity disorder. Conscious Cogn 7:27–41, 1998

Postma A: The influence of decision criteria upon remembering and knowing in recognition memory. Acta Psychol 103:65–76, 1999

Prince M, Peterson F: Experiments in psychogalvanic reactions from co-conscious ideal in a case of multiple personality. J Abnorm Psychol 3:114–131, 1908

Putnam FW, Guroff JJ, Silberman EK, et al: The clinical phenomenology of multiple personality disorder: 100 recent cases. J Clin Psychiatry 47:285–293, 1986

Ross CA, Norton GR, Wozney K: Multiple personality disorder: an analysis of 236 cases. Can J Psychiatry 34:413–418, 1989

Ross CA, Miller SD, Reagor P, et al: Structured interview data on 102 cases of multiple personality disorder from four centers. Am J Psychiatry 147:596–601, 1990

Schacter DL, Tulving E: Memory Systems 1994. Cambridge, MA, MIT Press, 1994

Schacter DL, Kihlstrom JF, Kihlstrom LC, et al: Autobiographical memory in a case of multiple personality disorder. J Abnorm Psychol 98:508–514, 1989

Silberman EK, Putnam FW, Weingartner H, et al: Dissociative states in multiple personality: a quantitative study. Psychiatry Res 15:253–260, 1985

Spiegel D, Frischholz EJ, Spira J: Functional disorders of memory. Rev Psychiatry 12:747–782, 1993

Steele K, van der Hart O, Nijenhuis ERS: Phasenorientierte Behandlung komplexer dissoziativer Störungen: Die Bewältigung Traumabezogener Phobien, in Dissoziative Störungen des Bewusstseins. Edited by Eckhart-Henn A, Hoffman SO. Stuttgart, Germany, Schattauer-Verlag, 2004, pp 357–394

Stroop JR: Studies of interference in serial verbal reactions. J Exp Psychol 18:643–662, 1935

Tipper SP, Bourque TA, Anderson SH, et al: Mechanisms of attention: a developmental study. J Exp Child Psychol 48:353–378, 1989

Tulving E: Memory and consciousness. Can Psychol 26:1–12, 1985

Tulving E: Introduction: memory, in The New Cognitive Neurosciences. Edited by Gazzaniga MS. Cambridge, MA, MIT Press, 2000, pp 727–732

Tulving E: Episodic memory: from mind to brain. Ann Rev Psychol 53:1–25, 2002

Tulving E, Thomson DM: Encoding specificity and retrieval processes in episodic memory. Psychol Rev 80:359–380, 1973

van der Hart O, Nijenhuis E, Steele K: The Haunted Self: Structural Dissociation and the Treatment of Chronic Traumatization. New York, Norton, 2006

Watts FN, McKenna FP, Sharrock R, et al: Colour naming of phobia-related words. Br J Psychology 77:97–108, 1986

Wegner DM: White Bears and Other Unwanted Thoughts. New York, Viking, 1989

Wilhelm S, McNally RJ, Baer L, et al: Directed forgetting in obsessive-compulsive disorder. Behav Res Ther 34:633–641, 1996

Williams JMG, Mathews A, MacLeod C: The emotional Stroop task and psychopathology. Psychol Bull 120:3–24, 1996

Wood J, Mathews A, Dalgleish T: Anxiety and cognitive inhibition. Emotion 1:166–181, 2001

C H A P T E R   4

RELATIONSHIPS BETWEEN DISSOCIATION AND POSTTRAUMATIC STRESS DISORDER

DAPHNE SIMEON, M.D.

The complexity of the relationship between dissociation and posttraumatic stress disorder (PTSD) is an area of unresolved controversy and one requiring more extensive research. Presently, four models can be put forth to reasonably account for the relationship between dissociative and PTSD symptoms: a comorbidity model, a shared risk factors model, a shared pathogenesis model, and a same disorder model.

MODEL 1: COMORBIDITY

Model 1, the comorbidity model, posits that traumatic dissociation and PTSD are merely commonly co-occurring nosological entities sharing a necessary prerequisite broadly conceptualized as a traumatic event. In this model, the two entities co-occur essentially by chance and not because of common vulnerabilities predating the trauma or common pathogenetic mechanisms set in motion by the traumatic event. Furthermore, in this model comorbidity between the two constructs could be partly explained by symptom overlap based on the current diagnostic criteria for these disorders. Therefore, to examine the utility of this model, we need to examine studies relating to the comorbidity of the two constructs, the types of traumas that give rise to each, and any shared symptomatology.

Comorbidity Between Posttraumatic Stress Disorder and Dissociative Disorders and Their Traumatic Antecedents

Only a small portion of the extensive PTSD research of the past two decades addresses comorbid dissociative symptoms. One of the earliest studies (Bremner et al. 1992) reported modest to moderate elevations in Dissociative Experiences Scale (DES) scores in a Vietnam veteran PTSD sample (mean, 27.0) and a large variance reflecting a wide range of dissociation severity. Similar elevations and large variances have been subsequently reported in other PTSD samples (Waller et al. 1996). Tampke and Irwin (1999) examined the degree to which anxiety and dissociation predicted the three PTSD symptom clusters in Australian war veterans. Contrary to expectation, intrusions and avoidance were predicted by anxiety symptoms alone, whereas the arousal cluster was predicted by both anxiety and dissociation, casting doubt on the conceptualization of chronic dissociation as an inherent feature of PTSD.

Turning to dissociative disorders, their comorbidity with PTSD ranges from almost ubiquitous in dissociative identity disorder (DID) to a very low 4% in depersonalization disorder (DPD) (Simeon et al. 2003b). DSM-IV-TR (American Psychiatric Association 2000) dissociative disorders are characterized by pathological dissociation (Waller et al. 1996) but differ in the dissociative domain in which symptoms are primarily manifested. Traumatic antecedents appear to play a major role in the pathogenesis of all dissociative disorders, although the onset age, type, and severity of the traumas involved vary greatly. In a meta-analysis (van IJzendoorn and Schuengel 1996), 26 studies ($N=2,108$) explored the relationship between abuse and dissociation; the effect size of this association ($d=0.52$) was highly significant ($P<0.001$) and essentially independent of the type of abuse (sexual abuse, $d=0.42$; physical abuse, $d=0.42$; both, $d=0.58$).

When examined by individual dissociative disorder, the role of trauma can be briefly summarized as follows. In DID several studies clearly document its relationship to childhood interpersonal trauma, in particular extreme and chronic early physical and/or sexual abuse (Braun 1984; Putnam 1985; Ross et al. 1990; Spiegel 1984). In dissociative amnesia, an acute traumatic event is typically identified (van der Hart and Nijenhuis 2001). In dissociative fugue, subacute chronic stress is typically described (Coons 1998). In DPD childhood interpersonal trauma of lesser severity than that encountered in the more severe dissociative disorders, particularly chronic emotional abuse and neglect, has been reported (Simeon et al. 2001b). In the more culturally bound dissociative disorders, such as ataque and possession/trance states, traumatic stressors are also typically described (Simeon and Hollander 2000).

There have been numerous attempts to dissect the salient characteristics of traumas that lead to particular types of symptoms, but these efforts have not been particularly fruitful in achieving diagnostic accuracy. Some studies have attempted to disentangle characteristics of an index trauma with regard to future propensity toward dissociation and PTSD. Johnson et al.'s (2001) thoroughly designed study addressed this matter in 89 female survivors of childhood sexual abuse. Most abuse characteristics correlated in the same direction and to similar degrees with both PTSD and dissociation. The only two variables that revealed a differential pattern across conditions were age at abuse onset and degree of trust in the perpetrator. Age at abuse onset correlated positively with PTSD (r=0.19) but negatively with dissociation (r=–0.24). Degree of trust in the perpetrator did not correlate with PTSD (r=0.008) but correlated negatively with dissociation (r=–0.19).

In other studies, early childhood onset and chronicity of trauma have been consistently associated with chronic dissociation (Chu 2000; Chu and Dill 1990; Kirby et al. 1993). In Holocaust survivors, Yehuda et al. (1997) found that younger age at the time of trauma was significantly related to amnesia and emotional detachment, whereas older age of trauma onset was positively correlated with the hallmark intrusive symptoms of PTSD. A longitudinal study of high-risk infants (N=168) strengthened retrospective correlational findings by showing that early age, chronicity, and severity of trauma predicted dissociation in adolescence (Ogawa et al. 1997).

With respect to trust in the perpetrator of a trauma, Freyd (1994, 1996) proposed an eloquent model that distinguishes between two types of trauma: betrayal and life threat. She described two primary dimensions of traumatic experience, a fear-inducing dimension that threatens survival and an interpersonal betrayal dimension that threatens attachment to important others (see Chapter 2 in this volume, "Attachment, Disorganization, and Dissociation"). Freyd argued that life threat traumas are more strongly associated with PTSD-type symptoms of hyperarousal and intrusiveness, whereas betrayal traumas are more strongly associated with numbing and dissociative symptoms.

Indeed, there is some evidence that violence, such as physical abuse or witnessing domestic violence, is predictive of PTSD severity (Silva et al. 2000), whereas sexual abuse may lead to more dissociative symptoms than other forms of childhood trauma (Putnam 1985). A cross-sectional study of adult psychiatric inpatients with widely varying histories of childhood abuse found that violent physical and violent sexual abuse were strong predictors of PTSD, whereas violent sexual abuse and neglect were strong predictors of dissociation (E.B. Carlson et al. 2001); this study then only partially supports a unique relationship between overwhelming fear of violence and PTSD. In the Johnson et al.

(2001) study, danger dimensions of the trauma such as belief that the self would be killed, belief that others would be killed, use of weapons, or sustaining injury demonstrated no symptom specificity, correlating to similar degrees with current PTSD and dissociative symptoms.

Freyd (1994, 1996) also indicated that trust is crucial in the maintenance of attachment to caregivers, which in turn is crucial to survival and adaptation. Traumatic acts that violate this trust tend to be more strongly dissociated in an attempt to maintain bonding. Empirical data supporting this formulation are limited, yet it merits more research. In the Johnson et al. (2001) study, degree of trust in the perpetrator correlated negatively, rather than positively, with dissociation severity, contradicting betrayal trauma theory. One plausible explanation may be that the relationship between trust and dissociation is more complex; thus, for example, in less severe trauma the power of a trusting relationship may be able to bring about reparation between victim and caregiver and protect against chronic symptoms. Alternatively, in more severe or chronic trauma the victim may have to resort more heavily to dissociative processes to preserve trust in an abusing caretaker.

Nosological Definitions and Symptom Overlap

The comorbidity between PTSD and dissociation might be artificially inflated or deflated by the particular symptoms assigned to each set of disorders under our current nosology. The definitions of *dissociation* and *dissociative disorders* presented in DSM-IV-TR do not make any reference to PTSD symptoms. However, dissociative symptoms and disorders in our current nosology are inadequately defined and may require major reevaluation. Dell (2002), for example, proposed a more detailed phenomenology for DID that includes some symptoms currently classified only under PTSD, such as flashbacks. Similarly, van der Hart et al.'s (2004) model of structural dissociation (reviewed later in this chapter) posits "positive" symptoms of dissociation such as the ones traditionally associated with classic PTSD.

On the other hand, a review of the 17 DSM-IV-TR symptom criteria for PTSD readily reveals that several criteria overlap to some degree with what are traditionally viewed as dissociative symptoms, including flashbacks (criterion 3, Cluster B) and amnesia, detachment, and restricted range of affect (criteria 3, 5, and 6, Cluster C). Flashbacks have been widely referred to, even in mainstream PTSD research, as dissociative phenomena (Krystal et al. 1998). Flashbacks involve varying degrees of a dreamlike state with immersion in past experience that effectively dissociates the self from present reality. The question of whether flashbacks compose a "core" dissociative symptom may be partly a question of semantics—whether we choose to define *intrusive* posttraumatic stress symptoms as dissociative. However, Lanius et al.'s (2002) innovative functional magnetic resonance imaging work has revealed that the majority (about 70%) of individuals with PTSD exposed to traumatic script-driven imagery respond with classic arousal and reliving symptoms. The remaining 30% respond with a dissociative blank state unassociated with heart rate increase. One way to interpret this research that is more in line with our current nosology would be to consider the former response as classic PTSD (intrusion and arousal) and the latter as dissociative (avoidance). Another interpretation, especially if these contrasting states occur at different points in time in the same individual, would be to say that such an individual has a more complex posttraumatic disorder that is not currently well-delineated in our diagnostic system, going under the name of complex PTSD or a dissociative disorder awaiting specification.

PTSD criterion C poses similar challenges. The criterion of detachment need not be dissociative and can range from frank depersonalization to a sense of alienation or disconnection from others that is harder to classify. The criterion of amnesia for portions of the original trauma is by definition dissociative in nature, but it only speaks to peritraumatic, not ongoing, dissociation. Finally, the criterion of emotional numbing, characterized by diminished experiencing of positive feelings such as love and happiness, is one that continues to elude precise classification. *Numbing* refers to a diminished intensity of affective experience, and although it could be interpreted to involve a "dissociation" of feelings, we still need to understand how it differs from the emotional blunting of depression or the anhedonia of schizophrenia.

In a thoughtful conceptual review of the dissociation construct, Holmes et al. (2005) proposed that all dissociative symptoms can be effectively grouped into two subtypes, detachment and compartmentalization. With respect to PTSD, numbing, disengagement from others, and flashbacks would all be conceptualized as dissociative "detachment," whereas amnesia for the traumatic event could be due either to dissociative detachment leading to poor encoding or to dissociative compartmentalization leading to retrieval difficulties.

The comorbidity between PTSD and dissociative disorders is too extensive, at least as far as the more extreme dissociative disorders are concerned, to be accounted for simply by shared traumatic antecedents and some overlap in diagnostic criteria.

MODEL 2: SHARED RISK FACTORS

Model 2 posits that PTSD and dissociative disorders are nosological entities that co-occur more commonly than dictated by their common traumatic antecedents, due to common vulnerabilities (biological, cognitive, or psychological) that predispose individuals to become symptomatic when challenged by trauma. In other words, this model presumes that PTSD and pathological dissociation share certain risk factors, with trauma being a necessary but not sufficient prerequisite for the development of both (Warshaw et al. 1993).

Twin studies suggest that there is clear genetic vulnerability to PTSD. Studying identical twins, Gilbertson et al. (2002) found that smaller hippocampal volume was a vulnerability factor for PTSD development in combat soldiers rather than an outcome either of trauma or of the disorder. Similarly, in a recent twin study, Gilbertson (2004) demonstrated that verbal memory, mental flexibility, and lower intelligence may heighten vulnerability for the disorder.

Two meta-analytical studies of PTSD, one by Brewin et al. (2000) and one by Ozer et al. (2003), assessed various predictors of PTSD, including factors that precede the index trauma and therefore can be construed as risk factors. Brewin et al. (2000) determined that age, gender, and race predicted PTSD in some populations but not in others; education, previous trauma, and childhood adversity predicted PTSD more consistently but to a varying extent; and psychiatric history, childhood abuse, and family psychiatric history had the most consistent predictive effects. Ozer et al. (2003) found that prior psychological adjustment, prior trauma history, and family history of psychopathology had only modest effects in predicting subsequent PTSD.

Turning to dissociation, there is debate as to whether pathological dissociation is a discrete entity (Waller et al. 1996) or lies on a continuum with normal dissociation. It is likely that a dissociative diathesis is in part genetically determined, only becoming expressed phenotypically in a pathological fashion in the face of later adversity. Three behavioral genetic studies have examined the heritability of dissociation, and findings are mixed. One twin study found no evidence for a genetic component to pathological dissociation (Waller and Ross 1997), with 45% of the variance attributable to shared environment and 55% to nonshared environment. Another twin study found a 48% genetic influence and a 52% nonshared environmental influence for pathological dissociation, and a similar 55% genetic and 45% nonshared environmental influence for nonpathological dissociation (Jang et al. 1998). Finally, a more recent twin and adoptee study (Becker-Blease et al. 2004) found that 59% of the variance in a nonpathological dissociation measure was accounted for by genetics and 41% by nonshared environmental influences. Taken together, the studies suggest that nonpathological dissociation, possibly the precursor to pathological dissociation, has a substantial—greater than 50%—heritability. This estimate is quite comparable with the approximately 50% heritability estimated for absorption, the perceptual capacity and disposition to enter internally generated experiential states (Tellegen et al. 1988).

Diathesis-stress models of dissociation have proposed that certain nonpathological heritable traits may lead to more pathological forms of dissociation if notable environmental stressors occur over the course of a lifetime. Based on theoretical and empirical lines of evidence, Butler et al. (1996) proposed that high hypnotizability may be a diathesis for pathological dissociation under conditions of acute traumatic stress. Hypnotizability includes several components: narrowed attention, absorption, and suggestibility. The relationship of these components to pathological dissociation has been explored in various studies. Some studies have not supported an association between hypnotizability and dissociation (Putnam et al. 1995; Ray 1996), whereas others have (Bryant et al. 2001; Frischholz et al. 1992). The dissociative trait of absorption has been proffered as a diathesis to acute dissociative reactions under severe stress (Sterlini and Bryant 2002), whereas fantasy proneness, a concept related to absorption, is another trait reportedly associated with pathological dissociation (Waldo and Merritt 2000).

Some empirical work in nonclinical samples (Ray 1996) suggests the traits of absentmindedness and forgetfulness may be dissociative diatheses. These traits involve lapses in awareness, possibly predisposing individuals with them to manifest more pronounced memory problems under the impact of traumatic stress. *Alexithymia*, the inability to identify and describe feelings, has also been identified as a potential dissociative diathesis and correlates strongly with pathological dissociation (Grabe et al. 2000). Irwin and Melbin-Helberg (1997) found that alexithymia, and in particular difficulty in identifying feelings, accounted for about 20% of the variance in dissociation scores in a student population. Alexithymia was the strongest predictor of dissociation from several personality and environmental variables in another student sample (Modestin et al. 2002).

Yet another powerful concept emerging is the unique association between backgrounds of emotional neglect and later dissociation (Brunner et al. 2000; Draijer and Langeland 1999), whereas positive parenting may be protective and has negative predictive value (Modestin et al. 2002). In 1992, Liotti proposed that parent–child disorganized attachment was an important factor in the etiology of dissociative disorders.

Compelling longitudinal studies have now borne out this formulation (E. A. Carlson 1998; Ogawa et al. 1997), highlighting that trauma is not a sufficient prerequisite for dissociative states (see Chapter 2). Simeon et al. (2002) reported that cognitive schemata reflective of overconnection and disconnection were associated with DPD and depersonalization symptom severity. Such risk factors of a disrupted early emotional environment appear to be powerfully related to dissociative processes but may not be unique to them. One study, for example, reported that attachment style was a stronger predictor of PTSD severity than trauma severity; dissociation was not measured (Dieperink et al. 2001).

Model 2 is only partly supported by empirical data, which indicate both shared but also unique risk factors associated with dissociation and PTSD.

MODEL 3: SHARED PATHOGENESIS

Model 3 posits that PTSD and dissociation share common pathogenetic mechanisms activated by the precipitating trauma. The traumatic event triggers a cascade of pathogenetic processes that—although by definition must vary in fundamental ways to result in different disease phenotypes—might also share some common pathways or features. Of note, Model 3 in part overlaps with Model 2 because preexisting risk factors may comprise some, but not the only, factors that determine pathogenetic pathways once trauma occurs.

The most definitive way to explore this model is to longitudinally examine in vivo or in experimental paradigms the early neurobiological processes involved in the genesis of posttraumatic stress versus dissociative symptoms. These kinds of studies are limited, but they offer some unique insights into the origins of the two conditions. Alternatively, some inferences about pathogenetic processes can be drawn from the end point neurobiological and neurocognitive findings that emerge as characteristic of the two conditions. These studies are much more abundant but have the shortcoming of not longitudinally tracking pathogenesis; similar end point neurobiological or neurocognitive deficits could either be epiphenomena of other shared abnormalities (i.e., not central to the pathogenesis of the conditions) or may have predated the trauma event and would be better conceptualized as vulnerabilities.

In examining the pathogenesis of PTSD and the possible role of dissociative processes in this pathogenesis, we turn to the peritraumatic dissociation literature. *Peritraumatic dissociation* is the acute dissociation that occurs during a traumatic event, and since the creation of the Peritraumatic Dissociative Experiences Questionnaire (Marmar et al. 1994), peritraumatic dissociation has been measured both retrospectively and prospectively in numerous studies (see Chapter 9 in this volume, "Peritraumatic Dissociation"). Although peritraumatic dissociation may be usefully mobilized as an escape from otherwise inescapable, overwhelming trauma, its continued use over the long term can hinder the emotional and cognitive processing of the original trauma, in effect perpetuating posttraumatic pathology (Foa and Hearst-Ikeda 1996).

Although initial studies consistently reported that peritraumatic dissociation was a strong predictor of subsequent PTSD, more recent studies and reviews have challenged this view. A critical review of the literature by R.D. Marshall et al. (1999) argued that acute stress disorder and PTSD are essentially the same disorder on a temporal continuum and that peritraumatic dissociation does not constitute a core feature of this unitary syndrome. In a methodologically sophisticated study, G.N. Marshall and Schell (2002) found that peritraumatic dissociation was not predictive of follow-up PTSD severity after controlling for baseline PTSD severity. Gershuny et al. (2003) showed that the predictive effect of peritraumatic dissociation on PTSD severity was eliminated after controlling for peritraumatic fears of death and losing control. Ozer et al. (2003), in the largest meta-analytic study of PTSD to date, reported that although peritraumatic dissociation was the strongest predictor of later PTSD, "the strength of the relationship of $r=0.35$ clearly does not support thinking about dissociative phenomena as an integral part of the phenomenology of the posttraumatic response" (p. 69). They concluded that the "subjective psychological response" to traumatic exposure may be the overall variable that best predicts later PTSD; different degrees of peritraumatic dissociation can be a component of this variable and may relate to the level of psychophysiological arousal during the trauma.

Beyond peritraumatic dissociation, a number of studies have attempted to quantify aspects of the subjective experience evoked by traumatic stressors and to determine their relationship to subsequent psychopathology. In the Ozer et al. (2003) meta-analysis, peritraumatic emotions and peritraumatic perceived life threat were both significant predictors of later PTSD. Psychometrically quantifying the concept of peritraumatic distress, Brunet et al. (2001) proposed that it encompasses various somatic and emotional aspects of the distress experience, including fears about safety, losing control, helplessness/anger, and guilt/shame. To date, particular distress components have not emerged as uniquely linked to later PTSD or dissociation. For example, in a study that prospectively followed a New York City convenience sample affected by the World Trade Center disaster, Simeon et al. (2005a) found that peritraumatic "loss of control" and "guilt/shame" feelings were strongly associated with both dissociation and posttraumatic stress at follow-up 1 year later.

Similarly, the ways in which traumatic events are cognitively processed, both initially and subsequently, are relevant to the evolution of trauma-spectrum symptomatology. Ehlers and colleagues (Clohessy and Ehlers 1999; Halligan et al. 2002, 2003; Mayou et al. 2002; Murray et al. 2002) have systematically studied cognitive processing factors that appear to relate to the initiation and perpetuation of PTSD symptoms, and they have consistently replicated their findings in various traumatized groups (e.g., motor vehicle accident survivors, ambulance workers, and victims of assault). These studies revealed that cognitive processes such as memory fragmentation, data-driven processing, rumination about the trauma, negative interpretation of intrusions, thought suppression, and angry cognitions contributed to PTSD severity from 3 months to 3 years posttrauma. Cognitive processes have also been implicated in the genesis of dissociation. Gershuny and Thayer (1999) proposed that the fear of death and fear of loss of control were central to triggering dissociative reactions. In one confirmatory study in novice skydivers, controllability was significantly negatively correlated with peritraumatic dissociation (Sterlini and Bryant 2002).

To better study the early evolution of PTSD, experimental paradigms looking at the induction of PTSD-like symptoms in the laboratory can be very informative. A series of such innovative studies has been conducted by Brewin and colleagues. These investigations have been designed to test the dual representation theory of PTSD (Brewin et al. 1996), which posits that PTSD is more likely to develop when stimuli are encoded as situationally accessible memories rather than as verbally accessible memories. Employing the screening of a traumatic video intended to induce intrusive memories over the ensuing weeks in normal volunteers, Holmes et al. (2004) showed that more intrusive recollections ensued when the linguistic encoding of the traumatic film was impeded by a competing verbal task that engaged the verbally accessible memory system. In contrast, a concurrent visuospatial tapping task during the video viewing led to fewer later intrusive recollections, presumably by engaging the situationally accessible memory system during the encoding process and impeding the formation of nonverbal PTSD-like memories. Increased dissociation and decreased heart rate during portions of the film viewing were associated with increased later intrusions of those portions.

The investigators hypothesized that if the volunteers viewed the tape in a dissociated state, they would be more likely to have later intrusive recollections. This prediction was not supported in a similar design in which participants were subjected to a 10-minute dot-staring task designed to induce dissociation prior to video viewing (Brewin and Holmes 2004). There are several possible interpretations of this null finding. One is that a modest laboratory stressor and a dot-staring task in otherwise normal volunteers do not sufficiently recreate either a traumatic stimulus or the peritraumatic phenomena often accompanying it. Another possibility is that the dot-staring paradigm is not a temporally adequate paradigm for assessing the impact of peritraumatic dissociation, because peritraumatic dissociation preceded the traumatic stressor rather than being a consequence of it. Finally, the finding could indicate that peritraumatic dissociation is irrelevant to the genesis of PTSD symptoms.

Further innovative studies are needed to empirically resolve whether dissociation or other peritraumatic variables are necessary components in the evolution of chronic PTSD and dissociative symptoms. Similarly, hardly any studies exist that examine the impact of peritraumatic dissociation on the later development of dissociative symptoms or disorders. One study prospectively followed disaster victims and found that peritraumatic dissociation was the strongest predictor of dissociation, but not PTSD, 1 year later (Simeon et al. 2004).

I turn now to end point neurobiological and cognitive alterations characteristic of both PTSD and dissociation. Such studies are abundant in PTSD, and despite some variations and inconsistencies they do delineate a fairly cohesive biological imprint for the disorder. In contrast, studies of dissociation are much fewer and have not yet yielded as cohesive a picture; this is further complicated by the fact that "dissociation" probably encompasses heterogeneous phenomena that are bound to have their own unique biological profiles. Still, from what is known, the biology of dissociation is emerging as quite distinct from that of PTSD in a number of different domains.

The hypothalamic-pituitary-adrenal (HPA) axis plays a central role in the regulation of the organism's response to stress. Preclinical and clinical studies to date are compellingly demonstrating that both early life stress and later adult trauma can result in lasting HPA axis dysregulation, thus affecting future stress responses to more minor life stressors and laying the foundation for future vulnerability and psychopathology. Conversely, *resilience*—that is, more intact psychobiological adaptation in light of major lifetime stress—is becoming an important area of research (Charney 2004).

Briefly summarized, and although not always consistent, HPA axis findings in PTSD tend to reveal normal or decreased basal urinary and plasma cortisol (Yehuda et al. 1990; Young and Breslau 2004); an altered cortisol circadian pattern with increased nadir-to-peak cortisol ratios and decreased cortisol in the evening and night hours (Bremner et al. 2003); elevated cerebrospinal fluid and corticotropin-releasing factor (CRF) (Bremner et al. 1997); blunted adrenocorticotropic hormone (ACTH) response to CRF challenge (Bremner et al. 2003; Smith et al. 1989); heightened ACTH response to metyrapone challenge (Yehuda et al. 1996); increased lymphocyte glucocorticoid receptors (Yehuda et al. 1991); and cortisol hypersuppression in response to low-dose dexamethasone challenge (Yehuda et al. 1993). These findings are all consistent with a highly sensitized HPA axis in PTSD (Yehuda 1997), characterized by hypothalamic CRF hypersecretion, downregulated pituitary CRF receptors, enhanced glucocorticoid negative feedback inhibition, and an unresolved question of adrenal insufficiency.

The HPA axis has, for the most part, not been examined in adult or child samples presenting primarily with dissociative disorders without major comorbidity. Stein et al. (1997) compared 19 adult women with childhood sexual abuse with nonvictimized control subjects. The victim group demonstrated enhanced cortisol suppression in response to low-dose dexamethasone compared with the control subjects, as is typically reported in PTSD. Of the 19 victims, 13 met criteria for PTSD and 15 met criteria for a dissociative disorder; only 2 dissociative disorder subjects did not have comorbid PTSD, therefore, a separate examination of the two diagnoses was not possible. Interestingly, Vermetten et al. (2003) studied a sample of adult DID patients with major PTSD comorbidity and reported resistance to dexamethasone suppression in most of the subjects, which is not consistent with the PTSD literature.

There is accumulating evidence that primary dissociative disorders, when examined in the absence of a major confounding comorbidity such as PTSD or major depression, are characterized by a unique profile of HPA axis dysregulation. Simeon et al. (2001a) conducted a pilot study of nine DPD subjects compared with nine healthy control subjects and found that depersonalized subjects presented with significantly elevated basal plasma cortisol when the authors controlled for depression scores. Most importantly, these depersonalized participants also demonstrated resistance to dexamethasone suppression. Similar findings have now been replicated in larger samples of depersonalized subjects compared with PTSD and normal control subjects (i.e., subjects free of lifetime psychopathology) (Simeon et al. 2005c).

Dissociation also differs from PTSD in its autonomic system profile, including physiological indexes such as blood pressure, heart rate, and galvanic skin responses as well as measures of noradrenergic activity. Norepinephrine plays a central role in arousal, attention, and emotional memory. In PTSD, a multitude of studies of basal catecholamines, noradrenergic challenges, and receptor binding have generally revealed heightened noradrenergic tone, consistent with the hyperarousal and intrusive symptomatology characteristic of the disorder (Southwick et al. 1999). Thus, the classic hypermnesia of PTSD, with its hallmark symptom of intrusive emotional recollections, appears to be at least partly related to the heightened basal catecholamine activity.

In contrast, given the "shut-down" amnesic symptomatology typically characteristic of dissociative disorders, one would predict basal autonomic hypoactivity in dissociation. Indeed, there exists limited support for this hypothesis. After rape, women experiencing high dissociation showed diminished heart rate and galvanic skin responses (Griffin et al. 1997). Sierra et al. (2002) showed that, compared with anxiety disorder and healthy control subjects, individuals with DPD exhibited reduced magnitude and increased latency of skin conductance responses to unpleasant stimuli compared with neutral stimuli. A study of motor vehicle accident victims found that peritraumatic dissociation was negatively associated with urinary norepinephrine and epinephrine collected in the emergency department soon after the trauma (Delahanty et al. 2003). Similarly, a significant inverse relationship between urinary norepinephrine and dissociation severity was reported in DPD (Simeon et al. 2003a) and in borderline personality disorder (Simeon et al. 2004).

With respect to other neurochemical systems, Morgan et al. (2000) examined the neurochemical profile of highly resilient Special Forces soldiers undergoing intensive military training in U.S. Army survival schools (see Chapter 8 in this volume, "Symptoms of Dissociation in Healthy Military Populations") and found that acute dissociation severity in response to overwhelming stress was significantly inversely correlated with plasma neuropeptide Y levels.

Neuroimaging studies are also revealing divergent findings between dissociative states and classic PTSD. Using functional magnetic resonance imaging with traumatic script-driven imagery, Lanius et al. (2002) studied women with PTSD secondary to childhood sexual abuse. Of the PTSD subjects, approximately 70% responded to the scripts with reliving, arousal, and increased heart rate, whereas 30% dissociated in response to the scripts and did not demonstrate heart rate increases (see Chapter 10 in this volume, "Posttraumatic Stress Disorder Symptom Provocation and Neuroimaging"). In this latter group, compared with a normal control group, the dissociative state was associated with increased activation in the medial prefrontal cortex (Brodmann's area [BA] 9,10), the inferior frontal gyrus (BA 47), the anterior cingulate (BA 24 and 32), the superior and middle temporal gyri (BA 38), the parietal lobe (BA 7), and the occipital lobe (BA 19). Interestingly, this pattern of activation was distinctly different from that found in the PTSD-reliving subgroup yet similar to the two published neuroimaging studies in non-PTSD DPD (Phillips et al. 2001; Simeon et al. 2000).

Finally, studies of cognition have revealed distinctly unique deficits characteristic of dissociative conditions versus PTSD. According to Yehuda et al. (1995), explicit memory in PTSD is generally intact, as exhibited on a variety of attention, immediate memory, and cumulative learning tasks, but when tasks involve interference conditions, the capacity for retention diminishes. Siegel (1995) proposed a resource allocation model to explain these disruptions of explicit memory in PTSD, according to which emotional reactivity resultant from the trauma leads to dividing attentional resources and disturbs focal attention and effortful learning. In a study by McNally et al. (2000), the severity of self-reported PTSD symptoms in participants with histories of sexual abuse positively predicted the magnitude of trauma-related interference on an emotional Stroop task. Interference effects on the emotional Stroop task in response to trauma-related words have been consistently documented in PTSD of various traumatic etiologies (Cassiday et al. 1992; Dubner and Motta 1999; Foa et al. 1991; McNally et al. 1990). These interference effects have not been demonstrated in control groups of trauma survivors without PTSD, suggesting that the abnormality is a feature of the disorder rather than a nonspecific sequel to trauma.

Less is known about attentional and memory processes in dissociative disorders (see Chapter 3 in this volume, "Memory and Attentional Processes in Dissociative Identity Disorder"). Studies of nonclinical student samples have found that high dissociators performed worse on the standard Stroop task compared with low dissociators, suggesting that high dissociators have deficits in selective attention (i.e., are more vulnerable to interference and distraction; Freyd et al. 1998). However, when tested on an emotional Stroop task that employed both neutral and negatively charged words, set up as a divided attention task with pretest instructions to not only respond to stimuli color but also remember the words in the test, high dissociators showed less interference than low dissociators, demonstrating superiority when dividing attention. In addition, high dissociators did worse than low dissociators in explicitly recalling negative words (DePrince and Freyd 1999). Similar findings were shown by Simeon et al. (2005b) in non-PTSD individuals with dissociative disorders who performed comparably with normal control subjects in a selective-attention emotional Stroop task but demonstrated less interference than control subjects in a divided-attention emotional Stroop task. Dissociative subjects were also found to explicitly recall more neutral words and fewer negative words than control subjects during a baseline explicit memory task.

Taken together, these findings suggest that individuals with PTSD present with a cognitive profile characterized by intrusion of and cognitive bias toward threatening material, whereas dissociative individuals present with a cognitive profile characterized by better performance at multitasking and a heightened capacity to dissociate negatively laden material. These dissociative cognitive strategies might be conceptualized as one type of adaptation to chronic trauma, facilitating distraction away from and poorer registration of affectively overwhelming experiences in an effort to preserve interpersonal attachment. Freyd et al. (1998) referred to this process as the *cognitive environments theory of trauma.*

In summary, there is not much evidence supporting Model 3 of a shared pathogenesis; the experiential, cognitive, and biological processes implicated in the development of PTSD versus dissociation are in many ways distinct.

MODEL 4: SAME DISORDER

In the final and most extreme model, dissociation and PTSD are essentially posited to be inseparable and artificially dissected by current nosological practices. In other words, if we broadened our diagnostic groupings, and in the process eliminated some of the complexity of the conditions resulting from traumatic stress, then we could more or less encompass in one uniform sweep the large range of posttraumatic psychopathological sequelae that are currently subsumed under PTSD, dissociative disorders, and possibly other disorders. There is some merit to this formulation, in that the various psychopathologies substantially linked to a traumatic etiology are now variably and rather arbitrarily classified into distinct groups that do not acknowledge their shared etiology and characteristics. In DSM-IV-TR, PTSD is classified with the anxiety disorders, dissociative disorders are classified together as a distinct group, and other trauma-related disorders, such as conversion, are classified under the somatoform disorders. On the other hand, it is difficult to imagine that the large and complex scope of psychopathological sequelae to trauma could all be lumped together in one category.

Bremner (1999) was one of the first mainstream PTSD researchers to acknowledge the importance and regularity of dissociative symptoms in posttraumatic phenomenology. He put forth the notion that there may be "two subtypes of acute trauma response, one primarily dissociative and the other intrusive/hyperarousal," both representing "unique pathways to chronic stress-related psychopathology" (p. 350). In terms of classification, he proposed that either a dissociative symptom cluster be added

to chronic PTSD or two separate chronic posttraumatic disorders be recognized: *chronic PTSD* (emphasizing intrusion and hyperarousal as currently found in ICD-10) and *chronic dissociative disorder*. This proposition
acknowledged the central importance that dissociative processes can
have in posttraumatic syndromes, yet in two ways this proposal falls
prey to reductionism. First, artificially dividing chronic PTSD from
chronic dissociative disorder ignores a large subgroup of individuals in
whom the two commonly co-occur. Second, collapsing chronic traumatic
dissociation into one disorder fails to capture the complexity of clinically
observed dissociative phenomena that can range from depersonalization to amnesia to DID.

Complex PTSD (Herman 1992), or disorders of extreme stress not
otherwise specified (DESNOS; van der Kolk et al. 1996), is a phenomenological presentation associated with chronic severe trauma that lies at
the interface of dissociation and PTSD and has not yet been satisfacto-
rily accounted for in our current classification systems. Theoretical conceptualization of complex PTSD transcends the narrow boundaries of
simple PTSD, emphasizing the profound impact of trauma, especially
chronic childhood trauma, on personality formation, the fundamental
sense of self, relatedness to others, and systems of meaning (Zlotnick
and Pearlstein 1997). The four core features of DESNOS include severe
affect and impulse dysregulation; pathological dissociation; somatization, including alexithymia; and fundamentally altered beliefs concerning the self and relationships (Ford 1999).

In the DSM-IV (American Psychiatric Association 1994) field trials,
the relationship between PTSD and DESNOS was investigated in approximately 500 traumatized individuals (van der Kolk et al. 1996). Probably due to selection criteria, more than 90% of participants with DES-
NOS also met criteria for PTSD, leading the investigators to recommend
that DESNOS was more likely to be an associated feature of PTSD than to
constitute a separate diagnosis. However, a later study of approximately
100 traumatized individuals revealed a distinctly different breakdown,
with 29% diagnosed as PTSD only, 26% as DESNOS only, 32% as both,
and 13% as neither (Ford 1999). In effect, about half the participants with
each diagnosis did not carry the other diagnosis, leading the investigator
to suggest that the dissection of PTSD and DESNOS warrants further
careful clinical and scientific investigation.

From the standpoint of dissociation, conceptual proposals have also
been put forth that attempt to unify PTSD and traumatic dissociation.
van der Hart et al. (2004) developed a structural dissociation model that
brings together trauma-related psychopathologies and frames their
manifestations in terms of positive and negative symptoms of dissocia-

tion (see Chapter 11 in this volume, "Psychobiology of Traumatization and Trauma-Related Structural Dissociation of the Personality"). *Positive symptoms* represent dissociative intrusions, such as hypermnesia (intrusion of traumatic memories) and various somatoform dissociative symptoms. *Negative symptoms* represent dissociative losses of function, such as memory (i.e., amnesia), motor control, or somatosensory perceptions. This model proposes that "simple" dissociative symptoms such as absorption, trance, and some examples of depersonalization/derealization are not dissociative symptoms at heart, because they are not manifestations of "structural" dissociation of the personality but rather reflect alterations of consciousness. Depersonalization of the ego-observing kind (i.e., a split between observing and experiencing ego) represents a manifestation of structural dissociation and is therefore included as a "true" dissociative symptom. In the simplest form of structural dissociation, two aspects of the personality are stipulated, an apparently normal part of the personality and an emotional part of the personality. The apparently normal aspect is dedicated to daily life functioning, whereas the emotional aspect is the segregated portion of the personality that is fixated on past trauma and responds to perceived danger. Secondary and tertiary dissociation represent more elaborate structural organizations involving further dissociated parts of the emotional and apparently normal aspects, respectively.

This is an ambitiously comprehensive model that offers the advantage of a conceptual foundation that extends beyond pure phenomenology. Its authors speculate a common neurobiological mechanism to all "structural dissociation," but such a mechanism has not been clearly articulated or empirically identified. The model best accounts for DID and its milder variants presently classified in the unfortunate DSM-IV-TR category of dissociative disorders not otherwise specified. However, the model fails to adequately incorporate a variety of "simple" dissociative presentations such as DPD, dissociative trance, and dissociative amnesia. These conditions are characterized by a more steady alteration in consciousness rather than by fluctuant positive and negative symptoms, yet they are undoubtedly dissociative in nature. In effect, using the terminology of Holmes et al. (2005), the structural model of dissociation retains the dissociative presentations that fall under "compartmentalization" while discarding those that fall under "detachment." The structural dissociation model also claims to encompass all of what is presently known as PTSD, arguing that the two parts of the personality (apparently normal and emotional) are operant even in classic simple PTSD. However, empirical evidence for this kind of structural segregation of the personality in simple PTSD or for temporal alterations between intrusive and dissociative states in most individuals with simple PTSD is limited at best.

CONCLUSION

The evidence presented here most strongly supports the conceptualization of dissociation and PTSD under Model 1, that is, as distinct entities that are often comorbidly associated yet differ in many of their predisposing vulnerabilities, as discussed in Model 2, and in their pathogenetic mechanisms, as discussed in Model 3. Certainly there exists no compelling evidence that the two constructs can be effectively combined in a single uniform model as posited by Model 4 without great sacrifice in diagnostic specificity and complexity. Clearly, many types of trauma can give rise to both PTSD and dissociative symptoms. Hardly any trauma characteristics have consistently emerged as unique to either construct, with the exception of early age and chronicity of trauma, which do appear to be more intimately linked to dissociation. Certain vulnerability factors associated with PTSD, including weaker verbal encoding of traumatic events, smaller hippocampi, and lower cognitive capacities in the areas of verbal memory, working memory, and cognitive flexibility, do appear to lead to a cognitive bias toward the intrusion of emotionally disturbing material. On the other hand, vulnerability to dissociation appears more linked to traits such as absorption, alexithymia, and forgetfulness, with a cognitive tendency toward multitasking and poorer registration and access to emotionally disturbing information. Neurobiological processes associated with the two constructs are emerging as quite distinct, including different patterns of HPA axis dysregulation, sympathetic activity, and regional brain activations and deactivations. There is little to suggest that PTSD should encompass most of traumatic dissociation, or the converse. It is clear that there exist both simple PTSD, characterized by intrusions and arousal with minimal dissociation, and simple dissociative conditions such as DPD that are mostly devoid of PTSD symptoms. There does, also, clearly exist an area of extensive overlap between the two constructs, variably referred to as PTSD with prominent dissociation, complex PTSD, disorders of extreme stress, dissociative disorder not otherwise specified, adult sequelae of serious childhood attachment disorders, or Axis II psychopathology associated with chronic trauma, that urgently needs more intensive investigation and accurate classification. This group of conditions composes a significant portion of the overlap between PTSD and dissociation, encompassing features of both as well as other features related to the chronic impingement of trauma and its consequences on personality and relatedness.

It is hoped that future research will be able to compare these entities head-to-head, by including samples with various presentations in the same studies and subjecting them to the same rigorous investigation rather than attempting to draw indirect comparisons and inferences from independent studies using different methodologies and measuring different descriptive, cognitive, or neurobiological characteristics.

REFERENCES

American Psychiatric Association: Diagnostic and Statistical Manual of Mental Disorders, 4th Edition. Washington, DC, American Psychiatric Association, 1994

American Psychiatric Association: Diagnostic and Statistical Manual of Mental Disorders, 4th Edition, Text Revision. Washington, DC, American Psychiatric Association, 2000

Becker-Blease KA, Deater-Deckard K, Eley T, et al: A genetic analysis of individual differences in dissociative behaviors in childhood and adolescence. J Child Psychol Psychiatry 45:522–532, 2004

Braun BG: Towards a theory of multiple personality and dissociative phenomena. Psychiatr Clin North Am 7:171–191, 1984

Bremner JD: Acute and chronic responses to psychological trauma: where do we go from here? Am J Psychiatry 156:349–351, 1999

Bremner JD, Southwick S, Brett E, et al: Dissociation and posttraumatic stress disorder in Vietnam combat veterans. Am J Psychiatry 149:328–332, 1992

Bremner JD, Licinio J, Darnell A, et al: Elevated CSF corticotropin-releasing factor concentrations in posttraumatic stress disorder. Am J Psychiatry 154:624–629, 1997

Bremner JD, Vythilingam M, Anderson G, et al: Assessment of the hypothalamic-pituitary-adrenal axis over a 24-hour diurnal period and in response to neuroendocrine challenges in women with and without childhood sexual abuse and posttraumatic stress disorder. Biol Psychiatry 54:710–718, 2003

Brewin C, Holmes E: The influence of encoding on the development of trauma memories. Presented at the 20th Annual Meeting of the International Society for Traumatic Stress Studies, New Orleans, LA, November 2004

Brewin CR, Dalgleish T, Joseph S: A dual representation theory of posttraumatic stress disorder. Psychol Rev 103:670–686, 1996

Brewin CR, Andrews B, Valentine JD: Meta-analysis of risk factors for posttraumatic stress disorder in trauma-exposed adults. J Consult Clin Psychol 68:748–766, 2000

Brunet A, Weiss DS, Metzler TJ, et al: The Peritraumatic Distress Inventory: a proposed measure of PTSD criterion A2. Am J Psychiatry 158:1480–1485, 2001

Brunner R, Parzer P, Schuld V, et al: Dissociative symptomatology and traumatogenic factors in adolescent psychiatric patients. J Nerv Ment Dis 188:71–77, 2000

Bryant RA, Guthrie RM, Moulds ML: Hypnotizability in acute stress disorder. Am J Psychiatry 158:600–604, 2001

Butler LD, Duran Ron EF, Jasiukaitis P, et al: Hypnotizability and traumatic experience: a diathesis-stress model of dissociative symptomatology. Am J Psychiatry 153:42–63, 1996

Carlson EA: A prospective longitudinal study of attachment disorganization/disorientation. Child Dev 69:1107–1128, 1998

Carlson EB, Dalenberg C, Armstrong J, et al: Multivariate prediction of posttraumatic symptoms in psychiatric inpatients. J Trauma Stress 14:549–567, 2001

Cassiday KL, McNally RJ, Zeitlin SB: Cognitive processing of trauma cues in rape victims with post-traumatic stress disorder. Cognit Ther Res 16:282–295, 1992

Charney DS: Psychobiological mechanisms of resilience and vulnerability: implications for successful adaptation to extreme stress. Am J Psychiatry 161:195–216, 2004

Chu JA: Psychological defense styles and childhood sexual abuse (letter). Am J Psychiatry 157:170, 2000

Chu JA, Dill DL: Dissociative symptoms in relation to childhood physical and sexual abuse. Am J Psychiatry 147:887–892, 1990

Clohessy S, Ehlers A: PTSD symptoms, response to intrusive memories, and coping in ambulance service workers. Br J Clin Psychol 38:251–265, 1999

Coons PM: The dissociative disorders: rarely considered and underdiagnosed. Psychiatr Clin North Am 21:637–648, 1998

Delahanty DL, Royer DK, Raimonde AJ, et al: Peritraumatic dissociation is inversely related to catecholamine levels in initial urine samples of motor vehicle accident victims. J Trauma Dissociation 4:65–79, 2003

Dell PF: Dissociative phenomenology of dissociative identity disorder. J Nerv Ment Dis 190:10–15, 2002

DePrince AP, Freyd JJ: Dissociative tendencies, attention and memory. Psychol Sci 10:449–452, 1999

Dieperink M, Leskela J, Thuras P, et al: Attachment style classification and posttraumatic stress disorder in former prisoners of war. Am J Orthopsychiatry 71:374–378, 2001

Draijer N, Langeland W: Childhood trauma and perceived parental dysfunction in the etiology of dissociative symptoms in psychiatric inpatients. Am J Psychiatry 156:379–385, 1999

Dubner AE, Motta RW: Sexually and physically abused foster care children and posttraumatic stress disorder. J Consult Clin Psychol 67:367–373, 1999

Foa EB, Hearst-Ikeda D: Emotional dissociation in response to trauma: an information-processing approach, in Handbook of Dissociation: Theoretical, Empirical, and Clinical Perspectives. Edited by Michelson LK, Ray WJ. New York, Plenum, 1996, pp 207–224

Foa EB, Feske U, Murdock TB, et al: Processing of threat-related information in rape victims. J Abnorm Psychol 100:156–162, 1991

Ford JD: Disorders of extreme stress following war-zone military trauma: associated features of posttraumatic stress disorder or comorbid but distinct syndromes? J Consult Clin Psychol 67:3–12, 1999

Freyd JJ: Betrayal-trauma: traumatic amnesia as an adaptive response to childhood abuse. Ethics and Behaviour 4:307–329, 1994

Freyd JJ: Betrayal Trauma: The Logic of Forgetting Childhood Abuse. Cambridge, MA, Harvard University Press, 1996

Freyd JJ, Martorello J, Alvarado SR, et al: Cognitive environments and dissociative tendencies: performance on the standard Stroop task for high versus low dissociators. Appl Cogn Psychol 12:S91–S103, 1998

Frischholz EJ, Lipman LS, Braun BG, et al: Psychopathology, hypnotizability, and dissociation. Am J Psychiatry 149:1521–1525, 1992

Gershuny BS, Thayer JF: Relations among psychological trauma, dissociative phenomena, and trauma-related distress: a review and integration. Clin Psychol Rev 19:631–657, 1999

Gershuny BS, Cloitre M, Otto MW: Peritraumatic dissociation and PTSD severity: do event-related fears about death and control mediate their relation? Behav Res Ther 41:157–166, 2003

Gilbertson M: Neurocognitive function in monozygotic twins discordant for PTSD. Presented at the 20th Annual Meeting of the International Society for Traumatic Stress Studies, New Orleans, LA, November 2004

Gilbertson M, Shenton ME, Ciszewski A, et al: Smaller hippocampal volume predicts pathologic vulnerability to psychological trauma. Nat Neurosci 5:1242–1247, 2002

Grabe HJ, Rainermann S, Spitzer C, et al: The relationship between dimensions of alexithymia and dissociation. Psychother Psychosom 69:128–131, 2000

Griffin MG, Resick PA, Mechnic MB: Objective assessment of peritraumatic dissociation: psychophysiological indicators. Am J Psychiatry 154:1081–1088, 1997

Halligan SL, Clark DM, Ehlers A: Cognitive processing, memory, and the development of PTSD symptoms: two experimental analogue studies. J Behav Ther Exp Psychiatry 33:73–89, 2002

Halligan SL, Michael T, Clark DM, et al: Posttraumatic stress disorder following assault: the role of cognitive processing, trauma memory, and appraisals. J Consult Clin Psychol 71:419–431, 2003

Herman J: Complex PTSD. J Trauma Stress 5:377–391, 1992

Holmes EA, Brewin CR, Hennessy RG: Trauma films, information processing, and intrusive memory development. J Exp Psychol 133:3–22, 2004

Holmes EA, Brown RJ, Mansell W, et al: Are there two qualitatively distinct forms of dissociation? A review and some clinical implications. Clin Psychol Rev 25:1–23, 2005

Irwin HJ, Melbin-Helberg EB: Alexithymia and dissociative tendencies. J Clin Psychol 53:159–166, 1997

Jang KL, Paris J, Zweig-Frank H, et al: Twin study of dissociative experience. J Nerv Ment Dis 186:345–351, 1998

Johnson DM, Pike JL, Chard KM: Factors predicting PTSD, depression, and dissociative severity in female treatment-seeking childhood sexual abuse survivors. Child Abuse Negl 25:179–198, 2001

Kirby JS, Chu JA, Dill DL: Correlates of dissociative symptomatology in patients with physical and sexual abuse histories. Compr Psychiatry 34:258–263, 1993

Krystal JH, Bremner DJ, Southwick SM, et al: The emerging neurobiology of dissociation: implications for treatment of posttraumatic stress disorder, in Trauma, Memory and Dissociation. Edited by Bremner DJ, Marmar CR. Washington, DC, American Psychiatric Press, 1998, pp 321–363

Lanius RA, Williamson PC, Boksman K, et al: Brain activation during script-driven imagery induced dissociative responses in PTSD: a functional magnetic resonance imaging investigation. Biol Psychiatry 52:305–311, 2002

Liotti G: Disorganized/disoriented attachment in the etiology of the dissociative disorders. Dissociation 4:196–204, 1992

Marmar CR, Weiss DS, Schlenger WE, et al: Peritraumatic dissociation and posttraumatic stress in male Vietnam theater veterans. Am J Psychiatry 151:902–907, 1994

Marshall GN, Schell TL: Reappraising the link between peritraumatic dissociation and PTSD symptom severity: evidence from a longitudinal study of community violence survivors. J Abnorm Psychol 111:626–636, 2002

Marshall RD, Spitzer R, Liebowitz MR: Review and critique of the new DSM-IV diagnosis of acute stress disorder. Am J Psychiatry 156:1677–1685, 1999

Mayou RA, Ehlers A, Bryant B: Posttraumatic stress disorder after motor vehicle accidents: 3-year follow-up of a prospective longitudinal study. Behav Res Ther 40:665–675, 2002

McNally RJ, Kaspi SP, Riemann BC, et al: Selective processing of threat cues in posttraumatic stress disorder. J Abnorm Psychol 99:398–402, 1990

McNally RJ, Clancy SA, Shachter DL, et al: Cognitive processing of trauma cues in adults reporting repressed, recovered or continuous memories of childhood sexual abuse. J Abnorm Psychol 109:355–359, 2000

Modestin J, Lotscher K, Erni T: Dissociative experiences and their correlates in young non-patients. Psychol Psychother 75:53–64, 2002

Morgan CA, Wang S, Southwick SM, et al: Plasma neuropeptide-Y concentrations in humans exposed to military survival training. Biol Psychiatry 47:902–909, 2000

Murray J, Ehlers A, Mayou RA: Dissociation and post-traumatic stress disorder: two prospective studies of road traffic accident survivors. Br J Psychiatry 180:363–368, 2002

Ogawa JR, Sroufe LA, Weinfield NS, et al: Development and the fragmented self: longitudinal study of dissociative symptomatology in a nonclinical sample. Dev Psychopathol 9:855–879, 1997

Ozer EJ, Best SR, Lipsey TL, et al: Predictors of posttraumatic stress disorder and symptoms in adults: a meta-analysis. Psychol Bull 129:52–73, 2003

Phillips ML, Medford N, Senior C, et al: Depersonalization disorder: thinking without feeling. Psych Res 108:145–160, 2001

Putnam FW: Dissociation as a response to extreme trauma, in The Childhood Antecedents of Multiple Personality. Edited by Kluft RP. Washington, DC, American Psychiatric Press, 1985, pp 65–97

Putnam FW, Helmers K, Horowitz LA, et al: Hypnotizability and dissociativity in sexually abused girls. Child Abuse Negl 19:645–655, 1995

Ray WJ: Dissociation in normal populations, in Handbook of Dissociation: Theoretical, Empirical, and Clinical Perspectives. Edited by Michelson LK, Ray WJ. New York, Plenum, 1996, pp 51–66

Ross CA, Miller SD, Reagor P, et al: Structured interview data on 102 cases of multiple personality disorder from four centers. Am J Psychiatry 147:596–601, 1990

Siegel DJ: Memory, trauma and psychotherapy: a cognitive science review. J Psychother Pract Res 4:93–122, 1995

Sierra M, Senior C, Dalton J, et al: Autonomic response in depersonalization disorder. Arch Gen Psychiatry 59:833–838, 2002

Silva RR, Alpert M, Munoz DM, et al: Stress and vulnerability to posttraumatic stress disorder in children and adolescents. Am J Psychiatry 157:1229–1235, 2000

Simeon D, Hollander E: Dissociative disorders not otherwise specified, in Comprehensive Textbook of Psychiatry, 7th Edition. Edited by Kaplan BJ, Sadock VA. Philadelphia, PA, Lippincott Williams & Wilkins, 2000, pp 1570–1576

Simeon D, Guralnik O, Hazlett E, et al: Feeling unreal: a PET study of depersonalization disorder. Am J Psychiatry 157:1782–1788, 2000

Simeon D, Guralnik O, Knutelska M, et al: Hypothalamic-pituitary-adrenal axis dysregulation in depersonalization disorder. Neuropsychopharmacology 25:793–795, 2001a

Simeon D, Guralnik O, Schmeidler J, et al: The role of childhood interpersonal trauma in depersonalization disorder. Am J Psychiatry 158:1027–1033, 2001b

Simeon D, Guralnik O, Knutelska M, et al: Personality factors associated with dissociation: temperament, defenses, and cognitive schemata. Am J Psychiatry 159:489–491, 2002

Simeon D, Guralnik O, Knutelska M, et al: Basal norepinephrine in depersonalization disorder. Psychiatry Res 121:93–97, 2003a

Simeon D, Knutelska M, Nelson D, et al: Feeling unreal: a depersonalization disorder update of 117 cases. J Clin Psychiatry 64:990–997, 2003b

Simeon D, Knutelska M, Hollander E: HPA axis function in borderline personality disorder as a function of dissociation. Paper presented at the 21st International Fall Conference of the International Society for the Study of Dissociation, New Orleans, LA, November 2004

Simeon D, Greenberg J, Nelson D, et al: Dissociation and posttraumatic stress 1 year after the World Trade Center disaster: follow-up of a longitudinal survey. J Clin Psychiatry 66:231–237, 2005a

Simeon D, Knutelska M, Putnam F, et al: Attention and emotional memory processes in individuals with dissociative disorders. Paper presented at the 22nd International Fall Conference of the International Society for the Study of Dissociation, Toronto, ON, Canada, November 2005b

Simeon D, Knutelska M, Yehuda R, et al: HPA axis function in dissociative disorders versus PTSD. Paper presented at the 21st Annual Meeting of the International Society for Traumatic Stress Studies, Toronto, ON, Canada, November 2005c

Smith MA, Davidson J, Ritchie JC, et al: The corticotrophin-releasing hormone test in patients with posttraumatic stress disorder. Biol Psychiatry 26:349–355, 1989

Southwick SM, Bremner DJ, Rasmusson A, et al: Role of norepinephrine in the pathophysiology and treatment of posttraumatic stress disorder. Biol Psychiatry 46:1192–1204, 1999

Spiegel D: Multiple personality as a posttraumatic stress disorder. Psychiatr Clin North Am 7:101–110, 1984

Stein MB, Yehuda R, Koverola C, et al: Enhanced dexamethasone suppression of plasma cortisol in adult women traumatized by childhood sexual abuse. Biol Psychiatry 42:680–686, 1997

Sterlini GL, Bryant RA: Hyperarousal and dissociation: a study of novice skydivers. Behav Res Ther 40:431–437, 2002

Tampke AK, Irwin HJ: Dissociative processes and symptoms of posttraumatic stress in Vietnam veterans. J Trauma Stress 12:725–738, 1999

Tellegen A, Lykken DT, Bouchard TJ, et al: Personality similarity in twins reared apart and together. J Pers Soc Psychol 54:1031–1039, 1988

van der Hart O, Nijenhuis E: Generalized dissociative amnesia: episodic, semantic, and procedural memories lost and found. Aust NZ J Psychiatry 35:589–600, 2001

van der Hart O, Nijenhuis E, Steele K, et al: Trauma-related dissociation: conceptual clarity lost and found. Aust NZ J Psychiatry 38:906–914, 2004

van der Kolk B, Pelcovitz D, Roth S, et al: Dissociation, somatization, and affect dysregulation: the complexity of adaptation to trauma. Am J Psychiatry 153:83–93, 1996

van IJzendoorn MH, Schuengel C: The measurement of dissociation in normal and clinical populations: meta-analytic validation of the Dissociative Experiences Scale (DES). Clin Psychol Rev 16:365–382, 1996

Vermetten E, Schmahl C, Wilson K, et al: Neurobiological correlates of DID in comparison with PTSD and BPD. Presented at the 19th Annual Meeting of the International Society for Traumatic Stress Studies, Chicago, IL, October 2003

Waldo TG, Merritt RD: Fantasy proneness, dissociation, and DSM-IV Axis II symptomatology. J Abnorm Psychol 109:555–558, 2000

Waller NG, Ross CA: The prevalence and biometric structure of pathological dissociation in the general population: taxometric and behavior genetic findings. J Abnorm Psychol 106:499–510, 1997

Waller NG, Putnam FW, Carlson EB: Types of dissociation and dissociative types: a taxometric analysis of dissociative experiences. Psychol Methods 1:300–321, 1996

Warshaw MG, Fierman E, Pratt L, et al: Quality of life and dissociation in anxiety disorder patients with histories of trauma or PTSD. Am J Psychiatry 150:1512–1516, 1993

Yehuda R: Sensitization of the hypothalamic-pituitary-adrenal axis in posttraumatic stress disorder. Ann NY Acad Sci 821:57–75, 1997

Yehuda R, Southwick SM, Nussbaum G, et al: Low urinary cortisol excretion in patients with posttraumatic stress disorder. J Nerv Ment Dis 178:366–369, 1990

Yehuda R, Lowy MT, Southwick SM, et al: Increased lymphocyte glucocorticoid receptor number in PTSD. Am J Psychiatry 149:499–504, 1991

Yehuda R, Southwick SM, Krystal JM, et al: Enhanced suppression of cortisol following dexamethasone administration in posttraumatic stress disorder. Am J Psychiatry 150:83–86, 1993

Yehuda R, Keefe RSE, Harvey PD, et al: Learning and memory in combat veterans with PTSD. Am J Psychiatry 152:137–139, 1995

Yehuda R, Levengood RA, Schmeidler J, et al: Increased pituitary activation following metyrapone administration in post-traumatic stress disorder. Psychoneuroendocrinology 21:1–16, 1996

Yehuda R, Schmeidler J, Siever LJ, et al: Individual differences in posttraumatic stress disorder symptom profiles in Holocaust survivors in concentration camps or in hiding. J Trauma Stress 10:453–463, 1997

Young EA, Breslau N: Cortisol and catecholamines in posttraumatic stress disorder. Arch Gen Psychiatry 61:34–401, 2004

Zlotnick C, Pearlstein T: Validation of the structured interview for disorders of extreme stress. Compr Psychiatry 38:243–247, 1997

C H A P T E R   5

PERCEPTUAL PROCESSING AND TRAUMATIC STRESS

Contributions From Hypnosis

ERIC VERMETTEN, M.D., PH.D.
DAVID SPIEGEL, M.D.

Trauma and a constitutional disposition to dissociate seem to be etiological contributors to dissociative disorders, together with a failure of working through traumatic memories and restorative soothing. Hypnosis is thought of as controlled dissociation and dissociation in turn as a form of spontaneous self-hypnosis The clinical notion that "parts of the body that previously experienced physical disease of trauma seem to be especially vulnerable to reactivation of that response with hypnosis" (D.S. Spiegel and Vermetten 1994, p. 202) requires identification of underlying mechanisms that can subsequently be integrated into a broader neurobiology knowledge base. Reciprocally, when these mechanisms are compatible with mainstream explanatory neurobiological circuits and systems, they may contribute to a shift in the body of established medical theory by emphasizing previously neglected factors (Rainville and Price 2004). This chapter briefly discusses contributions and challenges from the field of hypnosis as applicable to the study of traumatic dissociation.

HYPNOTIC RESPONSES IN TRAUMATIC STRESS SITUATIONS

It is well known that traumatic stress can mobilize responses that have hypnotic features, such that one's perception of one's body and of the environment is changed. These can be seen in a variety of situations, for example, the famous case report of Oliver Sacks when he breaks his leg, and his brain is "losing it" (Sacks 1984); in journalists watching an execution as an eyewitness (dissociation; Freinkel et al. 1994); in survivors of the Estonia ferry disaster who attempted to rescue other survivors in ice-cold water (numbing, in more than one sense; Eriksson and Lundin 1996); in people who witnessed the collapse of the World Trade Center on September 11, 2001 (verbal inhibition) or watched people jump from the building (visual distortions, e.g., "watching pigeons flying out of the tower"); the responses in orphaned Ruwandan children (stupor) or the survivors of the tsunami in Southeast Asia (dissociation, e.g., "feeling as though things were happening in slow motion"); and battered and abused children who create invisible identities so as not to feel the pain and humiliation (analgesia, time distortion, identity alteration, amnesia). Traumatic experiences can mobilize responses that resemble hypnotic phenomenology, a state during which intense absorption in the hypnotic focal experience (Tellegen and Atkinson 1974) can be achieved by means of a dissociation of other aspects of experience (E.R. Hilgard 1977; D. Spiegel et al. 1988; Vermetten and Bremner 2004).

MIND-BODY RELATIONSHIPS AND TRAUMA

Research in previous decades has provided considerable evidence for the importance of suggestion and hypnotic ability in the healing or amelioration of various somatic disorders (e.g., Bowers and Kelly 1979; D.S. Spiegel and Vermetten 1994). The phenomena of hypnotic influence are challenging and require a specific orientation to mind-body relations. Both hypnosis and dissociation could well be viewed as vehicles for altered control over neurophysiological and peripheral somatic functions. Several studies have suggested that highly hypnotizable individuals and those with dissociative symptoms are capable of an unusual degree of psychological control over various somatic functions or, conversely, demonstrate a loss of control over those functions. There seems an intensified relationship with the body in both extremes of highly hypnotizable persons and those with low hypnotizability, the former through a tendency to become intensely absorbed in noxious sensations and to develop dissociative or somatoform disorders, and the latter through an inability to block out noxious sensations with normal levels of concentration and absorption (Kirmayer et al. 1994). Individuals with low hypnotizability may be more prone to react with cognitions of control rather than cognitions of loss of control. These individuals may have a lack of words for feelings (Frankel et al. 1977); although their threat perception being relatively absent from verbal report or consciousness, it is present in measures of sympathetic activation or motor behavior. They "know the words but miss the music." Highly hypnotizable persons may spontaneously enter the hypnotic mode of information processing and experience "involuntary" changes in perception, memory, and mood that can amplify perception of fear and pain. They are prone to *surplus pattern recognition* or seeing meaning in events that seem randomly distributed or meaningless to persons with low hypnotizability, and they are at risk for threat-related disorders because they are prone to *surplus empathy*, involuntarily absorbing the pain or negative affect of others.

These notions relate to the long-standing clinical impression of an association between conversion, hysteria, and high hypnotizability (Brown 2004). It may take less severe stress or trauma to trigger a conversion symptom or other dissociative symptom in individuals who are highly hypnotizable. Highly hypnotizable individuals seem to be vulnerable to conversion symptoms or conversion disorder, suggesting that hypnotic states may be mobilized spontaneously or produce pseudosomatic conversion symptoms (Bliss 1984; Nemiah 1993). For example, in a review of special characteristics, Wilson and Barber (1981, 1983) observed that 60% of their study sample of high hypnotizable subjects had experienced pseudocyesis, with symptoms that included amenorrhea, breast changes, and abdominal enlargement. These subjects also experienced dramatic physical symptoms stimulated by stress. Patients with posttraumatic stress disorder (PTSD) show similar dissociative symptoms to dissociative disorder patients (Bremner et al. 1992; Hyer et al. 1993). Earlier findings have reported higher hypnotizability in patients with PTSD compared with patients with generalized anxiety disorder (D. Spiegel et al. 1988).

HYPNOSIS REVISITED

Hypnosis represents the first Western conception of a psychotherapy (Ellenberger 1970). Traditionally, hypnosis has a strong relation to suggestibility, and treatments using hypnosis have been regarded as especially applicable in cases of hysterical and neurotic complaints. Moreover, there is a long tradition of employing hypnotic capacity in the treatment of the hysterical and dissociative "psychoses" (see e.g., Kihlstrom 1994; D. Spiegel and Fink 1979). Early in the twentieth century (e.g., through the work of the Dutch psychiatrist Breukink) it was reported that hysterical psychoses were 1) trauma induced, 2) curable, and 3) most amendable to psychotherapy using hypnosis. Hypnosis was used for symptom-oriented therapy as both a comfortable and supportive mental state and for the uncovering and integrating of traumatic memories (van der Hart and Spiegel 1993).

Hypnosis has also been described as "artificial hysteria" (Bliss 1984). Ever since its discovery, hysteria has been linked with forgotten early traumas that were thought to be responsible for the symptoms. Information for which the individual was apparently amnesic could, at times, be revealed using hypnotic techniques such as age regression, although others have raised concerns that the information is more a response to suggestion than veridical recall. Now that hysteria as a diagnostic category has gone out of fashion, disorders that earlier would have been labeled hysterical are divided by DSM-IV-TR (American Psychiatric Association 2000) into, or among, a number of different categories: acute stress disorder, PTSD, somatoform disorder, conversion disorder, and dissociative disorder. In modern times, the explanations for these disorders has relied on different factors than those explaining and describing hysteria, although the psychodynamic explanation of the symptoms may well still be the same.

Hypnosis may be best described as consisting of three factors: absorption, dissociation, and automaticity/suggestibility (D. Spiegel 1990). Emphasis can be given to any one of the three factors, although no factor can explain the concept completely. Several attempts have been made to emphasize the different roles of these factors in their explanation of hypnotic responses. Lively debates about state and nonstate issues regarding hypnosis and hypnotic susceptibility or hypnotizability have ensued (Barber and Wilson 1977; Coe 1973; Orne 1977). In these discussions the controversy was not so much about the reality of the responses observed but whether the state was an explanation in itself or needed explanation.

THE HYPNOTIC DISPOSITION

A central theme in trauma-related psychopathology is that physical, emotional, or sexual trauma can play a major role in a shift of the dispositional control function of hypnosis manifesting psychological dysfunctions and/ or bodily or somatic problems (Kihlstrom et al. 1989; van der Kolk et al. 1996). This shift can be viewed as a disembodied process, with an emphasis on the information processing analysis of attention mechanisms, and also as a state of engagement of the body-self in the interaction with an object of consciousness, with emphasis on the biological substrate for the representation of self (Damasio 1999) and the property of selfhood (Metzinger 2003).

Hypnotizability has been described as the fundamental capacity to experience dissociation in a structured setting. It underlies the ability to enter trance and involves the ability to segregate and idiosyncratically encode experience into separate psychological or psychobiological structures (Janet 1898). Like dissociation, hypnotizability can be related to a lack of agency or control or loss of control over psychological and sometimes also physical functions. *Dissociation* is a dispositional term that points to its manifestation under certain circumstances, for example, hypnotic induction or traumatic stress. The critical alteration in these processes occurs in what Damasio (1999) called "feeling of knowing" (p. 82), which is a fundamental aspect of self-reflective consciousness that can be separated in hypnosis. Self-representation is a derivative of this fundamental function of consciousness. It is a kind of metaconsciousness that is more likely to be suspended during the intense absorption of the hypnotic state, especially among highly hypnotizable individuals (D. Spiegel 1990; Tellegen and Atkinson 1974). It is thought that in hypnosis, as well as in situations of traumatic stress, these representations can be disrupted or processed in separate (dissociated) streams of information. Self-representation is a hierarchically organized function, with activity in the brain that is necessary (but not sufficient) for higher-order representation of self (e.g., autobiographical self), regulation of cognition and behavior, and other more extended forms of consciousness. From these notions, hypnotic capacity can be considered to be both a liability and an asset: from the perspective of a defense strategy, it serves a protective purpose (e.g., *not* remembering or *not* feeling); however, it can also become maladaptive and lead to dysfunctions (e.g., time gaps, estrangement from inner feelings, flashbacks) and (psycho)pathology such as PTSD and dissociative or other trauma spectrum disorders. After trauma the disposition itself does not change but can be considered to be sensitized.

The symptoms of the dissociative and posttraumatic states have been hypothesized to fit in a diathesis-stress model that views pathological dissociation as originating from an interaction between innate hypnotizability and traumatic experience (Butler et al. 1996). If traumatic experiences involve a hypnotic process or induce a hypnotic state, then we should expect traumatized patients to show higher hypnotizability, in particular while still suffering from their trauma-induced disorder. One would expect these persons to have higher scores on classical hypnotizability scales than other psychiatric patient groups and healthy control subjects. Indeed, there is empirical support that patients with trauma spectrum disorder demonstrate higher scores on classic hypnotic susceptibility scales than other psychiatric patient groups and control subjects (Frischholz et al. 1992; D. Spiegel et al. 1988; Stutman and Bliss 1985). Josephine Hilgard (1970) observed that college students who were higher in measured hypnotizability had early life experiences typified by, on the one hand, "imaginative involvements" with parents and, on the other, a history of punishment unassociated with parental warmth, including physical punishment. Thus although positive identification seemed to lead to higher preserved hypnotizability in young adulthood, hypnosis as mechanism for escaping from an unpleasant childhood environment seemed to be another pathway.

As a result of trauma, attention and arousal systems are altered, rendering the traumatized individual prone to entering hypnotic states, with a relative uncoupling between irrelevant external events and mental (emotional) states during hypnotic episodes. What happens to hypnotic susceptibility after successful treatment in patients with disorders related to trauma is largely unknown. Although Janet observed that recovered patients became less hypnotizable (Janet 1898), this finding still awaits testing in systematic research.

HYPNOTIZABILITY SCALES

The methodology in the measurement of hypnotizability when hypnosis is introduced as a controlled and structured dissociation is a useful means for initiating therapeutic use of hypnosis while providing both therapist and patient with information about the patient's ability and style of response (H. Spiegel and Spiegel 2004). This can help the therapist assess the relative value of hypnosis in treatment and teach the patient how to best utilize his or her ability to control dissociative symptoms. Hypnotizability is described as a measurable concept with long-term personality characteristics, and various scales to measure it have been developed in the past 30 years. Although most research on hypnotizability was done in the 1970s and early 1980s, a new perspective on the relation between hypnosis and dissociation can evolve. Research in the 1980s provided a body of literature on correlations between scales, reliability studies, and developments of new scales, but research now focuses more on dissociation and dissociative disorders and their measurement through scales. Correlations between hypnotizability and dissociative symptoms are quite high (see Butler et al. 1996; Carlson and Putman 1989; Frischholz et al. 1992; D. Spiegel et al. 1988). This may have to do in part with control, with hypnotizability representing the mobilization of dissociated states under precise control, and dissociative symptoms occurring in an unbidden manner (Barrett 1992).

Hypnosis may account for many of the findings attributed to dissociation and dissociative disorders; the methodology of the measurements and the expertise built from previous research could serve a valuable purpose.

Different hypnotic susceptibility scales or hypnotizability scales have been developed in which the naming (i.e., susceptibility vs. hypnotizability) favors a conceptual standpoint regarding hypnosis. Hypnotizability is normally distributed in the general population and slowly declines with age (E.R. Hilgard 1965). A great deal of research has shown that hypnotizability is a fairly stable trait over time (E.R. Hilgard 1978–1979; Morgan et al. 1974). Test-retest correlation of 0.70 over periods of 10–25 years has been shown (Piccione et al. 1989). Hypnotizability seems to peak between the ages of 6 and 10 years and then begins a gradual decline until adulthood (Morgan et al. 1974). Approximately 10%–15% of the population are highly susceptible to hypnosis, 10%–15% are unresponsive, and the remaining 70%–80% are moderately susceptible to varying degrees (Perry et al. 1992). For a review of the measurement of hypnotizability see Perry et al. (1992). The following nine scales, in chronological order, can be considered most representative of the field of hypnotizability scales:

1. Stanford Hypnotic Susceptibility Scale forms A, B, and C (Weitzenhoffer and Hilgard 1959, 1962) and the Stanford Hypnotic Clinical Scale for Children (Morgan and Hilgard 1978–1979).
2. Harvard Group Scale of Hypnotic Susceptibility (Shor and Orne 1962)
3. Children's Hypnotic Susceptibility Scale (London 1962)
4. Barber Suggestibility Scale (Barber 1965)
5. Creative Imagination Scale (Wilson and Barber 1983)
6. Hypnotic Induction Profile (H. Spiegel 1977)
7. Carleton University Responsiveness to Suggestion Scale (Spanos et al. 1983).
8. Phenomenology of Consciousness Inventory (Forbes and Pekala 1993)
9. University of Tennessee Hypnotic Susceptibility Scale for the Deaf (Repka and Nash 1995).

EXPERIMENTAL STUDY OF HYPNOTIC RESPONSE PATTERNS

Several imaging studies in healthy populations have demonstrated differences in the neural circuitry that is involved in response patterns across hypnotic states, for example, alterations of pain affect and pain modulation (Faymonville et al. 2003; Rainville et al. 1997); alteration of visual processing (Kosslyn et al. 2000); hypnotic alteration of acoustic perception (Szechtman et al. 1998); and alteration of the Stroop color interference response (MacLeod and Sheehan 2003; Nordby et al. 1999; Raz 2005; Raz et al. 2002, 2003, 2005, 2006; Vermetten and Bremner 2004). Most of these studies have used subjects with high and low hypnotizability to gain insight in the neural mechanisms of perceptual alteration by measuring alteration in regional brain blood flow. From these studies, it appears that highly hypnotizable persons are capable of modifying their brain metabolisms in response to a specific set of instructions to alter affect, pain, or other experiences, and it has been pointed out that subjects can differentially alter (block or stimulate) certain perceptual functions (e.g., "taking the color out of a picture" that is presented in front of them [Kosslyn et al. 2000]. To a considerable extent, highly hypnotizable persons are capable of modifying the circuitry with which their brains process stimuli. Merely changing the words used in an hypnotic analgesia instruction from reducing pain intensity to reducing how much the pain is bothersome moves the locus of reduced cortical activity from somatosensory cortex to the anterior cingulated gyrus (Hofbauer et al. 2001; Rainville et al. 1997, 1999a, 1999b, 2001, 2002). Yet, to date, relatively few studies have used the cumulative power of combining these knowledge-based resources in functional neuroimaging studies in patient populations.

Hypnotic induction can mobilize a wide spectrum of responses, varying from increased anxiety to flashbacks that can occur with or without feelings of detachment. Other dissociative experiences, such as numbing or freezing, feelings of involuntariness, and loss of self-agency, may also be induced in hypnosis. The content of the emotion is also widespread and can change rapidly depending on the focus of attention (e.g., anger, shame, guilt, or disgust). These responses can have bimodal effects, such as enhanced attention versus lowering of attention or out-of-body experiences versus detailed focus on details, and can also be reflected on the level of psychophysiological alteration, for example, increased versus decreased heart rate. Although these may be related to hypnotic virtuosity, this has not been studied yet. Within a general framework of identification, production, and regulation of emotional recall (see Phillips et al. 2003a, 2003b), hypnotic response patterns are related to the involvement of different brain correlates (Lanius et al. 2002; see also Chapter 10 in this volume, "Posttraumatic Stress Disorder Symptom Provocation and Neuroimaging"). We propose that insight into these hypnotic response patterns needs to be taken into account when analyzing brain correlates of traumatic recall in trauma disorders, particularly PTSD but also dissociative identity disorder and borderline personality disorder. Moreover, hypnotic paradigms can provide additional information regarding the involvement of involuntary mechanisms in situations such as traumatic recall. In addition, we feel that by cross-correlating the phenomenology and neurophysiology of dissociation recall and hypnosis, results can be found that improve our understanding of hypnosis and basic elements of consciousness and emotion.

HYPNOSIS, INVOLUNTARINESS, AND THE SENSE OF AGENCY

One can think of the brain as being divided into an anterior effector portion and a posterior receptive portion (i.e., action vs. perception). Episodic memory retrieval commences in the frontal lobes with a search strategy and works its way downward to the hippocampus and posterior toward activation of images in the occipital lobes. This is controlled, desired activity accompanied by a willing sense of agency. By contrast, PTSD seems to move from back to front, with unbidden intrusive images that are experienced as uncontrolled and unwelcome (see Horowitz et al. 1999). Brain imaging in PTSD (Rauch and Shin 1997) shows hyperactivation of hippocampus (memory), amygdala (emotion), and occipital cortex (imagery) and hypoactivation of Broca's area (speech). Thus the deep and posterior portions of the brain are activated while the effector systems, especially speech, are inhibited, adding to the sense of helplessness and involuntariness in PTSD. Such individuals feel they are being retraumatized by their memories.

One would think that agency would be associated with efferent (motor) activity rather than passive perception. Yet it is not uncommon that people engaged in motor performance lack self-awareness (e.g., actors, athletes, people in states of flow [Csikszentmihalyi and Rathunde 1992]). Thus, strangely enough, a sense of agency does not uniformly accompany activity, even voluntary motor activity. One way to resolve this apparent paradox is to conceptualize self-awareness as a perception. Even if agency is best demonstrated by action, it may not be perceived as such if there is some inhibition of perception, for example, if perceptual processing is saturated with intrusive imagery or redirected through hypnotic instruction: the person is told that their hand will feel light and float up, and it seems to do so by itself, without conscious intent (H. Spiegel and Spiegel 2004). Motion can occur in hypnosis without the perception of agency. The well-established ability of hypnosis to alter perception may account for its less-well-understood ability to alter identity, memory, and consciousness (perception of self). Perception of motor activity is complex; it involves expectation of a response to a motor act initiated, hence we cannot tickle ourselves. Thus, hypnotically altering perception has great potential to alter the perception of agency in regard to our own actions, and action without agency can also be the way trauma is experienced.

Another way to think about the evidence is that in hypnosis, systems are affected that both respond to and manipulate perceptions. Typically, we respond to perceptions and manipulate words. In hypnosis, we seem to do the opposite: respond to words and manipulate perceptions. The majority of Stroop studies reviewed earlier indicate that words can be delexicalized by altering perception, but this is done in response to verbal instructions that in some ways do not make sense: the words are in English but they are perceived as unreadable, and Stroop interference decreases (MacLeod and Sheehan 2003; Nordby et al. 1999; Raz 2005; Raz et al. 2002, 2003, 2005, 2006). Relatively illogical instructions to alter perception thus are accepted uncritically, and perception is changed, with resulting alterations in primary association cortex (e.g., Kosslyn et al. 2000) or anterior cingulate gyrus (e.g., Crawford et al. 1993; Rainville et al. 1997). Perception is always a combination of raw sensory input and memory—stored images that facilitate pattern recognition (Kosslyn and Koenig 1992). Thus all perception is part hallucination, and in these hypnotic paradigms we seem to set up a competition between perception and imagination. Thus, analogous to the explication of dreaming as a kind of perceptual processing without the perceptions (Hobson and Stickgold 1995), the hypnotic state could be characterized as a different kind of perceptual processing without perception that results in hypnotic hallucination and alteration of perception, such as analgesia.

HYPNOSIS IN THE TREATMENT OF TRAUMATIC DISSOCIATION

The most distressing thing about a traumatic event is the sense of absolute helplessness that it engenders. It represents a sudden discontinuity of physical experience that is paralleled in dissociative discontinuities in mental experience. The events often seem unreal or dreamlike, and amnesia for components of them can occur (Classen et al. 1998; Freinkel et al. 1994; Koopman et al. 2001; D. Spiegel et al. 1994, 1996). This helplessness is reenacted in both acute stress disorder and PTSD through loss of control over one's state of mind in the aftermath of trauma, characterized by spontaneous dissociative states, startle reactions, or intrusive recollections of the event. Many trauma victims feel they have lost executive control over their minds and even after regaining control of their bodies, they experience nightmares, flashbacks, and intrusive memories. The process of the therapy, especially when employing a technique such as hypnosis, must be structured so that it enhances patients' sense of control. In this way the very hypnotic/dissociative mechanism that seems to induce a repetition of helplessness can be utilized to enhance control over traumatic memories and somatic responses. This approach can allow patients to integrate the image of themselves as victims with an ongoing image of themselves as coping effectively with severe stress, making the repressed material conscious and therefore less powerful and alien. The psychotherapy of PTSD contains elements of desensitization, in which reexposure to the traumatic stimulus may gradually deprive it of some of its emotional power. Indeed, the use of hypnosis in the psychotherapy of trauma was initially thought to be limited to abreaction, based on Freud's cathartic method (Breuer and Freud 1895). The idea was that some intense affect associated with the traumatic event needed to be released and that simple repetition of the memory of the event with its associated emotion in the trance state would discharge the energy producing the symptoms. However, it became clear to Freud that conscious, cognitive work must be done on the material for it to be successfully worked through and deprived of its symptomatic intrusion. Indeed, it is now clear that cognitive restructuring of the meaning of the traumatic event, coupled with a continued sense of being cared about by the therapist, enhances the effect of hypnosis in psychotherapy (H. Spiegel and Spiegel 2004).

Hypnosis can be used to provide controlled access to the dissociated or repressed memories of the traumatic experience and then to help patients restructure their memories of the events. The unusual characteristics of the hypnotic state provide reassurance that the distress associated with the traumatic memories can to some extent be put aside when the hypnotic state is ended. Also, the dissociation typical of hypnosis can be used to separate psychological from somatic distress. Patients can then find a condensation image that symbolizes some aspect of the trauma. It is often helpful to have them do this on an imaginary screen, giving them some sense of distance from the event. It is also useful to divide the screen in half, having the patient picture on one side of the screen some aspect of the event (e.g., a rape victim's image of the assailant) and on the other side some self-protective action (e.g., struggling with the assailant, talking with him, running away). This lets the patient restructure his or her view of the event, facing it, but not simply in the familiar terms of the humiliation, pain, and fear with which it was initially associated. Victims can better acknowledge their helplessness when they also recognize their efforts to protect themselves. Bereaved individuals can picture themselves at the graveside on one side of the screen and at an earlier moment of joy with the deceased on the other side. They can then be taught to practice a self-hypnosis exercise in

which they grieve and work through traumatic memories while enhancing their sense of control over the process.

CONCLUSION

The research reviewed here demonstrates that hypnotic phenomena
have many analogies to posttraumatic and dissociative phenomena.
The sudden discontinuity of experience that occurs with trauma can be
reflected in the discontinuities of experience in hypnosis: absorption,
dissociation, and suggestibility. The ability to alter perception in hypnosis can affect the sense of agency, which is disrupted as well (but with far
less control) during traumatic experience. It thus makes sense that controlled dissociation using hypnosis can be (and has been for more than a
century) a useful tool in treating the aftermath of traumatic experience,
including traumatic dissociation.

REFERENCES

American Psychatric Association: Diagnostic and Statistical Manual of Mental
    Disorders, 4th Edition, Text Revision. Washington, DC, American Psychiat-
    ric Association, 2000
Barber TX: Measuring "hypnotic like" suggestibility with and without "hypnotic
    induction": psychometric properties, norms, and variables influencing re-
    sponse to the Barber Suggestibility Scale (BSS). Psychol Rep 16:809–844, 1965
Barber TX, Wilson SC: Hypnosis, suggestions, and altered states of consciousness:
    experimental evaluation of the new cognitive-behavioral theory and the tra-
    ditional trance-state theory of "hypnosis." Ann N Y Acad Sci 296:34–47, 1977
Barrett D: Fantasizers and dissociaters: data on two distinct subgroups of deep
    trance subjects. Psychol Rep 71:1011–1014, 1992
Bliss EL: Hysteria and hypnosis. J Nerv Ment Dis 172:203–206, 1984
Bowers KS, Kelly P: Stress, disease, psychotherapy, and hypnosis. J Abnorm
    Psychol 88:490–505, 1979
Bremner JD, Southwick S, Brett E, et al: Dissociation and posttraumatic stress
    disorder in Vietnam combat veterans. Am J Psychiatry 149:328–332, 1992
Breuer J, Freud S: Studien über Hysterie. Leipzig, F. Deuticke, 1895
Brown RJ: Psychological mechanisms of medically unexplained symptoms: an
    integrative conceptual model. Psychol Bull 130:793–812, 2004
Butler LD, Duran RE, Jasiukaitis P, et al: Hypnotizability and traumatic experi-
    ence: a diathesis-stress model of dissociative symptomatology. Am J Psy-
    chiatry 153:42–63, 1996
Carlson E, Putnam FW: Integrating research on dissociation and hypnotizabil-
    ity: are there two pathways to hypnotizability? Dissociation 2:32–38, 1989

Classen C, Koopman C, Hales R, et al: Acute stress disorder as a predictor of posttraumatic stress symptoms. Am J Psychiatry 155:620–624, 1998

Coe WC: Experimental designs and the state-nonstate issue in hypnosis. Am J Clin Hypn 16:118–128, 1973

Crawford HJ, Gur RC, Skolnick B, et al: Effects of hypnosis on regional cerebral blood flow during ischemic pain with and without suggested hypnotic analgesia. Int J Psychophysiol 15:181–195, 1993

Csikszentmihalyi M, Rathunde K: The measurement of flow in everyday life: toward a theory of emergent motivation. Nebr Symp Motiv 40:57–97, 1992

Damasio AR: How the brain creates the mind. Sci Am 281:112–117, 1999

Ellenberger HF: The Discovery of the Unconscious. New York, Basic Books, 1970

Eriksson NG, Lundin T: Early traumatic stress reactions among Swedish survivors of the m/s Estonia disaster. Br J Psychiatry 169:713–716, 1996

Faymonville ME, Roediger L, Del Fiore G, et al: Increased cerebral functional connectivity underlying the antinociceptive effects of hypnosis. Brain Res Cogn Brain Res 17:255–262, 2003

Forbes EJ, Pekala RJ: Predicting hypnotic susceptibility via a phenomenological approach. Psychol Rep 73:1251–1256, 1993

Frankel FH, Apfel-Savitz R, Nemiah JC, et al: The relationship between hypnotizability and alexithymia. Psychother Psychosom 28:172–178, 1977

Freinkel A, Koopman C, Spiegel D: Dissociative symptoms in media eyewitnesses of an execution. Am J Psychiatry 151:1335–1339, 1994

Frischholz EJ, Lipman LS, Braun BG, et al: Psychopathology, hypnotizability, and dissociation. Am J Psychiatry 149:1521–1525, 1992

Hilgard ER: Hypnotic Susceptibility. New York, Harcourt, Brace & World, 1965

Hilgard ER: Divided Consciousness: Multiple Controls in Human Thought and Action. New York, Wiley, 1977

Hilgard ER: The Stanford Hypnotic Susceptibility Scales as related to other measures of hypnotic responsiveness. Am J Clin Hypn 21:68–83, 1978–1979

Hilgard J: Personality and Hypnosis: A Study of Imaginative Involvement. Chicago, IL, University of Chicago Press, 1970

Hobson JA, Stickgold R: Sleep. Sleep the beloved teacher? Curr Biol 5:35–36, 1995

Hofbauer RK, Rainville P, Duncan GH, et al: Cortical representation of the sensory dimension of pain. J Neurophysiol 86:402–411, 2001

Horowitz MJ, Wilner N, Kaltreider N, et al: Signs and symptoms of posttraumatic stress disorder, in Essential Papers on Posttraumatic Stress Disorder, Edited by Horowitz ML. New York, New York University Press, 1999, pp 22–41

Hyer LA, Albrecht JW, Boudewyns PA, et al: Dissociative experiences of Vietnam veterans with chronic posttraumatic stress disorder. Psychol Rep 73:519–530, 1993

Janet P: Névroses et Idées Fixes, Vol. 1. Paris, Félix Alcan, 1898

Kihlstrom JF: One hundred years of hysteria, in Dissociation: Clinical and Theoretical Perspectives. Edited by Lynn SJ and Rhue JW. New York, Guilford, 1994, pp 365–394

Kihlstrom JF, Register PA, Hoyt IP, et al: Dispositional correlates of hypnosis: a phenomenological approach. Int J Clin Exp Hypn 37:249–263, 1989

Kirmayer LJ, Robbins JM, Paris J: Somatoform disorders: personality and the social matrix of somatic distress. J Abnorm Psychol 103:125–136, 1994

Koopman C, Drescher K, Bowles S et al: Acute dissociative reactions in veterans with PTSD. J Trauma Stress 2:91–111, 2001

Kosslyn SM, Koenig O: Wet Mind: The New Cognitive Neuroscience. New York, Free Press, 1992

Kosslyn SM, Thompson WL, Costantini-Ferrando MF, et al: Hypnotic visual illusion alters color processing in the brain. Am J Psychiatry 157:1279–1284, 2000

Lanius RA, Williamson PC, Boksman K, et al: Brain activation during script-driven imagery induced dissociative responses in PTSD: a functional magnetic resonance imaging investigation. Biol Psychiatry 52:305–311, 2002

London P: The Children's Hypnotic Susceptibility Scale. Mountain View, CA, Consulting Psychologists Press, 1962

MacLeod CM, Sheehan PW: Hypnotic control of attention in the Stroop task: a historical footnote. Conscious Cogn 12:347–353, 2003

Metzinger T: Being No One: The Self-Model Theory of Subjectivity. Cambridge, MA, MIT Press, 2003

Morgan AH, Hilgard JR: The Stanford Hypnotic Clinical Scale for Children. Am J Clin Hypn 21:148–155, 1978–1979

Morgan AH, Johnson DL, Hilgard ER: The stability of hypnotic susceptibility: a longitudinal study. Int J Clin Exp Hypn 22:249–257, 1974

Nemiah JC: Dissociation, conversion and somatization, in Dissociative Disorders: A Clinical Review. Edited by Spiegel DS. Lutherville, MD, Sidran Press, 1993, pp 104–117

Nordby H, Hugdahl K, Jasiukaitis P, et al: Effects of hypnotizability on performance of a Stroop task and event-related potentials. Percept Mot Skills 88:819–830, 1999

Orne MT: The construct of hypnosis: implications of the definition for research and practice. Ann NY Acad Sci 296:14–33, 1977

Perry C, Nadon R, Button J: The measurement of hypnotic ability, in Contemporary Hypnosis Research. Edited by Fromm E, Nash MR. New York, Guilford, 1992, pp 459–491

Phillips ML, Drevets WC, Rauch SL, et al: Neurobiology of emotion perception, I: the neural basis of normal emotion perception. Biol Psychiatry 54:504–514, 2003a

Phillips ML, Drevets WC, Rauch SL, et al: Neurobiology of emotion perception, II: implications for major psychiatric disorders. Biol Psychiatry 54:515–528, 2003b

Piccione C, Hilgard ER, Zimbardo PG: On the degree of stability of measured hypnotizability over a 25-year period. J Pers Soc Psychol 56:289–295, 1989

Rainville P, Price DD: The neurophenomenology of hypnosis and hypnotic analgesia, in Psychological Methods of Pain Control: Basic Science and Clinical Perspectives. Progress in Pain Research and Management. Edited by Price DD, Bushnell MC. Seattle, WA, IASP Press, 2004, pp 235–267

Rainville P, Duncan GH, Price DD, et al: Pain affect encoded in human anterior cingulate but not somatosensory cortex. Science 277:968–971, 1997

Rainville P, Carrier B, Hofbauer RK, et al: Dissociation of sensory and affective dimensions of pain using hypnotic modulation. Pain 82:159–171, 1999a

Rainville P, Hofbauer RK, Paus T, et al: Cerebral mechanisms of hypnotic induction and suggestion. J Cogn Neurosci 11:110–125, 1999b

Rainville P, Bushnell MC, Duncan GH: Representation of acute and persistent pain in the human CNS: potential implications for chemical intolerance. Ann NY Acad Sci 933:130–141, 2001

Rainville P, Hofbauer RK, Bushnell MC, et al: Hypnosis modulates activity in brain structures involved in the regulation of consciousness. J Cogn Neurosci 14:887–901, 2002

Rauch SL, Shin LM: Functional neuroimaging studies in posttraumatic stress disorder. Ann NY Acad Sci 821:83–98, 1997

Raz A: Attention and hypnosis: neural substrates and genetic associations of two converging processes. Int J Clin Exp Hypn 53:237–258, 2005

Raz A, Shapiro T, Fan J, et al: Hypnotic suggestion and the modulation of Stroop interference. Arch Gen Psychiatry 59:1155–1161, 2002

Raz A, Landzberg KS, Schweizer HR, et al: Posthypnotic suggestion and the modulation of Stroop interference under cycloplegia. Conscious Cogn 12:332–346, 2003

Raz A, Fan J, Posner MI: Hypnotic suggestion reduces conflict in the human brain. Proc Natl Acad Sci USA 102:9978–9983, 2005

Raz A, Kirsch I, Pollard J, et al: Suggestion reduces the Stroop effect. Psychol Sci 17:91–95, 2006

Repka RJ, Nash MR: Hypnotic responsivity of the deaf: the development of the University of Tennessee Hypnotic Susceptibility Scale for the Deaf. Int J Clin Exp Hypn 43:316–331, 1995

Sacks O: A Leg to Stand On. London, Duckworth, 1984

Shor RE, Orne EC: Harvard Group Scale of Hypnotic Susceptibility. Palo Alto, CA, Consulting Psychologists Press, 1962

Spanos NP, Radtke HL, Hodgins DC, et al: The Carleton University Responsiveness to Suggestion Scale: normative data and psychometric properties. Psychol Rep 53:523–535, 1983

Spiegel D: Hypnosis, dissociation and trauma: hidden and overt observers, in Repression and Dissociation. Edited by Singer JL. Chicago, IL, University of Chicago Press, 1990, pp 121–142

Spiegel D, Fink R: Hysterical psychosis and hypnotizability. Am J Psychiatry 136:777–781, 1979

Spiegel DS, Vermetten E: Physiological correlates of hypnosis and dissociation, in Dissociation, Culture, Mind and Body. Edited by Spiegel DS. Washington, DC, American Psychiatric Press, 1994, pp 185–211

Spiegel D, Hunt T, Dondershine HE: Dissociation and hypnotizability in posttraumatic stress disorder. Am J Psychiatry 145:301–305, 1988

Spiegel D, Koopman C, Classen C: Acute stress disorder and dissociation. Australian Journal of Clinical and Experimental Hypnosis 22:11–23, 1994

Spiegel D, Koopman C, Cardeña E, et al: Dissociative symptoms in the diagnosis of acute stress disorder, in Handbook of Dissociation: Theoretical, Empirical, and Clinical Perspectives. Edited by Michelson KL, Ray JW. New York, Plenum, 1996, pp 367–380

Spiegel H: The Hypnotic Induction Profile (HIP): a review of its development. Ann NY Acad Sci 296:129–142, 1977

Spiegel H, Spiegel D: Trance and Treatment: Clinical Uses of Hypnosis. Washington, DC, American Psychiatric Publishing, 2004

Stutman RK, Bliss EL: Posttraumatic stress disorder, hypnotizability, and imagery. Am J Psychiatry 142:741–743, 1985

Szechtman H, Woody E, Bowers KS, et al: Where the imaginal appears real: a positron emission tomography study of auditory hallucinations. Proc Natl Acad Sci USA 95:1956–1960, 1998

Tellegen A, Atkinson G: Openness to absorbing and self-altering experiences ("absorption"), a trait related to hypnotic susceptibility. J Abnorm Psychol 83:268–277, 1974

van der Hart O, Spiegel D: Hypnotic assessment and treatment of trauma-induced psychoses: the early psychotherapy of H. Breukink and modern views. Int J Clin Exp Hypn 41:191–209, 1993

van der Kolk BA, Pelcovitz D, Roth S, et al: Dissociation, somatization, and affect dysregulation: the complexity of adaptation of trauma. Am J Psychiatry 153:83–93, 1996

Vermetten E, Bremner JD: Functional brain imaging and the induction of traumatic recall: a cross-correlational review between neuroimaging and hypnosis. Int J Clin Exp Hypn 52:280–312, 2004

Weitzenhoffer AM, Hilgard ER: Stanford Hypnotic Susceptibility Scale: Forms A and B. Palo Alto, CA, Consulting Psychologists Press, 1959

Weitzenhoffer AM, Hilgard ER: Stanford Hypnotic Susceptibility Scale: Form C. Palo Alto, CA, Consulting Psychologists Press, 1962

Wilson SC, Barber TX: Vivid fantasy and hallucinatory abilities in the life histories of excellent hypnotic subjects ("somnambules"): preliminary report with female subjects, in Imagery, Vol. 2: Concepts, Results and Applications. Edited by Klinger E. New York, Plenum, 1981, pp 133–149

Wilson SC, Barber TX: The fantasy prone personality: implication for understanding imagery, hypnosis, and parapsychological phenomena, in Imagery: Current Theory, Research and Application. Edited by Sheikh AA. New York, Wiley, pp 340–387, 1983

Part II

NEUROBIOLOGY OF TRAUMA
AND DISSOCIATION

CHAPTER 6

TRANSLATIONAL RESEARCH ISSUES IN DISSOCIATION

CHRISTIAN SCHMAHL, M.D.
MARTIN BOHUS, M.D.

The large field encompassed by brain science is currently undergoing an era of unpredicted developments. This applies not only to basic science, such as molecular and quantitative genetics, neurochemistry, and neurophysiology, but also to the fields of neuroimaging and experimental neuropsychology. With the fascinating progress in these research areas, the opportunity emerges to develop psychopathological concepts that are based on translations of knowledge from basic science rather than on pure clinical observation or hypothetical constructs. An example of this process is the use of D-cycloserine, a partial N-methyl-D-aspartate (NMDA) agonist, to facilitate extinction processes in humans (Ledgerwood et al. 2005). Here, several translational steps were made from cellular research to animal research before a potential treatment for anxiety disorders in humans finally was developed. In most other specialties of medicine it is obvious that clinical and laboratory scientists cooperate to solve major problems. However, in the field of neurobehavioral science, translational approaches are only beginning.

In this chapter, we first give an overview of the translational research steps required to study dissociation. These comprise operationalizing dissociation and developing a standardized induction of dissociative states in human and animal research. We then propose a translational research program for future investigation of dissociation. Finally, we describe general prerequisites and basic strategies of translational processes in neurobehavioral research.

OPERATIONALIZING DISSOCIATION

It took a long time to achieve the first step in a translational research process for dissociation: the definition of a distinct, highly consistent, and
measurable phenomenon. Now, several different ways of operationalizing dissociation exist. The term *dissociation* was developed concurrently
with the emergence of the concept of *hysteria* at the turn of the nineteenth
century (see Nemiah 1998). As outlined in Chapter 1, "Relationship Between Trauma and Dissociation," Pierre Janet (1907) described dissociation as "an inability of the personal self to bind together the various
mental components in an integrated whole under its control" (p. 23).
These components could be conceptualized as consisting of somatic (e.g.,
pain perception) as well as psychological (e.g., amnesia) representations.
In contrast, Freud and Breuer (1895/1977) came to consider dissociative
phenomena a result of active repression (e.g., repression of traumatic
memories) and introduced the concept of *defense hysteria*. This psychoanalytic understanding does not contribute much to an understanding of
true translational approaches, because it is clearly restricted to humans.

There are currently two models of nosological classification of dissociation: the dimensional and the categorical. The *dimensional model* describes
a continuum that ranges from mild experiences (e.g., nonreflective driving) that are relatively normative to more severe forms of dissociation,
such as amnesia. On the other hand, the *categorical model* divides the population into subjects who have pathological dissociative symptoms and
those who do not. A categorical model also underlies the current DSM-IV
(American Psychiatric Association 1994) and DSM-IV-TR (American Psychiatric Association 2000) conceptualization of dissociative disorders, and
this spectrum ranges from less severe conditions (e.g., depersonalization
disorder [DPD]) to the most extreme form of pathological dissociation as
represented by dissociative identity disorder (DID). Evidence for both dimensional and categorical models can be found, with nonpathological
dissociation (e.g., absorption) distributed dimensionally and pathological
dissociation (e.g., identity alterations) distributed categorically (Waller et
al. 1996).

A further nosological dichotomy concerns the temporal structure of
dissociation and distinguishes between dissociative *traits* (e.g., in DPD)
and dissociative *states*, which are of shorter duration (e.g., seconds to minutes). Dissociative states are a central feature of borderline personality disorder (BPD) and belong to the DSM-IV-TR diagnostic criteria. On the other
hand, dissociative symptoms are linked to a trauma history (Chu and Dill
1990). Patients with BPD frequently engage in self-injurious behavior,

TABLE 6–1. Dichotomies in dissociation research

• Dissociation as conditioned, biologically determined behavior	Dissociation as defense
• Dimensional dissociation model	Categorical dissociation model
• Dissociative traits	Dissociative states
• Dissociative disorders	Dissociative symptoms

which may function to terminate dissociative states (M. Bohus and Lieb 2001). Dissociative states in these patients comprise alterations of sensory processes (e.g., analgesia) and disturbances of the motor system, such as the phenomenon of tonic immobility, or freezing from an animal research perspective (Schmahl et al. 1999). These sensory and motor disturbances interfere with the coherence of the human sense of space and time and ultimately lead the individual to experience distortions in his or her perception of self (depersonalization) and his or her environment (derealization).

Another dichotomy of dissociation relates to the difference between dissociative *disorders* and dissociative *symptoms*. There exist several instruments for assessing DSM-IV-TR dissociative disorders (dissociative amnesia, dissociative fugue, DID, DPD) and dissociative symptoms. Well-validated measures of DSM-IV dissociative disorders include the Dissociative Disorders Interview Schedule (Ross et al. 1989) and the Structured Clinical Interview for DSM-IV Dissociative Disorders (Steinberg 1994). Trait and state measures of dissociative symptoms include the Dissociative Experiences Scale (Bernstein and Putnam 1986) and the Clinician-Administered Dissociative States Scale (Bremner et al. 1998), respectively (see also Chapter 13 in this volume, "Psychological Assessment of Posttraumatic Dissociation").

In summary, the operationalization of dissociation has been largely achieved. This opens the focus to physiological pathways underlying dissociative features. However, several dichotomies remain (see Table 6–1).

STANDARDIZED INDUCTION OF DISSOCIATIVE STATES IN HUMANS

On an observer-based behavioral level, severe dissociative states seem to be correlated with tonic immobility, often in combination with aphonia, bradycardia, and hypoventilation (M. Bohus and Lieb 2001). Consequently, investigating potential physiological correlates of dissociative states, such as the visceral nervous system, the endocrine system, respiration, movement coordination, and electrodermal activity, is an important enterprise.

Methods that enable us to induce dissociative states under experimental conditions will facilitate these investigations. Otherwise, we would have to depend on pure coincidence. For example, our group found a significant influence of dissociation on physiological reactivity measured by the startle response. Patients with self-reported low dissociative experiences during the experiment revealed enhanced startle responses, whereas patients with high dissociative experiences during the experiment showed reduced responses (Ebner-Priemer et al. 2005). Even if these data could be interpreted to suggest that dissociation is correlated with dampening amygdala reactivity, the fact that such findings can also be interpreted as an unspecific group effect renders this evidence problematic. Thus the development of methods to induce dissociative states has top priority. At least three different categories of induction can be defined: 1) pharmacological induction, 2) electrical stimulation, and 3) psychological induction.

Pharmacological Induction Methods

Several neurotransmitter systems have been implicated in dissociative symptoms, and these findings have been largely derived from studies using pharmacological induction of dissociative states. Tentatively, three classes of neurochemicals are suggested to be involved in the generation of dissociative states: NMDA antagonists, serotonergic hallucinogens, and opioid agonists.

Noncompetitive NMDA antagonists such as phenylcyclidine and ketamine, also known as the *dissociative anesthetic* and as the street drug Special K, produce a derealized and depersonalized state characterized by marked perceptual alterations at subanesthetic doses (Domino et al. 1965; Krystal et al. 1994). NMDA receptors are distributed widely in the cortex, as well as in the hippocampus and the amygdala, and are thought to mediate associative functioning and long-term potentiation of memory processes. Thus it is plausible that diminished NMDA neurotransmission may be related to dissociative states. The dissociative effects of cannabinoids such as marijuana, which consistently have been shown to induce depersonalization, might be mediated by their antagonistic action at NMDA receptors (Feigenbaum et al. 1989). Brain imaging studies stress the importance of the medial prefrontal cortex in the generation of dissociative symptoms. In healthy subjects, severity of tetrahydrocannabinol-induced depersonalization was correlated with blood flow increase in the right frontal cortex and the anterior cingulate (Mathew et al. 1999).

Serotonergic hallucinogens, such as lysergic acid diethylamide, mescaline, psilocybine, and dimethyltryptamine, also produce dissociative symptoms (Freedman 1968; Klee 1963; Simeon 2004). These substances stimulate 5-HT_{1A} and 5-HT_{2C} receptors (Rasmussen et al. 1986; Titeler et al. 1988). Neurochemical challenge studies with the 5-HT_{2C} receptor agonist *m*-chlorophenylpiperazine demonstrated the induction of significantly more depersonalization than placebo (Simeon et al. 1995) as well as the induction of flashbacks and dissociative symptoms in patients with posttraumatic stress disorder (PTSD; Southwick et al. 1991). Vollenweider et al. (1998) found increased metabolism on ^{18}F-fluorodeoxyglucose positron emission tomography in the anterior cingulate, striatum, and thalamus after amphetamine induced depersonalization.

The endogenous opioid system involves three classes of substances: endorphins, enkephalins, and dynorphins. In addition, a recently discovered neuropeptide, orphanin FQ, has anti-opioid properties (Griebel et al. 1999). The endogenous opioid system mediates stress-induced analgesia (Madden et al. 1977), and analgesia in response to combat stimuli in PTSD can be at least partially blocked by the opioid antagonist naloxone (Pitman et al. 1990). Surgical stress in humans is accompanied by β-endorphin release (Cohen et al. 1981; Dubois et al. 1981), and an increase of dynorphin A release was found with hypoxia stress, thus suggesting that not only β-endorphin is involved in the stress response (Chen 1998). Cerebral spinal fluid β-endorphin was found to be low in dissociative patients with eating disorders (Demitrack et al. 1993), and blood levels of noradrenaline, dopamine, and β-endorphin were elevated during trance states (Kawai et al. 2001). There are several conflicting reports showing alterations of endogenous opioid levels in disorders associated with elevated levels of stress, such as PTSD and BPD. Plasma β-endorphin immunoreactivity was low in patients with non-major depression, many of whom met criteria for BPD (Cohen et al. 1984). Also in patients with BPD, Coid et al. (1983) reported raised plasma met-enkephalin levels, whereas Pickar et al. (1982) reported low levels of opioid activity in cerebrospinal fluid. Low plasma levels of opioid activity have also been reported for patients with PTSD (Hoffman et al. 1989; Wolf et al. 1991), and one study reported a negative correlation between β-endorphin activity and intrusive and avoidant symptoms in PTSD (Baker et al. 1997).

The κ opioid receptor agonists ketocyclazocine, MR 2033, and enadoline can induce depersonalization, derealization, and perceptual alterations (Kumor et al. 1986; Pfeiffer et al. 1986; Walsh et al. 2001). Along these lines, opioid receptor antagonists have been reported to reduce dissociation, such as naltrexone in BPD (M. Bohus et al. 1999) and intravenous naloxone in chronic depersonalization (Nuller et al. 2001). In patients with BPD, however, naloxone was not superior to placebo in reducing acute dissociative symptoms (Philipsen et al. 2004).

The role of orphanin FQ in dissociation is unclear, although this substance has demonstrated anxiolytic as well as stress-reducing effects (Griebel et al. 1999; Jenck et al. 1997).

Electrical Stimulation

The evidence for electrical stimulation as a consistent and effective means for inducing dissociation is limited. Penfield and Perot (1963) elicited dreamlike states, memories, and complex experiential phenomena by direct electrical stimulation of structures in the temporal lobe, temporoparietal association areas, hippocampus, and amygdala. However, even if depersonalization is also common in temporal lobe epilepsy with left-sided foci (Devinsky et al. 1989; Sedman and Kenna 1963), the reported symptoms are quite vague, and there is little more than a hint that these areas may be even marginally involved.

Psychological Induction Paradigms

In analogy to the field of research on stress induction paradigms, one should distinguish between objective induction paradigms and subjective, biographically relevant induction paradigms. Because dissociation is usually triggered by biographically relevant aversive stimuli, the latter usually will be the first choice. Until recently, no standardized psychological induction paradigms were available. However, using the method of script-driven imagery with scripts depicting traumatic experiences, Lanius et al. (2002, 2005) induced dissociation in a subgroup of PTSD subjects and measured neuronal correlates of these induced states. Because subjective stimuli are very difficult to compare or assess and dissociation is not an on-off but rather a dimensional phenomenon, a method independent of subjective appraisal of the participant would be required to assess the level of dissociation under experimental conditions. Evoked potentials might be a possible approach. Patients report analgesia, numbness, and increased auditory thresholds during dissociative states, thus evoked sensory potentials might reveal electroencephalographic alterations correlated with the grade of dissociative states.

SYNTHESIS OF INDUCTION METHODS

One of the major fields of translational research in dissociation should compare pharmacological, electrical stimulation, and psychological induction paradigms. Given that the dependent variable, dissociative state, is a consistent entity, all three methods should lead to the same results. The psychological induction is clinically the most relevant and should be used as a positive control variable when searching for adequate pharmacological or electrical induction mechanisms.

Because standardized psychological induction methods are currently limited, one must examine spontaneous dissociative states in patients with a high probability of experiencing dissociative features under experimental conditions. This widespread approach has several intrinsic problems. Most important, and usually underestimated, is the simple clinical observation that psychiatric disorders are never monosymptomatic but rather are generally organized as a bundle of interlacing symptoms, with anxiety, stress, anger, and shame playing important roles either as primary or as secondary symptoms. Thus, any neurobiological finding within a specific group of patients can mean anything as long as it is not proven to be specific for a single symptom entity.

Concerning experiments based on comparisons between patients and healthy control subjects, translational research aims to clarify the specificity of the findings, requiring inclusion of subtype-differentiated controls not only among different patient groups (e.g., dissociative PTSD vs. dissociative borderline) but also among patients with the same diagnosis (e.g., PTSD patients with and without dissociative symptoms).

ANIMAL RESEARCH

In order to bridge the gap between human and animal research concerning dissociative features, one should be sure that the methodological domains are not confused. This means that behavioral manifestations in humans should be compared with behavioral manifestations in animals, physiological investigations in animals should be compared with such in human beings, and so on. An example for this approach is the analogy of freezing behavior in animals and tonic immobility in humans. Because of the problems with incomparability, intrapsychic observations or appraisals are not relevant to this method. In addition, models that switch between different levels of investigation (e.g., the learned helplessness paradigm for depression, which compares intrapsychic experience in humans with observable behavior in animals) are usually not valid and should be cautiously discussed.

The construct of dissociation has been derived from clinical experience as well as research in humans. There is to date no animal model for dissociation. Hence, animal research must rely on human analogues of this phenomenon. Animal research in this domain has two decisive advantages.

First, only in animals are real experimental designs possible in which only one independent variable in an experimental setting can be selectively changed, for example, by using genetically altered (knockout) animals. Second, intraspecies correlation analyses can be conducted on a more sophisticated level. On a neurobiological level, there are several decisive advantages of animal research. One is the higher spatial resolution in neuroanatomy (e.g., in the differentiation of subnuclei of the amygdala or the detection of the periaqueductal gray). A second advantage is the possibility of specific, experimentally derived pharmacological interventions that should throw light on the neurochemical pathways involved in dissociative experience. Thus, the animal model is the primary prerequisite for developing pharmacological interventions within human subjects.

One possible analogue of dissociation in animals can be derived from behavioral research using fear-conditioning paradigms. The *behavior systems approach* views an animal as having a set of several genetically determined, prepackaged behaviors that it uses to solve particular functional problems. If the problem has to be solved immediately, the animal's behavioral repertoire becomes restricted to those genetically hard-wired behaviors. This was outlined by Bolles (1970) in his species-specific defense reaction theory. When an animal is confronted by a natural environmental threat (e.g., a predator) or an artificial one (e.g., an electrical shock), its behavioral repertoire becomes restricted to its species-specific defense reaction. Freeze, fight, and flight are examples of such reactions. The *defensive behavior system* (Fanselow 1994) is organized by the imminence of a predator and can be divided into three stages: pre-encounter, post-encounter, and circa-strike. *Pre-encounter* defensive behaviors comprise reorganization of meal patterns and protective nest maintenance if the animal has to leave a safe nesting area. When the level of fear increases (e.g., because of actual detection of a predator), the *post-encounter* defensive behavior mode becomes active. This mode includes several dimensions (B. Bohus et al. 1996; Cleroux et al. 1985; Fanselow 1994; Mayer and Fanselow 2003; Nijsen et al. 1998; Overton 1993): 1) a motor component (freezing), 2) a sensory component (opiate analgesia), 3) an autonomic component (activity of the sympathetic and parasympathetic nervous system), 4) an endocrinological component (hypothalamic-pituitary-adrenal axis), and 5) an emotional component (anxiety). In the case of physical contact (e.g., by the experience of pain), the animal engages in more active defenses, such as biting and jumping. This is an example of *circa-strike* behavior. Analogies between these types of animal behavior and dissociation in humans have been discussed (Nijenhuis et al. 1998; see Chapter 11 in this volume, "Psychobiology of Traumatization and Trauma-Related Structural Dissociation of the Personality").

TABLE 6–2. Possible animal and human aspects of dissociation

	Animal	Human
Somatic aspects	Freezing	Tonic immobility
	Analgesia	Sensory deficits, including analgesia
	Parallel activation of sympathetic and parasympathetic nervous system	Reduction of respiration
Psychological aspects	Not applicable	Depersonalization Derealization

Translational research has to develop research designs to study these components in parallel with animals and human beings. Because the hypothesis is based on the assumption that dissociation is activated as part of a phylogenetically conservative pattern, there should be mechanisms common to all mammals. Dissociation is a phylogenetically evolved, complex behavioral pattern with species-specific modifications (see Table 6–2). It includes movement inhibition, sensory deficits, and vegetative and psychological aspects. Translational research has to dismantle these different components. For example, on the motor system level, freezing in animals can be compared with tonic immobility in humans. Psychological experience (e.g., depersonalization, derealization) can only be studied in humans and is therefore not valid phenomena for translational investigations.

Critical anatomical structures for post-encounter defensive behavior are the amygdala, the ventral periaqueductal gray, and the hypothalamus (see Figure 6–1). The amygdala has a central relay function for the mediation of post-encounter defensive behavior, with important glutamatergic input from the thalamus to the lateral amygdala (Fanselow 1994). Furthermore, the central amygdala mediates transfer of information about the threat level to the ventral periaqueductal gray, which in turn appears to mediate analgesia and freezing by opioidergic neurotransmission (Fanselow and Gale 2003; LeDoux 1992). Autonomic and endocrinological responses are mediated by connections from the amygdala to the hypothalamus (LeDoux et al. 1988). The exact localization of the emotional component is unclear but can be assumed to rely on amygdala–prefrontal cortex pathways (LeDoux 2002). Circa-strike behavior is mediated by the superior colliculus and the dorsolateral periaqueductal gray, which receives nociceptive input from the spinal cord and the trigeminal nucleus (Blomqvist and Craig 1991). In phylogenetically

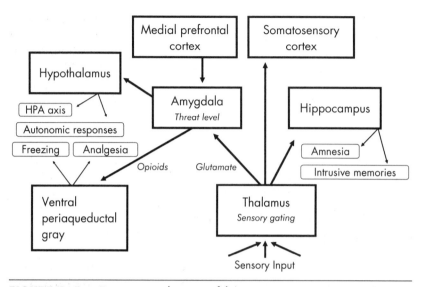

FIGURE 6–1.   Tentative neural circuitry of dissociation.

HPA = hypothalamic-pituitary-adrenal.

more recent species such as humans, these systems can be assumed to be usually controlled by higher cortical regions and to be activated under high levels of stress. It could be hypothesized that dissociation is the representation of the post-encounter defense mode in humans, comprising the same dimensions as described in animals but extended by an emotional-psychological component (depersonalization, derealization, and emotional numbness). In this model, self-destructive behavior, which can be observed frequently during dissociative states (e.g., in patients with BPD), may represent an analogue of the pain-induced switch of behavioral modes from post-encounter to the circa-strike in a human being faced with high levels of aversive stress. In patients with BPD, analgesia under high levels of stress, often in relation to dissociative symptoms, could be demonstrated (M. Bohus et al. 2000; Ludaescher et al., in press). It can be assumed that these patients use painful stimulation as a means to reduce stressful mental states. We recently demonstrated that heat stimulation above pain thresholds in hypoalgesic BPD patients is associated with a deactivation of the amygdala, a region where higher activity usually stands for elevated stress levels (Schmahl et al. 2006).

The development of this dissociative model exemplifies both the advantages and disadvantages of an animal model for mental disturbances. On the one hand, animal models enable the analysis and elucidation of components currently involved on physiological and neuroanatomical levels under experimental conditions. On the other hand, the relevance of these animal models to the human species is always one of analogy, insofar as psychological experience (depersonalization, derealization) cannot be simply made parallel. However, the validity of this analogy can be strengthened on the human level through experimental transfer, as gained, for example, through pharmacological interventions in the animal model.

PROPOSED TRANSLATIONAL RESEARCH PROGRAM FOR THE INVESTIGATION OF DISSOCIATION

Assessment of Psychophysiological Parameters of Dissociative States in Humans

Dissociative states are very frequent in the natural environment of patients with disorders related to stress, such as BPD, DID, and PTSD as well as in other Axis I (e.g., major depression) or Axis II (e.g., histrionic personality disorder) diagnoses. To assess psychophysiological correlates of acute dissociative states in these patient groups, a field study using ambulatory monitoring methods (e.g., assessing activity of the sympathetic and parasympathetic nervous system) could be used, and the results could be utilized to validate experimentally induced dissociative states.

Development of Standardized Methods to Induce Dissociative States

For the investigation of neural correlates of dissociative states it is necessary to induce these states in a safe and controlled way. Thus, the next step of the proposed program is to standardize psychological as well as pharmacological induction methods. For neurobiological research on dissociation to progress, researchers must develop methods to reliably induce and investigate dissociative states in an experimental setting.

Investigation of Neurobiological and Neuropsychological Correlates of Induced Dissociative States

As outlined earlier, there is to date no clear concept of the neurobiology and neurochemistry underlying dissociative states, although a variety of neurochemical, endocrinological, psychophysiological, and neuroimaging studies have been conducted. Using the established methods to induce dissociative states (e.g., pharmacological agents) and validating them by psychophysiological assessment, neurochemical as well as neurofunctional correlates of dissociative features could be directly investigated. These studies aim to determine which neurotransmitter systems and which brain regions are involved in the generation of dissociative states in humans.

Development of an Animal Model of Dissociation

Using shock-induced freezing in mice as an analogue of the human defense behavior system, one could investigate neural and psychophysiological responses in animals. If these responses are shown to be similar in animals and humans, animals may be tested further using experimental pharmacological interventions. In addition, genetically altered animals (e.g., knockout mice) could be studied to further elucidate genetic, neurochemical, and neuroanatomical aspects of dissociation. This would enable the utilization of the higher spatial resolution in neuroanatomy currently available in animal research.

Establishment of Pharmacological and Psychotherapeutic Treatments

To date, no established treatments for dissociative states or disorders are available. Translating findings directly derived from the animal research, new pharmacological treatment options (e.g., opioid antagonists or NMDA agonists) could be developed and evaluated for dissociative symptoms and disorders. In addition to the improvement in therapeutic options for these severely disordered patients, this research may also help to identify the underlying neurochemistry of dissociation.

General prerequisites and basic strategies of translational research in the neurobehavioral sciences underlie the proposals outlined in this chapter, and these are sketched in the following section.

PREREQUISITES AND BASIC STRATEGIES IN TRANSLATIONAL RESEARCH

The first prerequisite in translational research is to identify and differentiate clinically relevant phenotypes, independent of categorical diagnoses. Impulsivity, for example, plays an important role within a subgroup of patients with BPD, as well as in patients with antisocial personality disorder, histrionic personality disorder, and paranoid personality disorder. If we attempt to study the role of serotonergic dysfunctions in BPD using a mixed personality disorder comparison group, valid results would not be expected if we failed to control for concomitant impulsivity within the latter group. In addition, the construct of impulsivity comprises a heterogeneous cluster of lower-order traits. Depue and Lenzenweger (2001) postulated at least five different neurobehavioral systems that might underlie this trait complex: 1) positive, incentive motivation, 2) lack of fear of physical harm, 3) affective aggression, 4) instrumental aggression, and 5) disinhibition of impulse control. Thus, there is growing evidence that impulsivity emerges from the interaction of at least four to five independent neurobehavioral subsystems that should be carefully classified.

The second prerequisite in translational research is to break down the clinically based phenotypes into lower-order traits that can be studied on an experimental level. The next topic to be considered is that most behaviors are both dimensional and multifactorial. In this sense, individual differences and variations are considered normal, and certain psychopathological phenomena are thought to be the quantitative extreme of the normal distribution. This conceptualization has some far-reaching implications for research designs: rather than creating differences between experimental and control groups through manipulation, the individual difference perspective focuses on naturally occurring differences between individuals.

The third prerequisite in translational research is to focus on quantitative aspects rather than qualitative differences in the lower-order traits. As mentioned earlier, most behaviors have multifactorial and polygenic origins. Thus, even when the quantitative differentiation of the clinically defined phenotypes might be successful, studies of the neurobiological underpinnings are hampered by the etiological heterogeneity of psychopathologically defined behavioral alterations. An example is attention-deficit disorder, which can be related to dopaminergic depletion, serotonergic deficit, parasympathetic overdrive, or an interaction of these components. A phenotype always represents observable characteristics that are the joint product of both genotypic and environmental influences. Thus, the phenotypic output of the brain (i.e., behavior), is more than the sum of its parts. It appears reasonable that reduction of degrees of complexity should be a prerequisite to study underlying neurobiological and genetic mechanisms. To reduce complexity and bridge the gap between "the gene and the elusive disease," Gottesman and Gould (2003) suggested the term *endophenotype* or *internal phenotype*, discoverable by biochemical tests or microscopic examination. Endophenotypes should provide a means for identifying the downstream traits or facets of clinical phenotypes as well as the upstream consequences of genes and, in principle, could assist in the identification of aberrant genes in the hypothesized polygenetic systems conferring vulnerability to disorders. As such, they could mark the path between the genotype and the behavior of interest (Gottesman and Gould 2003).

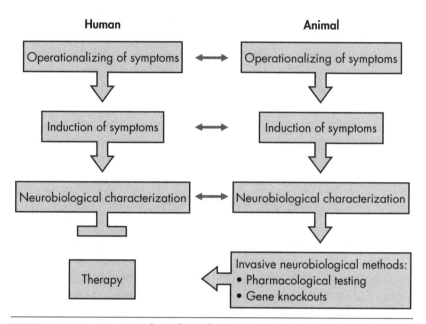

FIGURE 6–2.   Prototypical translational research program.

Once these prerequisites are fulfilled, researchers can begin with a translational research program, which may be conducted in the following way (see Figure 6–2): First, in humans, well-operationalized endophenotypes may be studied if they occur naturally or, if this is too difficult to achieve, they may have to be induced in a standardized and reliable way. Then neurochemical and neuroanatomical correlates of these endophenotypes can be investigated using the whole spectrum of modern neurobiological methods, such as functional neuroimaging. In a parallel fashion, animal analogues of these endophenotypes should also be operationalized, and induction (e.g., pharmacologically) of states resembling human endophenotypes should be accomplished. If neuroanatomical and neurochemical substrates of these states in animals and humans are comparable, then animals may be tested further using novel genetic (e.g., gene knockouts) or more invasive pharmacological methods, which are not possible to conduct in human subjects. The overall goal of such a translational research program is the search for potent pharmacological or psychological interventions to treat severe psychopathological states in humans.

Dissociation research has only started to make inroads into the prerequisites just described, and translational research in dissociation is at its very beginning. Identification of relevant phenotypes in humans can be considered to have been accomplished to a certain degree, and development of induction methods has recently progressed. However, operationalizing dissociation-like animal behavior is still a major stumbling block for further progress in translational research in this field.

CONCLUSION

In a nutshell, translational research processes in the field of dissociation can be summarized as a circular procedure. Initially, the most precise and concise operationalization of the clinical symptoms is achieved on the phenomenological level. This enables the parallel analysis of physiological and neuroanatomical variables, in which one fundamentally strives on this level to arrive at experimental induction methods. This enables the development of animal analogues of human dissociation. On this level, experimental pharmacological and molecular-genetic operations can be conducted. The transfer back ensues through the application of the methods of intervention acquired in the animal model, and an examination of whether the clinical phenomena have been influenced by it.

REFERENCES

American Psychiatric Association: Diagnostic and Statistical Manual of Mental Disorders, 4th Edition. Washington, DC, American Psychiatric Association, 1994

American Psychiatric Association: Diagnostic and Statistical Manual of Mental Disorders, 4th Edition, Text Revision. Washington, DC, American Psychiatric Association, 2000

Baker DG, West SA, Orth DN, et al: Cerebrospinal fluid and plasma β-endorphin in combat veterans with posttraumatic stress disorder. Psychoneuroendocrinology 22:517–529, 1997

Bernstein E, Putnam FW: Development, reliability and validity of a dissociation rating scale. J Nerv Ment Dis 174:727–735, 1986

Blomqvist A, Craig AD: Organization of spinal and trigeminal input to the PAG, in The Midbrain Periaqueductal Grey Matter: Functional, Anatomical and Immunohistochemical Organization. NATO ASI Series A, Vol 213. Edited by Depaulis A, Bandler R. New York, Plenum, 1991, pp 345–363

Bohus M, Lieb K: Zum Verständnis von Selbstverletzung bei Patientinnen mit Borderline-Persönlichkeitsstörungen. Z Allgemeinmed 77:539–547, 2001

Bohus B, Koolhaas JM, Korte SM, et al: Forebrain pathways and their behavioural interactions with neuroendocrine and cardiovascular function in the rat. Clin Exp Pharmacol Physiol 23:177–182, 1996

Bohus M, Landwehrmeyer GB, Stiglmayr CE, et al: Naltrexone in the treatment of dissociative symptoms in patients with borderline personality disorder: an open-label trial. J Clin Psychiatry 60:598–603, 1999

Bohus M, Limberger MF, Ebner-Priemer UW, et al: Pain perception during self-reported distress and calmness in patients with borderline personality disorder and self- mutilating behavior. Psychiatry Res 95:251–260, 2000

Bolles RC: Species-specific defense reactions and avoidance learning. Psychol Rev 77:32–48, 1970

Bremner JD, Krystal JH, Putnam FW, et al: Measurement of dissociative states with the Clinician-Administered Dissociative States Scale (CADSS). J Trauma Stress 11:125–136, 1998

Chen D: Changes of plasma level of neurotensin, somatostatin, and dynorphin A in pilots under acute hypoxia. Mil Med 163:120–121, 1998

Chu JA, Dill DL: Dissociative symptoms in relation to childhood physical and sexual abuse. Am J Psychiatry 147:887–892, 1990

Cleroux J, Peronnet F, De Champlain J: Sympathetic indices during psychological and physical stimuli before and after training. Physiol Behav 35:271–275, 1985

Cohen M, Pickar D, Dubois M, et al: Surgical stress and endorphins. Lancet 1:213–214, 1981

Cohen M, Pickar D, Extein I, et al: Plasma cortisol and β-endorphin immunoreactivity in nonmajor and major depression. Am J Psychiatry 141:628–632, 1984

Coid J, Allolio B, Rees LH: Raised plasma metenkephalin in patients who habitually mutilate themselves. Lancet 2:545–546, 1983

Demitrack MA, Putnam FW, Rubinow DR, et al: Relation of dissociative phenomena to levels of cerebrospinal fluid monoamine metabolites and beta-endorphin in patients with eating disorders: a pilot study. Psychiatry Res 49:1–10, 1993

Depue RA, Lenzenweger MF: A neurobehavioral dimensional model, in Handbook of Personality Disorder. Edited by Livesley JW. New York, Guilford, 2001, pp 136–177

Devinsky O, Putnam F, Grafman J, et al: Dissociative states and epilepsy. Neurology 39:835–840, 1989

Domino EF, Chodoff P, Corssen G: Pharmacologic effects of CI-581, a new dissociative anesthetic in man. Clin Pharmacol Ther 6:279–291, 1965

Dubois M, Pickar D, Cohen MR, et al: Surgical stress in humans is accompanied by an increase in plasma beta-endorphin immunoreactivity. Life Sci 29:1249–1254, 1981

Ebner-Priemer UW, Badeck S, Beckmann C, et al: Affective dysregulation and dissociative experience in female patients with borderline personality disorder: a startle response study. J Psychiatr Res 39:85–92, 2005

Fanselow MS: Neural organization of the defensive behavior system responsible for fear. Psychon Bull Rev 1: 429–438, 1994

Fanselow MS, Gale GD: The amygdala, fear, and memory. Ann NY Acad Sci 985:125–134, 2003

Ludaescher P, Bohus M, Lieb K, et al: Elevated pain thresholds correlate with dissociation and aversive arousal in patients with borderline personality disorder. Psychiatry Res (in press)

Madden J, Akil H, Patrick RL, et al: Stress-induced parallel changes in central opioid levels and pain responsiveness in the rat. Nature 265:358–360, 1977

Mathew RJ, Wilson WH, Chiu NY, et al: Regional cerebral blood flow and depersonalization after tetrahydrocannabinol administration. Acta Psychiatr Scand 100:67–75, 1999

Mayer EA, Fanselow MS: Dissecting the components of the central response to stress. Nat Neurosci 6:1011–1012, 2003

Nemiah JC: Early concepts of trauma, dissociation, and the unconscious: their history and current implications, in Trauma, Memory, and Dissociation. Edited by Bremner JD, Marmar CR. Washington, DC, American Psychiatric Press, 1998, pp 1–26

Nijenhuis ER, Vanderlinden J, Spinhoven P: Animal defense reactions as a model for trauma-induced dissociative reactions. J Trauma Stress 11:243–260, 1998

Nijsen MJMA, Croiset G, Diamant M, et al: Conditioned fear-induced tachycardia in the rat: vagal involvement. Eur J Pharmacol 350:211–222, 1998

Nuller YL, Morozova MG, Kushnir ON, et al: Effect of naloxone therapy on depersonalization. J Psychopharmacol 15:93–95, 2001

Overton JM: Influence of autonomic blockade on cardiovascular responses to exercise in rats. J Appl Physiol 75:155–161, 1993

Penfield W, Perot P: The brain's record of auditory and visual experience: a final summary and discussion. Brain 86:595–696, 1963

Pfeiffer A, Brantl V, Herz A, et al: Psychotomimesis mediated by κ opiate receptors. Science 233:774–776, 1986

Philipsen A, Schmahl C, Lieb K: Naloxone in the treatment of acute dissociative states in female patients with borderline personality disorder. Pharmacopsychiatry 37:196–199, 2004

Pickar D, Cohen MR, Naber D, et al: Clinical studies of the endogenous opioid system. Biol Psychiatry 17:1243–1276, 1982

Pitman RK, van der Kolk BA, Orr SP: Naloxone-reversible analgesic response to combat-related stimuli in posttraumatic stress disorder. Arch Gen Psychiatry 54:749–758, 1990

Rasmussen K, Glennon RA, Aghajanian GK: Phenethylamine hallucinogens in the locus coeruleus: potency of action correlates with rank order of 5-HT$_2$ binding affinity. Eur J Pharmacol 32:79–82, 1986

Ross CA, Heber S, Norton GR, et al: The Dissociative Disorders Interview Schedule: a structured interview. Dissociation 2:169–189, 1989

Schmahl C, Stiglmayr CE, Boehme R, et al: Behandlung von dissoziativen symptomen bei borderline-persönlichkeitsstörungen mit naltrexon. Nervenarzt 70:262–264, 1999

Schmahl C, Bohus M, Esposito F, et al: Neural correlates of antinociception in borderline personality disorder. Arch Gen Psychiatry 63:659–667, 2006

Sedman G, Kenna JC: Depersonalization and mood changes in schizophrenia. Br J Psychiatry 109:669–673, 1963

Simeon D: Depersonalization disorder: a contemporary overview. CNS Drugs 18:343–353, 2004

Simeon D, Hollander E, Stein DJ: Induction of depersonalization by the serotonin agonist meta-chlorophenylpiperazine. Psychiatry Res 58:161–164, 1995

Southwick SM, Krystal JH, Bremner JD, et al: Noradrenergic and serotonergic function in posttraumatic stress disorder. Arch Gen Psychiatry 54:749–758, 1991

Steinberg M: Interviewer's Guide to the Structured Clinical Interview for DSM-IV Dissociative Disorders. Washington, DC, American Psychiatric Press, 1994

Titeler M, Lyon RA, Glennon RA: Radioligand binding evidence implicates the brain 5-HT$_2$ receptor as a site of action for LSD and phenylisopropylamine hallucinogens. Psychopharmacology 94:213–216, 1988

Vollenweider FX, Maguire RP, Leenders KL, et al: Effects of high amphetamine dose on mood and cerebral glucose metabolism in normal volunteers using positron emission tomography (PET). Psychiatry Res 83:149–162, 1998

Waller NG, Putnam FW, Carlson EB: Types of dissociation and dissociative types: a taxometric analysis of dissociative experiences. Psychol Methods 1:300–321, 1996

Walsh SL, Geter-Douglas B, Strain EC, et al: Enadoline and butorphanol: Evaluation of κ-agonists on cocaine pharmacodynamics and cocaine self-administration in humans. J Pharmacol Exp Ther 299:147–158, 2001

Wolf ME, Mosnaim AD, Puente J, et al: Plasma methionine enkephalin in PTSD. Biol Psychiatry 29:305–307, 1991

C H A P T E R 7

NEUROENDOCRINE MARKERS OF EARLY TRAUMA

Implications for Posttraumatic Stress Disorders

E. RONALD DE KLOET, PH.D.
THOMAS RINNE, M.D., PH.D.

Dissociation challenges the individual's perception of being in control, which is correlated with self-esteem and a sense of identity. Recently, the extent of self-esteem was found to be a predictor of the activity of the hypothalamic-pituitary-adrenal (HPA) axis (Pruessner et al. 2005). The HPA axis is a neuroendocrine system that links experience and behavior with the secretion and action of cortisol. Another predictor of lasting changes in HPA activity is a traumatic early life experience. In this chapter we focus on the mechanism underlying the effect of early trauma on the HPA axis and the consequences of early trauma in later life. This is of relevance for the field of posttraumatic stress disorder (PTSD) because it touches on questions as to whether dissociation alters the incidence of PTSD and what pattern of HPA responses evolves in patients with dis-

The research described in this review was supported by the Netherlands Organisation for Scientific Research (NWO) and the Royal Netherlands Academy for Arts and Sciences.

139

sociative symptomatology. The answers to these questions are important for understanding the role of the HPA axis and cortisol in programming the brain after adverse early life events, because this can have important implications for understanding the pathogenesis of dissociative disorders and PTSD.

The role of the HPA axis and cortisol is also of interest because recently it has become apparent that a neuroendocrine hallmark of PTSD is a low circulating cortisol concentration in the face of high central stress system activity as reflected by elevated corticotropin-releasing hormone (CRH) levels (Yehuda 2002). This finding raised the question of whether low cortisol may be a risk factor for PTSD or a consequence of the disorder (Vermetten and Bremner 2002; Yehuda 2002). If low cortisol is a risk factor in the precipitation of PTSD, neuroendocrine markers may exist that identify a vulnerable phenotype. In contrast, if low cortisol develops after the adverse experience it may be either an epiphenomenon or a factor that aggravates the onset and progression of trauma-related emotional and cognitive dysregulation.

To address these questions we briefly summarize the stress system, focusing on the neuroendocrine rather than the autonomic branch during development and in adult life. Subsequently, we discuss an animal model for neglect and abuse (i.e., the maternally deprived rodent). This model is frequently used to study the chain of events taking place in the brain and stress system after an early adverse event (de Kloet et al. 2005a; Levine et al. 2000; McEwen 2003; Parker et al. 2004; Sanchez et al. 2001). We briefly consider preliminary studies on trauma-related dissociative phenomena, such as amnesia, and circulating cortisol concentrations. Finally, we formulate a number of questions in an attempt to define a conceptual framework of stress system operation in those with an endophenotype vulnerability for PTSD. Recent reports suggest that such a conceptual framework may provide a promising step toward treatment of patients with the disorder (Aerni et al. 2004).

THE HYPOTHALAMIC-PITUITARY-ADRENAL AXIS

The stress response proceeds through interacting acute and recovery phases (de Kloet et al. 2005a). The acute phase involves the CRH-1 receptor–driven sympathetic, neuroendocrine, and behavioral fight-or-flight response, which is activated via specific neuronal pathways conveying physical and psychological information. The recovery phase represents a slower system promoting adaptation and recovery that is governed by the recently discovered urocortins II and III acting via the CRH-2 receptor system (Reul and Holsboer 2002). The CRH-1 and CRH-2 receptor systems have a partly overlapping central nervous system distribution in the hypothalamus, brain stem, and limbic system that matches their CRH and urocortin terminal fields. CRH administered in the bloodstream mimics the initial stress response and produces anxiogenesis, whereas urocortins have anxiolytic properties. Thus, CRH and the urocortins with their cognate receptors form interacting signaling networks that are involved in the acute and recovery phases of the stress response, respectively.

The stress response can be monitored by measuring the activity of the sympathetic nervous system and the HPA axis. In the case of the HPA axis, exposure to a brief stressor ultimately causes up to a hundredfold rise in the concentration of circulating corticosteroid hormone—cortisol in humans and corticosterone in rats and mice—that is reached after 15–30 minutes and returns to baseline 60–120 minutes later. The corticosteroids can modulate the initial stress reaction as well as the recovery response. The initial reaction is illustrated in recent work in rats showing that corticosterone facilitates aggressive behavior either triggered by an opponent or evoked by electrical stimulation of the hypothalamic attack area near the periventricular nucleus (PVN; Kruk et al. 2004). It is a feedforward loop because stimulation of that area triggers corticosterone, which then lowers the threshold for agonistic behavior that further stimulates corticosterone secretion. In the slower recovery mode, the elevated corticosteroid concentrations block the initial stress reaction in the very same pathways that have led to HPA axis activation. Thus, cortisol prevents the primary stress reactions from overactivating. These primary stress reactions are of course essential for survival, but if not controlled, they become damaging themselves (Sapolsky et al. 2000). Cortisol exerts this essential control irrespective of whether the stressor is physical or purely psychological in nature.

The reaction to a psychological stressor depends on the appraisal of the experience for its destabilizing potential as well as the choice of an appropriate coping response. The most powerful psychological stressors are conditions in which the individual cannot exert control. As a consequence, the adrenal gland persists in secreting very high amounts of cortisol. Because of the inability to shut off the stress reaction there is apparently resistance to the feedback action of cortisol during severely stressful conditions. Resistance may occur in various parts of the limbic circuitry, such as the hippocampus, amygdala, septum, and frontal cortical areas that participate in emotional and cognitive processing of the event (Herman et al. 2003). Naturally, resistance also may occur on the level of the synthesis of vasopressin (arginine vasopressin [AVP]) and

CRH itself or the synthesis of pituitary pro-opiomelanocortin and release of adrenocorticotropic hormone (ACTH) and endorphins.

CORTICOSTEROID HORMONE AND RECEPTORS

Corticosteroid hormone is secreted from the adrenal gland in pulsatile fashion in 20 bursts of about 20-minute durations over the 24-hour period (Tempel et al. 1993; Young et al. 2004). The hormone operates as a zeitgeber in the coordination and synchronization of daily and sleep-related events as well as the onset and termination of the stress reaction. In coordinating the stress reaction in the body and brain, corticosteroids have a dual mode of action: 1) modulation of the appraisal process and facilitation of initial stress reactions; and 2) termination of stress reactions and facilitation of behavioral adaptation. In order to exert these actions, corticosteroids target cortical neurons, the limbic circuitry, the PVN neurons, and the pituitary corticotrophs. Corticosteroids control intermediary metabolism to provide the energy substrates for dealing with stressful situations. As is the case in the integrated response to stress, corticosteroid control also proceeds in integrated fashion from appetite and choice of macronutrients to energy mobilization and disposition. Coping with stress and energy metabolism are therefore intertwined and coordinated, with corticosteroids as one of the principal integrating signals.

These actions exerted by the steroids are mediated by two types of intracellular receptors, mineralocorticoid receptors (MRs) and glucocorticoid receptors (GRs). These receptors function as transcriptional regulators (de Kloet et al. 1998), and they bind the naturally occurring corticosteroids with a large difference in affinity. This implies that under basal conditions only the high-affinity receptor, MR, is activated, whereas when steroid levels are high (i.e., after stress), both receptors are in operation. The stress receptor, GR, is expressed in every cell, but unevenly, with highest concentrations in the PVN, corticotrophs, and cortical and limbic neurons as well as in the ascending serotonergic and catecholaminergic neurons. The MR occurs only in high amounts in limbic neurons, where they are co-localized with GR. Pharmacological and genetic manipulations have revealed that the MR is important for an optimal appraisal process and the threshold or sensitivity of the initial stress reactions. Thus, MR manipulation affects macronutrient choice (Tempel et al. 1993) and also aspects of anxiety and aggression regulation (Korte 2001; Kruk et al. 2004). The GR facilitates recovery from stress and promotes the consolidation of fear-motivated and spatial memories in preparation for future events.

These MR- and GR-mediated processes proceed in concert with other stress mediators (e.g., norepinephrine, CRH, vasopressin) over different time domains. The rapid actions are probably nongenomic, involving reaggregation of receptor complexes and membrane events at the moment of steroid binding. The slower actions involving both receptor types are genomic processes in which the GR and the MR activate and/or repress partially overlapping gene patterns. The latter steroid effects are conditional. This implies that they change the excitability of cells and circuits, but the nature of the responses is determined by the context (de Kloet et al. 1999). This conditional effect may explain why memories will be more lasting when a situation is particularly arousing (Sandi 2004). It was demonstrated that corticosteroid effects on consolidation of memory in fear conditioning require concomitant norepinephrine input and that interactions between basolateral amygdaloid nucleus, hippocampus, and frontal cortex are crucial in this respect. Cortisol is claimed to impair retrieval of information if administered prior to testing (McGaugh and Roozendaal 2002). However, rather than impairment of the acquisition of new (traumatic) information, an alternative interpretation is behavioral extinction through active learning of new, more appropriate information rather than as loss of prior memory, very similar to the current view on extinction of Pavlovian conditioning (Myers and Davis 2002).

CORTISOL LEVELS AND PATHOGENESIS OF POSTTRAUMATIC STRESS DISORDER

These findings have important implications for understanding the pathogenesis of PTSD. Recent reports suggest that, in PTSD, cortisol exerts too strong a feedback action on the core of the HPA axis, resulting in a lower set point of the axis (Yehuda 2002). The resultant lower cortisol tone leaves the circuits that control fear and emotions underexposed to the hormone, which allows excessive retrieval of traumatic memories. This hypothesis calls for studies in which cortisol is administered in an attempt to facilitate extinction of the traumatic memory. Indeed, in a recent preliminary study low-dose cortisol alleviated cardinal symptoms of PTSD (Aerni et al. 2004).

Interestingly, reports of two preliminary studies suggest that dissociative amnesia after an inescapable traumatic event is correlated with high circulating cortisol levels (Delahanty 2004; Morgan et al. 2001). The patients who were acutely amnesic for a traumatic incidence excreted more cortisol in 24-hour urine samples and were less likely to meet PTSD criteria than the nonamnesic patients. Moreover, the feedback resistance observed in patients with a dissociative disorder hints at a pathophysiology distinct from PTSD (Simeon et al. 2001). These observations raise new, somewhat provocative questions. For instance, does dissociation decrease the incidence of PTSD, and what are the cortisol dynamics if PTSD develops in patients with dissociative symptomatology?

EARLY LIFE EXPERIENCE AND THE HYPOTHALAMIC-PITUITARY-ADRENAL AXIS

Immediate Effects

Newborn rodents experience a so-called stress hyporesponsive period (SHRP), which implies that mild common stressors are unable to trigger an ACTH or corticosterone response from postnatal days 4–14 in the rat. For instance, exposure to a mild stressor (e.g., novelty or a saline injection) hardly produces a response in the immature animal, whereas the same procedure triggers a profound response in the adult. The pituitary and adrenal glands are hyporesponsive, but mild stressors trigger in the pup a profound CRH heterogeneous nuclear ribonucleic acid (RNA) response, whereas in the adult this takes about 4 hours. More severe stressors such as infection are capable of breaking through the quiescence of the peripheral HPA axis (Levine et al. 2000).

The most powerful effect is achieved when the pup is deprived of the dam's care (e.g., lacks feeding, licking, and grooming). The separation of mother and pup for 24 hours not only activates the HPA axis to a higher set point but also sensitizes the axis to the very same stressors that did not evoke a corticosterone response in the well-groomed infant. The high set point after 24 hours of maternal deprivation is achieved during a series of adaptive changes. In the first 8 hours during deprivation circulating ACTH and corticosterone rise, then feedback action of corticosterone starts to suppress ACTH and CRH messenger RNA (mRNA). The adrenal gland becomes sensitized, and the higher corticosterone level—the corticostat—can be maintained (Figure 7–1) (de Kloet et al. 2005b).

After maternal deprivation, mild stressors are capable of triggering an HPA response. Anogenital stroking of the pup with a warm, wet artists' brush every 8 hours for 45 seconds (which forces the pups to urinate) reinstates quiescence on the level of pituitary ACTH release and also normalizes the exaggerated stress-induced hypothalamic CRH and c-Fos responses. Additional feeding also normalizes adrenal sensitivity and

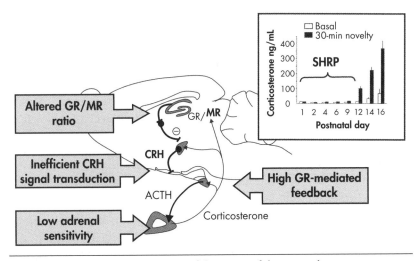

FIGURE 7–1. Schematic overview of the activity of the neonatal stress system.

Peripheral hypothalamic-pituitary-adrenal (HPA) axis activity is low due to a high inhibitory tone of corticosterone on the pro-opiomelanocortin gene via the glucocorticoid receptors (GRs) and the low adrenal sensitivity to adrenocorticotropic hormone (ACTH). In contrast, the activity of central HPA components such as corticotropin-releasing hormone (CRH) is high due to the lack of efficient negative feedback. MR=mineralocorticoid receptors; SHRP=stress hyporesponsive period.

Source. Reprinted from de Kloet ER, Sibug RM, Helmerhorst FM, et al.: "Stress, Genes and the Mechanism of Programming the Brain for Later Life." *Neuroscience Behavioral Reviews* 29:271–281, 2005. Copyright 2005, with permission from Elsevier.

circulating corticosterone back to SHRP status. The data suggest that metabolic signals as well as sensory signals are important for maintenance of the SHRP. The underlying mechanism to maintain the SHRP appears to be glucocorticoid feedback at the level of the pituitary gland. This is because systemic (Schmidt et al. 2005) rather than central glucocorticoid antagonist application (Yi et al. 1993) disrupts the SHRP and produces a profound ACTH and corticosterone response. In contrast, CRH mRNA expression in response to the GR antagonist does not change, further reinforcing a pituitary site of action. Maternal deprivation increases responsiveness of the neural stress circuitry. MRs and GRs in the hippocampus, as well as GRs in the PVN, are downregulated. In contrast, the hippocampal GR is upregulated irreversibly under conditions of intensified maternal care. This irreversible upregulation is due to demethylation of a cysteine residue at the early gene transcription factor 5'NGFI-A binding region in the exon 1–7 promoter (Weaver et al. 2004).

In light of the strong corticosterone response to maternal deprivation, it seems logical that in the literature this hormone is held responsible for most effects of mother–pup separations. Nevertheless, caution
should be taken in the interpretation of these data, because firm proof
for the causality of corticosterone is lacking. For instance, pretreatment
of pups with dexamethasone completely abolished the corticosterone
response to maternal deprivation but did not affect the central effects of
mother–pup separation (Van Oers et al. 1998b).

Long-Term Consequences

In the 1950s, Seymour Levine demonstrated that handling of rat pups
(removing the animals daily for 15 minutes) during their postnatal development produced a lasting suppression of emotional and neuroendocrine reactivity (Levine 1957). In subsequent studies this finding has
proved robust. Adult rats handled during infancy show a reduced
ACTH and corticosterone response to stress in the hippocampus as well
as lower levels of CRH and AVP expression and immunoreactivity
when compared with nonhandled animals (Meaney et al. 1988). Furthermore, handling has been shown to reduce anxiety-like behavior.
However, as was recently pointed out in a cautious note, the nonhandled animals, which are commonly used as control group, also present
an experimental extreme (Pryce and Feldon 2003).

The control group problem has been elegantly overcome by Meaney's
group, who introduced the model of low versus high grooming mothers.
In this model, naturally occurring differences in maternal care are scored
in a population of Long-Evans rat mothers and used as a criterion for sub-
grouping the females according to the intensity of their maternal care
(Meaney et al. 1998). The offspring of high grooming mothers had significantly lower ACTH and corticosterone responses to stress, a lower CRH
mRNA expression in the PVN, and a higher GR mRNA expression in the
hippocampus (Liu et al. 1997). In addition, these rats from high grooming
mothers also displayed a higher spatial learning and memory ability compared with the offspring of low grooming mothers. Taken together, these
data underscore that maternal care matters and that alterations of maternal care during development affect the function of the individual during
adulthood. However, it should be pointed out that such outcome differences in pups exposed to low versus high grooming mothers represent
correlational rather than causal findings. For causality, cross-fostering
studies are essential.

Long-term effects on the receptors for corticosteroids also have been
measured. In handled animals, Meaney and colleagues always reported

elevated expression levels of the GR solely for the hippocampus. In studies using maternal deprivation for 24 hours, downregulation of the hippocampal GR was reported in adult male rats. This was enhanced if the adrenals were further stimulated with ACTH at the time of maternal deprivation (Sutanto et al. 1996). Downregulation of MR also was observed in the deprived males. In contrast, GRs were increased in adulthood for females deprived as pups, and this increase was further enhanced with neonatal ACTH injection. MRs were not affected in females by any of the neonatal manipulations.

We must point out that the timing of these acute treatments is crucial for the long-term effects. Some of the applied paradigms aiming for a disruption of HPA function circumvent this problem by simply extending the treatment throughout postnatal development (Plotsky and Meaney 1993). It seems logical that if increased maternal care is beneficial for the development of the infants, then a prolonged maternal absence or neglect is unfavorable or even harmful. One of the best-studied models employs a separation paradigm of 3 hours daily throughout the SHRP. The repeated separations produced a phenotype in later life characterized by enhanced emotional and HPA responses to stress and elevated hypothalamic and amygdaloid CRH mRNA expression. MR expression was enhanced in the hippocampus, but GR expression was not affected. Accordingly, the repeated separations do produce lasting changes in the stress system, but only partly the PTSD phenotype. However, the strategy underlying the repeated separation paradigm is based on the assumption that the induced effects are cumulative and unidirectional, and this may not be the case at all. In other words, maternal separation at the beginning of the SHRP may have very different long-term consequences from the same treatment applied toward the end of the SHRP. Studies with a single 24-hour separation period indicated that, especially at the beginning of the SHRP, the stress system of the pups is vulnerable to external disturbances (Van Oers et al. 1998a). Thus, the stage of development is crucial for the effect of maternal neglect.

One question that has not yet been addressed directly but is nevertheless of great importance is the role of the genetic background on the possible long-term consequences of disrupted stress system development. Although virtually all mice (and rats) subjected to maternal deprivation of more than 4 hours will react with an activation of the HPA axis, the long-term consequences of maternal deprivation are much more subtle. Besides the duration of the separation, they depend also on the time point of the separation during the SHRP and the gender of the mouse as well as the genetic background. A study of brown Norway rats subjected to maternal deprivation at postnatal days 3–24 showed that some deprived animals aged successfully in regard to their learning ability, whereas others did not (Oitzl et al. 2000). Compared with control subjects the maternally deprived animals were mostly either good or bad learners, with only a few (12% of the animals) partially impaired. This implied that, after deprivation, the number of good performers increased twofold at senescence and the number of bad performers increased 1.5-fold. This dissociation in good and bad performers correlated with the expression of brain-derived neurotrophic factor in the hippocampus (Schaaf et al. 2001). The higher the expression of this factor, the better the animals learned.

What is the role of the stress system and of genetic background in this dichotomization of cognitive performance at senescence as a result of maternal deprivation? In the same study by Oitzl et al. (2000), parameters of HPA activity were measured. If exposed to novelty, the response of corticosterone slowly attenuated during the aging process and was lowest at senescence. In deprived rats, peak levels of stress-induced corticosterone levels were far higher at midlife than in the control subjects but were much lower at a younger age. At senescence, particularly after exposure to more severe stressors, the corticosterone response was attenuated (Workel et al. 2001). It would be of interest, therefore, to examine whether the extent of midlife stress is a determinant in selecting a trajectory toward either successful aging or senility and, if so, which gene patterns are being activated under such conditions.

IMPLICATIONS AND PERSPECTIVES

Do Humans Have a Stress Hyporesponsive Period?

An SHRP has recently been proposed in human children (Davidson et al. 2004), developing gradually during the first year of life, but its duration is unclear. Children ages 12–18 months exhibit a clear behavioral response to novel events but do not respond with a rise in circulating cortisol levels (Gunnar and Donzella 2002).

Is Stress System Operation in Newborn Children Affected by Maternal Signals?

In humans, the quality of child care has been described to influence the cortisol response to mild stressors, especially during the SHRP. Eighteen-month-old children showed a cortisol response to novelty only if the attachment to the mother was insecure (Nachmias et al. 1996). Childhood trauma appears associated with a permanently altered HPA axis as a risk factor for psychiatric diseases during adulthood (Heim and Nemeroff 2001; Rinne et al. 2002).

Are All Individuals Affected in the Same Direction by Early Events?

Early experiences appear capable of enhancing or suppressing the expression of certain genetic traits and, by doing so, may change the outcome of behavioral performance in later life. The outcomes of the studies of early handling seem to suggest that individuals will be affected in the same mode and direction (Liu et al. 1997; Meaney et al. 1988). Other studies, however, clearly demonstrate that the maternal deprivation paradigm amplifies genetically determined individual differences (some people gain from trauma, others lose the ability to cope), much like the variation in PTSD development in those exposed to trauma (i.e., 10%–40% develop PTSD) (Oitzl et al. 2000).

Which Are Candidate Vulnerability Genes for Mediating Long-Term Effects of Early Trauma?

In favor of the gene-by-environment interaction for individual variation in coping with stress, a recent report demonstrated that individuals carrying the long allele of the 5-HT transporter are resistant to depression (Caspi et al. 2003). Other important candidates are the ER22/23EK polymorphism located at the beginning of exon 2 of the GR gene. Individuals carrying this polymorphism have a healthier metabolic profile, better cognitive function, and more favorable treatment outcome with antidepressants than the general population. In contrast, individuals with N363S—located at the end of exon 2 and the Bcl-I restriction site, a probable marker of a large allele, or haplotype, spanning almost the entire intron B—have negative prospects. They have more body fat, less lean mass, hypersensitive insulin secretion, and increased cholesterol levels (Van Rossum and Lamberts 2004). These GR polymorphisms have not been tested in relation to PTSD and dissociative disorders.

What Is the Mechanism Underlying the Programming of Brain and Behavior by Adverse Experience?

Ample evidence suggests that the stress hormones are key mediators, because glucocorticoid feedback in the anterior pituitary and consequent adrenal hyporesponsiveness maintain the SHRP. During the SHRP the brain's stress system is, however, fully capable of responding.

In the mother–pup interaction in rodents the quiescent HPA axis is only disrupted if the infant is deprived once for several hours of maternal care. It is reasonable to assume that the activated CRH and corticosteroid systems then are the primary signals engaged in programming the brain, and a role for the hippocampal GR has been advocated. In a series of elegant studies, Meaney and coworkers demonstrated that the upregulation of the GR is due to demethylation of a cysteine residue at the 5'NGFI-A binding region in the exon 1–7 promoter of the GR (Meaney et al. 1998; Weaver et al. 2004). It is reasonable to assume that GR-mediated actions affect the wiring and synaptic organization of the brain's stress circuitry, as has been shown by the long-term effects of perinatal dexamethasone treatment (Welberg et al. 2001).

What Is the Mechanism Underlying the Outcome of Early Life Events in the Precipitation of Posttraumatic Stress Disorder?

The underlying belief is that genetic predisposition generates a vulnerable phenotype that is sensitive to adverse childhood experiences as a risk factor for the precipitation of PTSD during adulthood (Bremner et al. 1993; Carlson et al. 2001). Chronic childhood adversity appears to render HPA axis function permanently hyperresponsive, resulting in a strongly increased ACTH and cortisol output to a combined dexamethasone/CRH challenge test as well as to a psychological stress challenge in female victims of sustained childhood abuse (Figure 7–2) (Heim et al. 2002; Rinne et al. 2003). These effects are due to an increased responsivity of the hypothalamic CRH/AVP drive and turn out to be independent of a concurrent PTSD.

However, a concurrent PTSD mitigates the net ACTH and cortisol output in chronically abused and nonabused subjects (Rinne et al. 2003). This finding hints at two different and independent pathophysiological mechanisms underlying the neuroendocrine sequelae of chronic childhood abuse and PTSD. On the one hand, chronic childhood abuse is likely to be correlated with an increased CRH/AVP drive. Frequent exposure to high cortisol levels may facilitate the development of dissociation under very stressful conditions in genetically predisposed, chronic traumatized patients. On the other hand, PTSD appears to be associated with an increased glucocorticoid feedback inhibition and low cortisol levels (Heim et al. 2002; Newport et al. 2004). If individuals with increased feedback inhibition (glucocorticoid hypersensitivity) are at risk for PTSD and those with decreased feedback inhibition (glucocorticoid resistance) are at risk for dissociative disorders, this apparent dichotomy would call for studies on possible associations with genetic polymorphisms in MR and GR signaling.

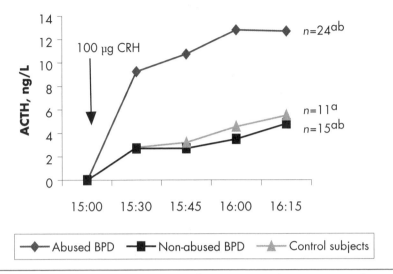

FIGURE 7–2. Mean adrenocorticotropic hormone (ACTH) plasma response to the combined dexamethasone/corticotropin-releasing hormone (CRH) challenge over time.

[a] Analysis of variance of the areas under curve (chronically abused, nonabused patients with borderline personality disorder [BPD], and healthy control subjects): $P=0.002$.

[b] Stepwise backward analysis of covariance in BPD sample (posttraumatic stress disorder [PTSD], major depressive disorder, childhood abuse): childhood abuse, $P=0.001$; PTSD, $P=0.049$.

Source. Reprinted from Rinne T, de Kloet ER, Wouters L, et al.: "Hyperresponsiveness of Hypothalamic-Pituitary-Adrenal Axis to Combined Dexamethasone/Corticotropin-Releasing Hormone Challenge in Female Borderline Personality Disorder Subjects With a History of Sustained Childhood Abuse." *Biological Psychiatry* 52:1102–1112, 2002. Copyright 2002, with permission from the Society of Biological Psychiatry.

What Are the Implications of Our Current Knowledge for Treatment Outcome of Traumatic Stress-Related Disorders Such as Posttraumatic Stress Disorder?

In general, broad-spectrum agents such as the selective serotonin reuptake inhibitors (SSRIs) are a good first choice for treatment. In a meta-analysis of the double-blind, placebo, controlled studies, SSRIs appear to have reasonably robust effects, defined as "much improved" or even "very much improved" (Asnis et al. 2004; Stein et al. 2000). Moreover, SSRIs normalize the HPA axis hyperresponsiveness in patients who were exposed to sustained childhood abuse (Caspi et al. 2003) or those with

PTSD (Vermetten et al. 2006). This effect occurs only during treatment; HPA hyperreactivity reappears upon cessation of treatment (Stout et al. 2002). An interesting new twist in treatment strategy is directly targeting the stress system. Low dosages of cortisol (10 mg/day for 1 month) appeared effective in reducing excessive retrieval of traumatic memories (Aerni et al. 2004). In future, new drugs may be developed that more directly and effectively target hyperresponsivity to traumatic stress.

CONCLUSION

A frequent misconception is that trauma automatically causes PTSD (see Chapter 8 in this volume, "Symptoms of Dissociation in Healthy Military Populations," for further discussion). Yet only a minority of about 10%–40% of persons who are exposed to a single severe trauma or to repetitive traumatic events develop PTSD. Others may develop different forms of (psycho)pathology, such as depression (Davidson et al. 2004) or somatic complaints. Early childhood adverse experiences are thought to sensitize for traumatic stressors during adult life, with consequences for neuroendocrine alterations either with or without PTSD and/or dissociative disorders (Newport et al. 2004; Rinne et al. 2002). Nevertheless, the overview provided in this chapter generates a number of questions about the role stress hormones play in programming the brain after adverse early events—questions that may have implications for understanding the pathogenesis of posttraumatic stress–related disorders. The interplay between genetic background and developmental stage is not only an important factor in the regulation of the stress response in adult life but also may serve as a strong antecedent factor for dysregulations observed in stress-related disorders.

REFERENCES

Aerni A, Traber R, Hock C, et al: Low-dose cortisol for symptoms of posttraumatic stress disorder. Am J Psychiatry 161:1488–1490, 2004

Asnis GM, Kohn SR, Henderson M, et al: SSRIs versus non-SSRIs in post-traumatic stress disorder: an update with recommendations. Drugs 64:383–404, 2004

Bremner JD, Southwick SM, Johnson DR, et al: Childhood physical abuse and combat-related posttraumatic stress disorder in Vietnam veterans. Am J Psychiatry 150:235–239, 1993

Carlson EB, Dalenberg C, Armstrong J, et al: Multivariate prediction of posttraumatic symptoms in psychiatric inpatients. J Trauma Stress 14:549–567, 2001

Caspi A, Sugden K, Moffitt TE, et al: Influence of life stress on depression: moderation by a polymorphism in the 5-HTT gene. Science 301:386–389, 2003

Davidson JR, Stein DJ, Shalev AY, et al: Posttraumatic stress disorder: acquisition, recognition, course, and treatment. J Neuropsychiatry Clin Neurosci 16:135–147, 2004

de Kloet ER, Vreugdenhil E, Oitzl MS, et al: Brain corticosteroid receptor balance in health and disease. Endocr Rev 19:269–301, 1998

de Kloet ER, Oitzl MS, Joëls M: Stress and cognition: are corticosteroids good or bad guys? Trends Neurosci 22:422–426, 1999

de Kloet ER, Joëls M, Holsboer F: Stress and the brain: from adaptation to disease. Nat Rev Neurosci 6:463–475, 2005a

de Kloet ER, Sibug RM, Helmerhorst FM, et al: Stress, genes and the mechanism of programming the brain for later life. Neurosci Biobehav Rev 29:271–281, 2005b

Delahanty D: Peritraumatic amnesia, PTSD and cortisol levels after trauma. Ann NY Acad Sci 1032:183–184, 2004

Gunnar MR, Donzella B: Social regulation of the cortisol levels in early human development. Psychoneuroendocrinology 27:199–220, 2002

Heim C, Nemeroff CB: The role of childhood trauma in the neurobiology of mood and anxiety disorders: preclinical and clinical studies. Biol Psychiatry 49:1023–1039, 2001

Heim C, Newport DJ, Wagner D, et al: The role of early adverse experience and adulthood stress in the prediction of neuroendocrine stress reactivity in women: a multiple regression analysis. Depress Anxiety 15:117–125, 2002

Herman JP, Figueiredo H, Mueller NK, et al: Central mechanisms of stress integration: hierarchical circuitry controlling hypothalamo-pituitary-adrenocortical responsiveness. Front Neuroendocrinol 24:151–180, 2003

Korte SM: Related corticosteroids in relation to fear, anxiety and psychopathology. Neurosci Biobehav Rev 25:117–142, 2001

Kruk MR, Halász J, Meelis W, et al: Fast positive feedback between the adrenocortical stress response and a brain mechanism involved in aggressive behavior. Behav Neurosci 118:1062–1070, 2004

Levine S: Infantile experience and resistance to physiological stress. Science 126:405, 1957

Levine S, Dent GW, de Kloet ER: Stress-hyporesponsive period, in Encyclopedia of Stress. Edited by Fink G. San Diego, CA, Academic Press, 2000, pp 518–526

Liu D, Diorio J, Tannenbaum B, et al: Maternal care, hippocampal glucocorticoid receptors, and hypothalamic-pituitary-adrenal responses to stress. Science 277:1659–1662, 1997

McEwen BS: Early life influences on life-long patterns of behavior and health. Ment Retard Dev Disabil Res Rev 9:149–154, 2003

McGaugh JL, Roozendaal B: Role of adrenal stress hormones in forming lasting memories in the brain. Curr Opin Neurobiol 12:205–210, 2002

Meaney MJ, Aitken DH, van Berkel C, et al: Effect of neonatal handling on age-related impairments associated with the hippocampus. Science 239:766–768, 1988

Morgan CA, Wang S, Rasmusson A, et al: Relationship among plasma cortisol, catecholamines, neuropeptide Y, and human performance during exposure to uncontrollable stress. Psychosom Med 63:412–422, 2001

Myers KM, Davis M: Behavioral and neural analysis of extinction. Neuron 36:567–584, 2002

Nachmias M, Gunnar M, Mangelsdorf S, et al: Behavioral inhibition and stress reactivity: the moderating role of attachment security. Child Dev 67:508–522, 1996

Newport DJ, Heim C, Bonsall R, et al: Pituitary-adrenal responses to standard and low-dose dexamethasone suppression tests in adult survivors of child abuse. Biol Psychiatry 55:10–20, 2004

Oitzl MS, Workel JO, Fluttert M, et al: Maternal deprivation affects behaviour from youth to senescence: amplification of individual differences in spatial learning and memory in senescent Brown Norway rats. Eur J Neurosci 12:3771–3780, 2000

Parker KJ, Buckmaster CL, Schatzberg AF, et al: Prospective investigation of stress inoculation in young monkeys. Arch Gen Psychiatry 61:933–941, 2004

Plotsky PM, Meaney MJ: Early, postnatal experience alters hypothalamic corticotropin-releasing factor (CRF) mRNA, median eminence CRF content and stress-induced release in adult rats. Brain Res Mol Brain Res 18:195–200, 1993

Pruessner JC, Baldwin MW, Dedovic K, et al: Self-esteem, locus of control, hippocampal volume, and cortisol regulation in young and old adulthood. Neuroimage 28:815–826, 2005

Pryce CR, Feldon J: Long-term neurobehavioural impact of the postnatal environment in rats: manipulations, effects and mediating mechanisms. Neurosci Biobehav Rev 27:57–71, 2003

Reul JM, Holsboer F: Corticotropin-releasing factor receptors 1 and 2 in anxiety and depression. Curr Opin Pharmacol 2:23–33, 2002

Rinne T, de Kloet ER, Wouters L, et al: Hyperresponsiveness of hypothalamic-pituitary-adrenal axis to combined dexamethasone/corticotropin-releasing hormone challenge in female borderline personality disorder subjects with a history of sustained childhood abuse. Biol Psychiatry 52:1102–1112, 2002

Rinne T, de Kloet ER, Wouters L, et al: Fluvoxamine reduces responsiveness of HPA axis in adult female BPD patients with a history of sustained childhood abuse. Neuropsychopharmacology 28:126–132, 2003

Sanchez MM, Ladd CO, Plotsky PM: Early adverse experience as a developmental risk factor for later psychopathology: evidence from rodent and primate models. Psychopathology 13:419–449, 2001

Sandi C: Stress, cognitive impairment and cell adhesion molecules. Nat Rev Neurosci 5:917–930, 2004

Sapolsky RM, Romero LM, Munck AU: How do glucocorticoids influence stress responses? Integrating permissive, suppressive, stimulatory, and preparative actions. Endocr Rev 21:55–89, 2000

Schaaf MJ, Workel JO, Lesscher HM, et al: Correlation between hippocampal BDNF mRNA expression and memory performance in senescent rats. Brain Res 915:227–233, 2001

Schmidt M, Levine S, Oitzl MS, et al: Glucocorticoid receptor blockade disinhibits pituitary-adrenal activity during the stress hyporesponsive period of the mouse. Endocrinology 146:1458–1464, 2005

Simeon D, Guralnik O, Knutelsa M, et al: Hypothalamic-pituitary-adrenal axis dysregulation in depersonalization disorder. Neuropsychopharmacology 25:793–795, 2001

Stein DJ, Seedat S, van der Linden GJ, et al: Selective serotonin reuptake inhibitors in the treatment of post-traumatic stress disorder: a meta-analysis of randomized controlled trials. Int Clin Psychopharmacol 15(suppl):S31–S39, 2000

Stout SC, Owens MJ, Nemeroff CB: Regulation of corticotropin-releasing factor neuronal systems and hypothalamic-pituitary-adrenal axis activity by stress and chronic antidepressant treatment. J Pharmacol Exp Ther 300:1085–1092, 2002

Sutanto W, Rosenfeld P, de Kloet ER, et al: Long-term effects of neonatal maternal deprivation and ACTH on hippocampal mineralocorticoid and glucocorticoid receptors. Brain Res Dev Brain Res 92:156–163, 1996

Tempel DL, McEwen BS, Leibowitz SF: Adrenal steroid receptors in the PVN: studies with steroid antagonists in relation to macronutrient intake. Neuroendocrinology 57:1106–1113, 1993

Van Oers HJ, de Kloet ER, Levine S: Early vs. late maternal deprivation differentially alters the endocrine and hypothalamic responses to stress. Brain Res Dev Brain Res 111:245–252, 1998a

Van Oers HJ, de Kloet ER, Whelan T, et al: Maternal deprivation effect on the infant's neural stress markers is reversed by tactile stimulation and feeding but not by suppressing corticosterone. J Neurosci 18:10171–10179, 1998b

Van Rossum EF, Lamberts SW: Polymorphisms in the glucocorticoid receptor gene and their associations with metabolic parameters and body composition. Recent Prog Horm Res 59:333–357, 2004

Vermetten E, Bremner JD: Circuits and systems in stress, I: preclinical studies. Depress Anxiety 15:126–147, 2002

Vermetten E, Vythilingam M, Schmahl C, et al: Alterations in stress reactivity after long-term treatment with paroxetine in women with posttraumatic stress disorder. Ann NY Acad Sci 1071:184–202, 2006

Weaver ICG, Cervoni N, Champagne FA, et al: Epigenetic programming by maternal behavior. Nat Neurosci 7:847–854, 2004

Welberg LA, Seckl JR, Holmes MC: Prenatal glucocorticoid programming of brain corticosteroid receptors and corticotrophin-releasing hormone: possible implications for behaviour. Neuroscience 10:71–79, 2001

Workel JO, Oitzl MS, Fluttert M, et al: Differential and age-dependent effects of maternal deprivation on the hypothalamic pituitary-adrenal axis of brown Norway rats from youth to senescence. J Neuroendocrinol 13:569–580, 2001

Yehuda R: Posttraumatic stress disorder. N Engl J Med 346:108–114, 2002

Yi SJ, Masters JN, Baram TZ: Effects of a specific glucocorticoid receptor antagonist on corticotropin releasing hormone gene expression in the paraventricular nucleus of the neonatal rat. Brain Res Dev Brain Res 73:253–259, 1993

Young EA, Abelson J, Lightman SL: Cortisol pulsatility and its role in stress regulation and health. Front Neuroendocrinol 25:69–76, 2004

C H A P T E R 8

SYMPTOMS OF DISSOCIATION IN HEALTHY MILITARY POPULATIONS

*Why and How Do War Fighters Differ in
Response to Intense Stress?*

C. ANDREW MORGAN III, M.D., M.A.
STEVEN M. SOUTHWICK, M.D.
GARY HAZLETT, PSY.D.
GEORGE STEFFIAN, PH.D.

This chapter examines the prevalence, nature, and impact of dissociation in healthy humans. Historically, many clinicians and researchers have viewed symptoms of dissociation as being tightly associated with illness or disease. Most mental health professionals are not aware that such symptoms are commonly experienced by healthy people exposed to situations entailing high levels of stress and that the presence of such symptoms does not necessarily indicate poor outcome or vulnerability to illness. Currently, however, we know that dissociation is both a normal response to stress and is associated with stress vulnerability and illness.

In this chapter we present and discuss a number of prospective studies that were systematically designed to help us understand how healthy people respond psychologically to personally relevant, highly stressful events. All studies were conducted in populations of healthy active-duty military personnel from the United States, Canada, and

Norway in various types of military training. Some individuals had just begun military careers, whereas others were experienced, elite soldiers.

Although the various research sites differed in location or the focus of military training, they each entailed a level of stress that was extremely realistic and intense. Indeed, the military venue chosen for each study was primarily based on whether the stress experienced by personnel was realistic and comparable with the stress associated with real-world military operations such as engaging with the enemy, awaiting ambushes, and landing on aircraft carriers. Our decision to focus exclusively on high-stress military training programs was driven by the fact that laboratory stress (what researchers can typically do to increase stress in participants coming to a university-based laboratory) is not comparable with the stress experienced by military personnel. Studying people in environments that best approximated real-world conditions would provide ethologically valid data regarding dissociation and its relationship to a person's performance and ability to cope under conditions of high stress.

Participants were recruited from several military training programs, including Combat Diving, Special Forces, Hostage Rescue, Joint Task Force, and U.S. Navy and Army survival schools.

Assuming that many readers are not familiar with these military training programs, we provide a brief description of each training environment before discussing findings. Descriptions of the training will provide a sense of the various physical and mental challenges participants experience while enrolled in the training and will offer a context for the research findings. The studies discussed range from published papers to manuscripts currently being prepared for scientific review. After presenting the findings, we attempt to synthesize them into a coherent model of dissociation. We conclude the chapter with suggestions and comments about future directions in dissociation research with healthy subjects.

WHY STUDY DISSOCIATION?

Although many people are exposed to trauma, only a small percentage develop posttraumatic stress disorder (PTSD) (Breslau et al. 1991; Davidson et al. 1991; Kessler et al. 1995; Kulka et al. 1991). Furthermore, a large portion of individuals who do develop the disorder fully remit over time. These data suggest that chronic PTSD may represent a specific type of adaptation in individuals who have a unique vulnerability to stress. To date, a number of specific psychosocial risk factors for PTSD have been identified, such as history of exposure to traumatic events, exposure to multiple traumatic events, exposure to childhood sexual or physical trauma, and the subjective experience of fearing for one's life (Breslau et al. 1999; Duncan et al. 1996; Freedy et al. 1994). However, because these factors still leave a great deal of variance in outcome unexplained, much work remains in evaluating specific risk factors for the development of PTSD.

Since the 1990s, a number of research groups have examined the relationship between trauma, symptoms of dissociation, and the development of PTSD. Overall, the data from these studies suggest that peritraumatic dissociation (i.e., symptoms of dissociation experienced during, and for a short period immediately after, exposure to a traumatic event) represents a significant risk factor for the subsequent development of PTSD (Bremner and Brett 1997; Bremner et al. 1992; Cardeña and Spiegel 1993; Carlson and Rosser-Hogan 1991; Holen 1993; Koopman et al. 1994; Marmar et al. 1994, 1999; Shalev et al. 1996; Spiegel et al. 1988). Symptoms of dissociation also appear to be significantly related to somatic complaints in victims of trauma and may play an influential role in the reported relationship between PTSD and physical health (Farley and Keaney 1997; Schnurr and Spiro 1999).

Although the findings from these studies are interesting and valuable, they cannot be interpreted with a high degree of certainty because most were retrospective or longitudinal in nature. Study results that rely on hindsight may be limited by poor memory or the tendency of people to reinterpret the past based on how they feel in the present. As a result, researchers interested in dissociation were unclear about 1) whether dissociation was a risk factor for the development of PTSD, 2) whether trauma exposure independently caused dissociation and PTSD, and 3) whether people with chronic symptoms of dissociation overreported the presence and severity of such symptoms when asked about previously experienced traumatic events. Prospective studies are able to address these issues. Moreover, these methodological designs can address whether the propensity to dissociate is the result of trauma exposure or represents a trait that predisposes a person to dissociate more during stress and, in so doing, causes greater vulnerability to PTSD development (e.g., see Butler et al. 1996). The implications of each of these possibilities are significant because depending on the relationship between dissociation and health or illness, one might propose different intervention and treatment models.

We reasoned that one way to increase our understanding about the relationship between trauma, stress, and dissociation would be to examine people before exposure to stress. This strategy would provide much-needed information about whether dissociation is a relatively common response to realistic threat and whether there is a relationship between a person's history of trauma exposure and his or her propensity to dissociate when confronted with high stress. This type of information may help clarify the relationship between dissociation and PTSD.

PROSPECTIVE STUDIES OF DISSOCIATION IN MILITARY PERSONNEL

Healthy Subjects Participating in Military Survival School Training

Military survival school training is one of the most difficult and rigorous programs offered to U.S. military personnel. Those enrolled in such training represent healthy, nonclinical individuals at high risk for exposure to military-related trauma—and consequently at increased risk for the development of combat-related stress disorders such as PTSD. Moreover, personnel are exposed to a highly controlled and uniform application of stress, with the training scenario representing a reliable analogue to multidimensional military operational stress (i.e., participants experience psychological, physical, and environmental stress). Thus, from a research perspective, survival school is a unique laboratory where the stress is realistic and uniformly applied across subjects.

Survival school training consists of a low-stress didactic (classroom) phase followed by a highly stressful experiential phase. During the experiential phase, participants are confronted with two broad tasks or challenges: 1) to survive in the wilderness and avoid "capture" by "enemy" forces and 2) to endure the stress of captivity in a mock prisoner-of-war setting following capture. The goal of this second challenge is to help service personnel adhere to a military code of conduct while "removed" from the field of battle.

The types of stress experienced by military personnel in survival school include semistarvation, sleep deprivation, lack of control over personal hygiene, and external control over movement, social contact, and communication. Exposure to these types of stress gives war fighters an opportunity to apply what they have learned in the didactic phase of the course in a controlled but challenging environment. The principle in training is the same as for other types of military training: "Train as you will fight." The goal is to equip military personnel with the skills and abilities needed to do their jobs and return home with honor.

Prior to studying dissociation, we examined several neurobiological factors known to be affected by stress (Morgan et al. 2000a, 2000b, 2001b). The results showed that compared with the classroom phase of training, the mock captivity phase caused significant alterations in neuroendocrine responses (glucocorticoids, catecholamines, and the gonadal steroid neuropeptide Y). The magnitude of these responses has been shown to be analogous to those exhibited by people experiencing real-world life-threatening situations and to demanding military environments such as nocturnal landings on an aircraft carrier, military free-fall training, and Ranger training. Moreover, soldiers rate the training as one of the most rigorous experienced.

When carefully considering how we would measure symptoms of dissociation, we elected to use an instrument that assessed "state" symptoms of dissociation in response to a specific stressor: the Clinician-Adminstered Dissociative States Scale (CADSS; Bremner et al. 1998). Unlike most dissociation instruments that examine longstanding, stable (trait) symptoms, the CADSS allowed us to achieve our goal of assessing changes from baseline to conditions of stress in symptoms of dissociation.

Participants were instructed to complete the CADSS using the 4 days previous to the course as their reference point. To exclude people with symptoms of dissociation related to a recent stressor, participants were also instructed to inform the research team (orally and in writing) if during the previous 4 days they had experienced any traumatic or highly stressful events. The CADSS is composed of 19 self-report items and 8 observer (i.e., clinician) rated items. The 8 observer items were omitted because the large number of subjects enrolled made it impossible to individually rate each subject in an accurate or reliable manner. This modification did not alter the validity or reliability of the CADSS.

Exposure to the stress of mock captivity and confinement resulted in significant increases in symptoms of dissociation in all subjects. However, in our first study ($N=120$) we found that stress-induced symptoms of dissociation were significantly lower in elite compared with general troop soldiers (Morgan et al. 2001a). This was an intriguing finding because we knew from our neurobiological data that these elite troops also exhibited significantly different hormonal responses to stress—specifically stress-induced levels of the neurotransmitter neuropeptide Y. Many animal studies have shown that neuropeptide Y reduces anxiety and animal freezing behavior. Here we observed that soldiers with high levels of neuropeptide Y were the very people who reported fewer symptoms of dissociation (Morgan et al. 2000b, 2001b, 2002). This finding suggested a potentially important neurobiological factor for how and why people differ in their vulnerability to stress-induced symptoms of dissociation.

To understand how and why elite troops differed from general troops, our next study assessed CADSS at baseline and after stress exposure (Morgan et al. 2001b). We found that elite and general troops differed in both the total score on the CADSS and also on many of the subscale items on the instrument both before and after exposure to stress. We also found that the soldiers' trauma history (on the Brief Trauma

Questionnaire [P.P. Schnurr, M.J. Viieilhauer, F. Weathers, et al., "Brief Trauma Questionnaire," unpublished instrument, National Center for PTSD, 1999]) explained why people differed in their symptoms of dissociation at baseline and in response to stress. Findings were generally in line with expectations. General troop soldiers who reported a history of traumatic stress exposure reported more symptoms of dissociation at baseline and in response to stress. Surprisingly, however, elite troops with a history of trauma reported increased symptoms of dissociation at baseline but reduced symptoms of dissociation in response to stress relative to general troops. These data suggested that elite and general troops represented two different groups of people. The elite troops appeared to have higher histories of trauma exposure compared with general troops but fewer symptoms of dissociation in response to stress. Therefore, the possibility is raised that the elite troops represented a stress-inoculated or stress-hardy group.

In our original publications (Morgan et al. 2001a), we only studied men due to the small numbers of women available for recruitment. However, we are currently recruiting a cohort of women enrolled in survival school, and with 40 now assessed, tentative conclusions are possible. First, as a group, women in survival school training do not appear to exhibit significantly more or fewer symptoms of dissociation compared with general troop soldiers. Yet their rates of symptom endorsement are higher than those reported by men in elite units. In addition, as we found in men, the data from these women suggest that symptoms of dissociation during stress are significantly associated with increased health complaints at the conclusion of the military training. Although tentative at present, these findings counter a commonly held view in the army that women are not able to tolerate high-stress training as well as men. Insofar as these findings replicate the association between physical health complaints and stress-induced symptoms of dissociation observed in men, the data underscore the need for further research into the biological basis of psychosomatic complaints and into the ways in which military populations may present psychological issues to physicians (Morgan et al. 2001a).

The findings from the initial studies highlighted several important questions: Why did stress-induced symptoms differ between elite and general troops? Why did neuropeptide Y differences exist between the two groups? Were these differences primarily due to a weed-out effect of the selection and assessment programs conducted by the military for elite troop membership? With the aim of examining these questions, we recruited soldiers from the U.S. Army Special Forces Assessment and Selection (SFAS) program and the Canadian Joint Task Force-2 Selection and Assessment program.

Special Military Selection Programs

To assess the role selection and assessment might play in creating differences between elite and general troops, we studied soldiers applying for entry into U.S. Special Forces units. The selection course (SFAS) is a physically and psychologically demanding 3-week program. In order to pass, applicants must 1) demonstrate a sufficient ability to cope with the physical endurance demands of the course, 2) demonstrate skill and aptitude in executing operational tasks (such as land navigation during day- and nighttime conditions), and 3) successfully negotiate challenges designed to test their capacities for leadership and decision making under conditions of stress (e.g., team building, leadership, cohesion). Of the 300 applicants who enroll in each cycle of SFAS, approximately 90–100 complete the course, with approximately 40–60 selected for elite training programs.

For the baseline measure, subjects completed the CADSS during the initial psychological assessment phase of the course. At this stage they also completed personality inventories as well as IQ and aptitude tests. We instructed participants to complete the CADSS using the week prior to arrival at SFAS as their baseline, and as in our previous studies we asked soldiers to indicate stressful or traumatic events within the past week that might influence their responses.

Although this study is ongoing, early analysis ($N=450$) suggests that the distribution of baseline symptoms of dissociation is similar to what we observed in our studies at survival school. Approximately 35% of subjects endorse experiencing some symptoms of dissociation prior to starting SFAS. A preliminary chi-square analysis suggests that those who endorsed *any* symptoms of dissociation differ significantly in their pass rates at SFAS compared with those who did not experience dissociation symptoms. Those who endorsed *any* symptoms of dissociation at baseline were significantly less likely to pass the course.

As this study progresses, we aim to assess the likelihood of passing the course relative to specific scores on the CADSS. Preliminary analyses of this type, using receiver operating characteristics (ROC) analyses, suggest that this can be of potential use in predicting, for any given score, how likely it is that a person who obtains such a score on the CADSS will successfully complete and graduate from SFAS. For example, preliminary ROC analyses indicate error in fewer than 5 out of 100 cases when predicting that a student who endorsed 11 or more CADSS items at baseline would fail the course. Although mental health researchers might be excited about the news that a psychological instrument significantly predicts success or failure in a military program, military officials have not warmed to the thought. The idea of being able to predict how well a soldier may do strikes many as unfairly depriving a person of the chance to prove to him- or herself and others whether he or she is eligible for the elite units.

Predictive ability of dissociation measures aside, it is clear that in a selection and assessment program there are multiple reasons why a person may fail the course: physical injury, low IQ, inability to get along well with others, and so on. However, based on our research findings in survival school (i.e., general troops who endorsed symptoms of dissociation at baseline were more likely to dissociate under stress), we are curious about the relationship between baseline propensity to dissociation in SFAS candidates and their performance in a specific skill set of the course. Because it is a stressful task that requires a soldier to remain acutely aware of his or her surroundings (especially when conducted at night), land navigation may be one task where individuals with a greater propensity to dissociate have difficulties. Land navigation requires orienteering skills for which soldiers must have the ability to correctly use a compass and a map and arrive at a specific site in a timely manner. Our preliminary data suggest that soldiers who report a propensity to dissociate at baseline experience greater difficulty when performing land navigation (unpublished observations by C. A. Morgan and G. Hazlett based on review of military performance data with SFAS instructors, 2002–2003). However, since soldiers may differ in their experience with land navigation prior to SFAS program entry, future analyses must control for this factor before the degree to which dissociation plays a negative role in such skills is determined. At this point, however, the evidence suggests that soldiers who endorse symptoms of dissociation at baseline are significantly disadvantaged in successfully completing SFAS.

These early findings suggest that selection programs such as SFAS tend to weed out people who are prone to dissociate at baseline and during stress. This would appear to explain, in part, the findings of less dissociation in response to stress in elite versus general troops when enrolled in survival school. Elite soldiers looked different because they represent a prescreened group of low dissociating persons.

Moving to neuropeptide Y release, we hypothesized that those soldiers who exhibit a return to baseline neuropeptide Y values following the stressful selection course would be selected to the elite programs, whereas those with depleted neuropeptide Y values (lower than pre-stress, baseline values) after the course would not. This hypothesis was based on the survival school findings that elite troops return to baseline at the end of stressful training, whereas general troops show depleted neuropeptide Y levels at the end of the course. A study of troops attending a Canadian elite training group program offered an assessment of this hypothesis.

The Canadian selection program was structured along similar lines as the U.S. program. Applicants to the 1-week course participate in a psychological assessment phase and then are confronted with various challenges and stressors (physical endurance, ability to execute operational tasks, and decision making). Of the 120 applicants, we randomly selected 30 to participate in our study. All subjects completed baseline assessment on the CADSS and provided a blood sample (for neuropeptide Y analysis) prior to starting the course. Moreover, the 12 subjects in our sample who completed the course provided a blood sample and also completed the CADSS at the conclusion of the course.

Similar to our preliminary findings at SFAS, a significant negative relationship between baseline dissociation and success in the course was found in the Canadian selection program. Indeed, no subject who endorsed dissociation at baseline completed the course. Of the 12 successful soldiers, only 7 were accepted for admission to the elite units. Although small, the sample size did permit an analysis of neuropeptide Y before and after the course. A significant difference was found between selected and non-selected soldiers, with those selected for elite training showing a smaller baseline-to-recovery difference in neuropeptide Y values compared with those who were not selected ($n=5$). This result was consistent with our previous findings that people who returned to their pre-stress levels of neuropeptide Y once stress exposure had ceased were more likely to be successful in the military training programs.

These results support the idea that military selection programs weed out individuals who exhibit certain psychological and biological factors. People who are prone to dissociation or who have less capacity for neuropeptide Y responses are deselected. Taken together, these early findings indicate that the association between neuropeptide Y and low dissociation is real. People who are less vulnerable to stress-induced dissociation are likely to be those with greater levels of a neurotransmitter known to attenuate the negative effects of high arousal in mammalian brains. Selection programs[1] serve to sort these stress-hardy individuals from the rest of the group.

---

[1]At the time of writing this chapter we received communication from other researchers who found similar relationships between baseline dissociation and success in U.S. Navy selection programs for aviators (A. O'Donnel, personal communication, February 2000) and in recruits for the Norwegian Army (J. Eid, personal communication, November 2000).

Combat Diver and Hostage Rescue Training Programs

The findings from the aforementioned studies raised questions regarding whether dissociation exerted its influence through a generalized negative effect on attention and concentration or affected specific areas of the brain devoted to problem solving. One limitation of our previous studies was that military performance measures were assessed by military personnel, making the observed relationship between increased dissociation, lower neuropeptide Y, and poorer performance somewhat subjective. To further explore the relationship between dissociation and military performance, we elected to hunt for training venues where performance scores were more objective and standardized. Using the Combat Diver Qualification Course (CDQC) and Hostage Rescue Training (HRT) for the next set of studies offered such measures of performance.

CDQC is designed to select and train military personnel for combat dive operations in a highly stressful 1-month program. Participants know that there is a real threat-to-life risk during the course. The performance assessment is clear: in addition to written examinations, participants must demonstrate their competence in underwater navigation. Because underwater navigational ability determines whether a soldier arrives accurately and on time at his target destination without being detected by enemy troops, this skill represents 90% of the final CDQC grade. A brief description of the underwater navigation exercise may clarify the nature of stress confronted by soldiers in the course.

A student is placed in the water approximately 2 miles offshore at night. After having the target on the beach pointed out to him by the instructor, the student submerges and should not resurface until arrival on the beach. In order to perform the task correctly, students must remain aware of rules and risks involved and of the timed nature of the task. The penalty for resurfacing prematurely or traveling parallel to the shore is expulsion from the course (under actual combat conditions, a soldier who resurfaces is likely to be detected by the enemy and betray the location of U.S. military personnel). All participants are well aware that if they descend below 25 feet while using the oxygen rebreather devices, they will be at risk of serious medical injury or death. Finally, students know that failure to arrive on the beach in a timely way will result in them running out of oxygen or failing the course. Thus, the challenge for individuals in CDQC is to remain mentally focused on direction, depth, speed of travel, and supply of oxygen in order to successfully attain the target landing site on the beach.

To determine the relationship between neurohormones, dissociation, and military performance, we assessed dissociation symptoms and collected plasma samples at baseline and after the final underwater navigation exercise in 41 soldiers enrolled in CDQC. As in our previous studies, approximately 30% of subjects at CDQC endorsed at least one symptom in the week prior to starting the course. Preliminary analyses using ROC indicated that soldiers who endorsed more than six symptoms on the CADSS were significantly less likely to complete the course. These data are extremely similar to those from our research at SFAS and add weight to the argument that people who experience dissociation under conditions of low stress are unlikely to cope well with situations that entail a high degree of stress. Because so many subjects who endorsed symptoms of baseline dissociation were dropped from CDQC, it was not possible to examine the relationship between dissociation at baseline and objective performance on the course.

However, subjects who remained in the course ($n=25$) did endorse stress-induced symptoms of dissociation, and we found a trend toward a negative relationship between these symptoms and underwater navigation accuracy. The absence of a significant finding may have been due to the fact that one-half of the subjects who completed the course did not endorse any symptoms of dissociation in response to the stress of underwater navigation. This perhaps is not surprising given the high likelihood of a selection bias for low dissociation people who elect to apply for CDQC. Interestingly, preliminary analyses of the hormone data collected in subjects during the course suggest a significant negative relationship between dissociation and the neurosteroid dehydroepiandrosterone (DHEA). If true, this would replicate our previously published data (Morgan et al. 2004), which are not discussed in this chapter, showing that subjects high in DHEA relative to cortisol had few symptoms of dissociation during stress. Suffice it to say that people in whom dissociation was low (or absent) appeared to fare better during the underwater navigation task.

Before discussing the neurochemistry and brain regions potentially related to stress-induced symptoms of dissociation, a discussion of our HRT study is necessary. HRT is designed to prepare elite troops for entering buildings in order to rescue hostages held by hostile forces or terrorists. When performing hostage rescue operations, soldiers are exposed to many challenges, including entering a building while avoiding detection by the enemy, avoiding being shot by enemy forces, working in an environment with low visibility, and shooting the hostage-takers, not the hostages. These challenges place great demands on physical endurance, perceptual/situational awareness, and the ability to inhibit impulses so as to shoot the correct targets (stimulus discrimination). HRT requires soldiers to enter a building one at a time (or in pairs) for a total of 15 minutes to apprehend the terrorists and rescue the hostages.

Soldiers have a limited supply of ammunition and typically wear body armor to protect them from "enemy" fire directed toward them.[2]

We studied 12 U.S. Army Special Forces soldiers in HRT training. These soldiers completed CADSS questionnaires at baseline and after the exercise. The soldiers' performance was videotaped and objectively rated by the instructor teams on several categories that made up a total performance score. These categories were presence of mind (how well the soldier discriminated between targets, avoided being shot or ambushed, and kept track of ammunition supply); performance concentration (how well the soldier was able to execute a sequence of 10 specific tasks during the exercise); physical fitness (whether the soldier was physically able to continue throughout the exercise without stopping to catch his[3] breath or slowing down to such a degree that he became trapped by the enemy); and aggressiveness (a measure of force used and risks taken in order to find and rescue the hostages and kill the terrorists). The scores from each of these categories were summed for a total performance score.

A significant negative relationship ($r=-0.59$, $P=0.01$) betwee stress-induced symptoms of dissociation and military performance scores was found. A closer examination of the data suggests that the specific performance skills most strongly and negatively associated with dissociation were those of performance concentration and presence of mind. These data suggest that dissociation (or its primary cause) may disrupt performance via a negative effect on brain areas responsible for attention/concentration and for the ability to maintain spatial awareness. If a person experiencing dissociation is not able to orient him- or herself within the environment or follow a prescribed sequence of behaviors or tasks, it is less likely that he or she will successfully cope under conditions where action or decision making is required.

Cognitive Operations During Stress

Our findings from CDQC and HRT suggested that stress-induced symptoms of dissociation might be disrupting military performance in soldiers by disrupting brain systems involved in spatial mapping, working memory, and concentration. From a real-world perspective, the need to

---

[2]Participants in HRT use simulated ammunition similar to paintball pellets. The discomfort associated with being hit is thought to keep trainees serious in their efforts to avoid being shot during the exercise.

[3]At the time of this writing, women are not permitted to participate in the U.S. Army HRT.

understand why and how stress disrupts performance is very important, because other researchers (Belenky et al. 1994) have reported that many battlefield errors (e.g., friendly-fire incidents, collateral damage) are linked to a decline in cognitive operations in soldiers.

To better define and characterize stress-induced dissociation, we (C.A. Morgan, G. Hazlett, S.M. Southwick, et al., unpublished data, March 2004) used the Rey-Osterrieth Complex Figure (ROCF) drawing task with survival school soldiers (Osterrieth 1944). The ROCF is a standardized neuropsychological test that indexes visual perception, visuospatial organization, motor functioning, and memory (Loring et al. 1990). It is a complex figure incorporating 36 different elements that participants are instructed to copy as accurately as possible (i.e., copy phase). Normative data suggest that postpubertal children and adults typically copy the figure using a configurational approach (i.e., the large central rectangle is drawn first, followed by the addition of details).

After the copy phase, participants are asked to reproduce the figure from memory (i.e., recall phase). Normative data have been established for recall performance at 1 minute, 3 minutes, and 25 minutes. Factor analytic studies suggest that the copy phase of the ROCF measures a person's visuo-constructive ability, whereas the recall phase taps into memory functions.

When we conducted our study, very few data existed on the impact of acute psychological stress on ROCF performance in healthy humans. Hoffman and Al'Absi (2004) found that the social stress test (i.e., public speaking task) elicited significant alterations in measures of psychophysiology and mood but not in ROCF performance. These null ROCF findings may be the result of the low levels of stress generated in the laboratory task. Military stress experienced by soldiers undergoing survival school training is significantly greater than traditional laboratory stress (e.g., the social stress test).

Based on our previous findings, we hypothesized that 1) ROCF recall performance, but not copy performance, would be significantly reduced by exposure to acute stress; and 2) ROCF recall during stress would be negatively associated with stress-induced symptoms of dissociation.

Preliminary analyses show that stress exposure results in altered performance on ROCF copy and ROCF recall tasks. In addition, there was a significant negative relationship between ROCF recall during stress and stress-induced symptoms of dissociation ($r=-0.57$, $P=0.01$). Finally, the data seem to indicate that baseline symptoms of dissociation predict which people exhibit ROCF deficits during stress.

In interpreting these findings, we found that a stress-induced reduction in ROCF recall scores indicated that memory was adversely affected by acute stress. The 1-minute delay interval used in the protocol suggests that the reduction in ROCF recall scores is most likely due to an impairment in working memory (the short-term capacity to retain and manipulate information required for executive cognitive operations—see Chapter 3 in this volume, "Memory and Attentional Processes in Dissociative Identity Disorder"). Within the context of battlefield activity, soldiers have to rely on working memory for a number of tasks. For example, when receiving and relaying target coordinates via radio communications, military personnel must utilize working memory to retain the sequence of numbers that correspond to the grid locations on a map. An inability to do this accurately may result in missing the enemy targets or even mistakenly bombing allies or one's own troops (i.e., friendly fire).

The ability to hold in mind and recall ROCF information is dependent, in large part, on the prefrontal cortex (PFC), a region of the brain critical to working memory. In both rats and monkeys, high levels of dopamine and norepinephrine turnover in the PFC have been shown to induce cognitive impairment, including deficits in spatial working memory (Henry et al. 1995; Zahrt et al. 1997). Consistent with these preclinical findings, the soldiers exposed to interrogation stress in our study—a stimulus known to elicit high turnover of catecholamines—exhibited the greatest deficits on ROCF recall, a task dependent on intact spatial working memory.

Thus our finding that stress-induced symptoms of dissociation are significantly negatively related to working memory helps determine how stress may specifically affect perception, cognition, and memory, all of which are necessary for optimal battlefield performance. Little is known about the neuropsychological and biological mechanisms involved in symptoms of dissociation. However, if dissociation, like altered ROCF recall during stress, reflects the consequences of high states of arousal, we would speculate that brain areas underpinning dissociation and stress-induced cognitive deficits are regions such as the PFC and the hippocampus.

In our study (C.A. Morgan, G. Hazlett, S.M. Southwick, et al., unpublished data, March 2004) we also found that people who endorsed experiencing baseline symptoms of dissociation were significantly more likely to exhibit stress-induced ROCF deficits. Not only did this suggest that a common neurobiology may link the phenomena of dissociation at baseline and during stress, it also highlighted the need to acquire a better understanding of baseline symptoms of dissociation. It is currently unclear why the specific CADSS items at baseline that best predicted ROCF deficits were "feeling disconnected from your own body," "other people seem motionless, dead, or mechanical," "objects look different than you would expect," "things seem to be very real as if there is a special sense of clarity," and "looking at the world through a fog so that people and objects appear far away or unclear." These items refer to alterations in perceptions about one's body, others, and the environment but do not appear to reflect a homogeneous factor. Clearly, additional work remains to be done in this arena.

Simultaneously with our study of dissociation and ROCF performance, we collaborated to study baseline symptoms of dissociation and ROCF performance in Norwegian cadets participating in survival school training (Eid and Morgan 2006). In replicating the aforementioned findings, subjects who endorsed baseline symptoms of dissociation exhibited significant deficits in ROCF recall during stress. Interestingly, the baseline symptoms that best accounted for the variance in ROCF performance during stress were nearly identical to those just mentioned: "feeling disconnected from your own body," "other people seem motionless, dead, or mechanical," "objects look different than you would expect," "things seem to be very real as if there is a special sense of clarity." Again, these symptoms did not, at face value, appear to represent a single construct. However, they do suggest that some individuals are different *prior* to stress exposure and that this difference puts them at risk of difficulties under stress.

When we conducted our first study of ROCF performance and dissociation, we also assessed history of trauma. In our early studies at survival school we had found that history of traumatic stress exposure was associated with increased baseline symptoms of dissociation ($r=0.45$), but there was no indication of a significant relationship between history of traumatic stress and military performance. In this instance, however, an examination of the relationships among the variables of history of traumatic stress exposure, baseline dissociation, and ROCF performance during stress revealed that history of traumatic stress was the greatest predictor of poor ROCF performance during stress.

This is a valuable clue regarding what might happen in people who experience stress-induced ROCF performance problems. It is well known in preclinical studies that early exposure to uncontrollable stress can cause sensitization of noradrenergic and dopaminergic systems. Animals with histories of trauma exposure may respond to subsequent stress with enhanced catecholamine synthesis and release (Abercrombie and Zigmond 1995). Analogously, neurochemical challenge studies in humans have provided evidence for stress sensitization in individuals who have been exposed to uncontrollable stress (Heim et al. 2000; Southwick et al. 1993, 1997). It is possible that exaggerated noradrenergic release in subjects with a sensitized sympathetic nervous system leads to an impairment in the PFC and working memory. We think that poor performance under stress and dissociation may both reflect the negative effects of heightened catecholamine turnover in the PFC. Thus, a working hypothesis is that the significant relationship between dissociation and poor performance (in both training and ROCF) may be due to the fact that each is caused by an impairment of PFC functioning and working memory.

NEUROBIOLOGY AND DISSOCIATION

In our studies with military personnel, we have consistently found that people who exhibit a propensity to dissociate before or during stress are those with a low capacity for neuropeptide Y release or a low ratio of DHEA-sulfate (DHEA-S) to cortisol (Morgan et al. 2002, 2004). These findings are exciting because they appear to be compatible with the data from nonhuman animals: Animals that have an increased capacity for neuropeptide Y or an increased ratio of DHEA-S to glucocorticoids are significantly better at tolerating stress (Kimonides et al. 1999). That said, our current understanding about the neurobiology of dissociation is very limited. One of the biggest obstacles researchers face is the lack of a clear animal model of dissociation (see Chapter 6 in this volume, "Translational Research Issues in Dissociation"). Some scientists have assumed that dissociation is to humans what freezing behavior is to infrahuman animals (Krystal et al. 1995). Others have assumed that stress-induced neurotoxicity at the level of the hippocampus is akin to dissociation (Kimonides et al. 1999). Although these are reasonable hypotheses, we simply do not know how well the different constructs overlap. Given the findings of recent drug-challenge studies in humans, it is likely that dissociative symptoms are mediated, in part, through N-methyl-D-aspartate (NMDA) receptors and through modulation of the γ-aminobutyric acid (GABA)-benzodiazepine receptor complex at the level of the hippocampus (Krystal et al. 1994, 1998, 1999). Although the neurobiology of dissociation is extremely limited, we discuss in more detail our current thinking about the issue in the following section.

A WORKING MODEL OF THE NEUROBIOLOGY OF DISSOCIATION

Glutamate is an amino acid and the brain's primary excitatory neurotransmitter. It is rapidly released in response to arousing and dangerous situations and mediates nearly all fast excitatory point-to-point synaptic transmission in the brain. GABA, the brain's primary inhibitory neurotransmitter, regulates excitatory glutamatergic synaptic transmission. During resting, nonstressful states, GABA exerts tonic inhibition on glutamate transmission in numerous brain regions such as the thalamus and amygdala, allowing the brain to filter out a continuous flow of irrelevant and extraneous sensory information. However, when excitation is increased in response to stress or danger, elevated levels of glutamate have the capacity to overcome tonic inhibition by GABA and thereby trigger a cascade of protective responses (i.e., freeze, flight, fright) (for review, see Krystal et al. 1994; Morgan et al. 2003).

Although stress-induced elevations of glutamate facilitate the cortical and subcortical communication necessary for effective responses to danger, failure to modulate heightened glutamatergic activation can lead to extreme changes in intracellular calcium, toxicity, and even cell death (Krystal et al. 1995). To protect the brain from its own unchecked glutamatergic excitation, additional GABA is released during stress. Thus, GABA provides tonic central nervous system inhibition during nonstressful states and enhanced inhibition during stressful states.

GABA and glutamate both possess two classes of receptors: 1) ionotropic receptors (GABA$_A$ and the glutamatergic NMDA and non-NMDA receptors) that enhance membrane ion conductance and 2) metabotropic receptors (GABA$_B$ and metabotropic glutamate receptors) that increase intracellular second-messenger activity. In addition to its site for binding GABA, the GABA$_A$ receptor complex has binding sites for alcohol, barbiturates, and benzodiazepines. GABA increases the permeability of chloride ions through the GABA$_A$ chloride ion channel, which decreases neuronal excitability by hyperpolarizing the neuronal membrane.

Preclinical research points to GABA as a key neurotransmitter in stress-induced behavioral deficits that mirror depression and PTSD (i.e., the learned helplessness animal model). These data suggest that decreasing GABA transmission renders naïve, nonstressed rats helpless. Conversely, increasing GABA in selective brain regions ameliorates many of the harmful effects of stress.

In humans with trauma-related disorders, very little research has specifically focused on GABA. In a study of accident victims, Vaiva et al. (2004) reported significantly lower plasma GABA levels in subjects who developed PTSD compared with subjects who did not. The authors suggested that low plasma GABA might have increased vulnerability for development of PTSD, whereas normal or high levels may have served a protective role. In another study, Bremner et al. (2000) found that benzodiazepine receptor density and/or affinity was reduced in the medial PFC among patients with PTSD compared with control subjects. This reduction may have been secondary to stress-related alterations in GABAergic transmission. On the other hand, Fujita et al. (2004) did not find a difference in prefrontal cortical benzodiazepine receptor density in Desert Storm veterans .with PTSD compared with healthy control subjects.

Although decreased GABA activity in a number of brain regions (e.g., medial PFC, amygdala) has been suggested as a potential neurobiological factor associated with PTSD, excessive glutamatergic activity may also play a role in the pathophysiology of PTSD. Investigations in healthy subjects have provided evidence that the NMDA glutamate receptor plays a central role in symptoms of dissociation commonly seen in individuals with PTSD (Krystal et al. 1999). In a series of studies, Krystal et al. (1994, 1998, 1999) produced significant dose-dependent increases in dissociative symptoms with the administration of the NMDA antagonist ketamine, which increases glutamate release. Low doses of ketamine caused alterations in the form and content of thought (such as paranoia, loosening of associations, tangentiality, and ideas of reference), whereas high doses caused dissociative symptoms commonly reported by trauma victims. Administration of a GABA agonist benzodiazepine prior to infusion with ketamine resulted in a significant reduction in some, but not all, dissociative symptoms (Krystal et al. 1994, 1998, 1999). Similarly, pretreatment administration of lamotrigine, an anticonvulsant that attenuates glutamate release via inhibition of sodium, calcium, and potassium channels, significantly decreased dissociative and cognitive effects of ketamine. The findings represent exciting early steps in elucidating the neurobiology of dissociation.

In medicine it is often the case that a better understanding of the physiology and pathophysiology of a clinical condition has led to improved treatments. We believe the same principle may apply to treating dissociative disorders. However, our understanding of the neurobiology of dissociation is quite limited. This is primarily due to the fact that there is a significant gap between what we know from studies conducted in nonhuman animals and what we know from studies of dissociation in humans. Preclinical studies deal specifically with neurobiological factors related to neurotoxicity. Although neurotoxicity is not equivalent to symptoms of dissociation, much is known about the regulation of hormones such as cortisol, DHEA-S, and glutamate and noradrenergic regulation and the relationship of these hormones to the phenomenon of stress-induced neurotoxicity. The findings of recent studies in humans showing a relationship between dissociation and specific hormones that are known to be involved in neurotoxicity studies in animals lead us to believe that these data may inform us about the nature of dissociation and about possible future interventions for symptoms of dissociation.

CONCLUSION

Symptoms of dissociation were observed in all of our healthy subjects when they were exposed to high-intensity stress. This observation suggests that the mere presence of stress-induced symptoms of dissociation, per se, cannot be a significant predictor of illnesses such as PTSD. After all, if everyone might be expected to experience dissociation in response to very stressful events, the statement "stress-induced symptoms of dissociation represent a risk factor for PTSD" is akin to saying "being human is a risk factor for PTSD." This would not make clinical decisions any easier, nor would it enhance how we might think about such symptoms.

Taken together, the results of our prospective studies in military personnel suggest it may be more useful to think about symptoms of dissociation that occur at baseline (prior to stress exposure) and in response to stress as two separate phenomena. We consistently observed that soldiers who endorsed symptoms of dissociation at baseline were at increased risk for experiencing problems coping with high stress. These subjects were more likely to exhibit cognitive deficits, performance deficits, increased health complaints, and increased symptoms of dissociation under stress. The consistent association between baseline dissociation and history of traumatic stress exposure suggests that people who exhibit baseline symptoms of dissociation may represent a group of individuals who have been sensitized by previous trauma and who are at risk for difficulties coping under highly stressful circumstances. Our findings also underscore the value to clinicians of taking a trauma history as well as assessing baseline dissociation when performing clinical evaluations. Based on the present data, we suggest that individuals who report symptoms of dissociation indicative of a shift in the sense of their own body—or their perception of others—prior to stress are at increased risk for illnesses such as PTSD following stress.

Although stress-induced symptoms of dissociation were observed, to varying degrees, in all subjects, soldiers successful in elite selection programs exhibited fewer such symptoms. They also demonstrated greater performance and coping skills during stress. Moreover, these selected individuals also exhibited significant neurobiological differences compared with nonselected soldiers during and after stress exposure (i.e., a greater capacity for neuropeptide Y release during stress and more rapid return to prestress baseline; greater baseline and stress-induced release of DHEA). This suggests that many people who self-select for high-stress types of work (policemen, firefighters, Federal Bureau of Investigation, Secret Service, military special operations groups) may be at

lower risk for stress-related illness such as PTSD. Indeed it may be confusing to some clinicians why these individuals appear to cope well with
stress in spite of having experienced significant rates of early trauma. We
suggest that the perspective of most clinicians is the result of a selection
bias in which people present to the hospital (or clinic) for treatment.
Many people who experience early trauma survive their experience and
move on to successful careers. They do not present to the clinic. While
dealing with the people who, due to trauma, have experienced difficulties coping, most clinicians remain unaware of the numbers of people
who experience significant trauma yet lead healthy, productive lives.

The present studies have provided valuable clues about the psychological and neurobiological differences between people who tolerate
stress well and those who do not. Although our understanding at this
time is limited, the present data provide important insights for future
studies designed to test whether specific psychological or neurobiological interventions will buffer or protect people from the negative effects
of highly intense stress.

REFERENCES

Abercrombie ED, Zigmond MJ: Modification of central catecholaminergic sys-
    tems by stress and injury, in Psychopharmacology: The Fourth Generation
    of Progress. Edited by Bloom FE, Kupfer DJ. New York, Raven Press, 1995,
    pp 355–361
Belenky G, Penetar DM, Thorne D, et al: The effects of sleep deprivation on per-
    formance during continuous combat operations, in Food Components to
    Enhance Performance: An Evaluation of Potential Performance Enhancing
    Food Components for Operational Rations. Edited by Marriott BM. Wash-
    ington, DC, National Academy Press, 1994, pp 127–136
Bremner JD, Brett E: Trauma-related dissociative states and long-term psycho-
    pathology in posttraumatic stress disorder. J Trauma Stress 10:37–49, 1997
Bremner JD, Southwick S, Brett E, et al: Dissociation and posttraumatic stress
    disorder in Vietnam combat veterans. Am J Psychiatry 149:328–332, 1992
Bremner JD, Krystal JH, Putnam FW, et al: Measurement of dissociative states
    with the Clinician-Administered Dissociative States Scale (CADSS).
    J Trauma Stress 11:125–136, 1998
Bremner JD, Innis RB, Southwick SM, et al: Decreased benzodiazepine receptor
    binding in prefrontal cortex in combat-related posttraumatic stress disor-
    der. Am J Psychiatry 157:1120–1126, 2000
Breslau N, Davis GC, Andreski P, et al: Traumatic events and posttraumatic
    stress disorder in an urban population of young adults. Arch Gen Psychia-
    try 48:216–222, 1991

Breslau N, Chilcoat HD, Kessler RC, et al: Previous exposure to trauma and PTSD effects of subsequent trauma: results from the Detroit Area Survey of Trauma. Am J Psychiatry 156:902–907, 1999

Butler LD, Duran RE, Jasiukaitis P, et al: Hypnotizability and traumatic experience: a diathesis-stress model of dissociative symptomatology. Am J Psychiatry 153:42–63, 1996

Cardeña E, Spiegel D: Dissociative reactions to the San Francisco Bay Area earthquake of 1989. Am J Psychiatry 150:474–478, 1993

Carlson EB, Rosser-Hogan R: Trauma experiences, posttraumatic stress, dissociation, and depression in Cambodian refugees. Am J Psychiatry 148:1548–1551, 1991

Davidson JRT, Hughes D, Blazer D, et al: Posttraumatic stress disorder in the community: an epidemiological study. Psychol Med 21:1–9, 1991

Duncan RD, Saunders BE, Kilpatrick DG, et al: Childhood physical assault as a risk factor for PTSD, depression, and substance abuse: findings from a national survey. Am J Orthopsychiatry 66:437–448, 1996

Eid J, Morgan III CA: Dissociation, hardiness and performance in military cadets participating in survival training. Mil Med 171:436–42, 2006

Farley M, Keaney JC: Physical symptoms, somatization, and dissociation in women survivors of childhood sexual assault. Women Health 25:33–45, 1997

Freedy JR, Resnick HS, Kilpatrick DG, et al: The psychological adjustment of recent crime victims in the criminal justice system. J Interpers Violence 9:450–468, 1994

Fujita M, Southwick SM, Denucci CC, et al: Central type benzodiazepine receptors in Gulf War veterans with posttraumatic stress disorder. Biol Psychiatry 56:95–100, 2004

Heim C, Newport DJ, Heit S, et al: Pituitary-adrenal and autonomic responses to stress in women after sexual and physical abuse in childhood. JAMA 284:592–597, 2000

Henry C, Guegant G, Arnauld E, et al: Prenatal stress in rats facilitates amphetamine-induced sensitization and induces long-lasting changes in dopamine receptors in the nucleus accumbens. Brain Res 685:179–186, 1995

Hoffman R, Al'Absi M: The effect of acute stress on subsequent neuropsychological test performance. Arch Clin Neuropsychol 19:497–506, 2004

Holen A: The North Sea oil rig disaster, in International Handbook of Traumatic Stress Syndromes. Edited by Wilson JP, Raphael B. New York, Plenum, 1993, pp 471–478

Kessler RC, Sonnega E, Bromet A, et al: Posttraumatic stress disorder in the national comorbidity survey. Arch Gen Psychiatry 52:1048–1060, 1995

Kimonides VG, Spillantini MG, Sofroniew MV, et al: Dehydroepiandrosterone antagonizes the neurotoxic effects of corticosterone and translocation of stress-activated protein kinase 3 in hippocampal primary cultures. Neuroscience 89:429–436, 1999

Koopman C, Classen C, Spiegel D: Predictors of posttraumatic stress symptoms among survivors of the Oakland/Berkeley, Calif, firestorm. Am J Psychiatry 151:888–894, 1994

Krystal JH, Karper LP, Seibyl JP, et al: Subanesthetic effects of the noncompetitive NMDA antagonist, ketamine, in humans: psychotomimetic, perceptual, cognitive, and neuroendocrine responses. Arch Gen Psychiatry 51:199–214, 1994

Krystal JH, Bennett AL, Bremner JD, et al: Toward a cognitive neuroscience of dissociation and altered memory functions in posttraumatic stress disorder, in Neurobiological and Clinical Consequences of Stress: From Normal Adaptation to PTSD. Edited by Friedman MJ, Charney DS, Deutch AY. Philadelphia, PA, Lippincott-Raven Publishers, 1995, pp 293–269

Krystal JH, Karper LP, Bennett A, et al: Interactive effects of subanesthetic ketamine and subhypnotic lorazepam in humans. Psychopharmacology (Berl) 135:213–229, 1998

Krystal JH, D'Souza DC, Karper LP, et al: Interactive effects of subanesthetic ketamine and haloperidol in healthy humans. Psychopharmacology (Berl) 145:193–204, 1999

Kulka RA, Schlenger WE, Fairbank JA, et al: Trauma and the Vietnam War Generation: Report of Findings From the National Vietnam Veterans' Readjustment Study. New York, Brunner/Mazel, 1991

Loring DW, Martin RC, Meador KJ, et al: Psychometric construction of the Rey-Osterrieth Complex Figure: methodological considerations and interrater reliability. Arch Clin Neuropsychol 5:1–14, 1990

Marmar CR, Weiss DS, Schlenger WE, et al: Peritraumatic dissociation and posttraumatic stress in male Vietnam theater veterans. Am J Psychiatry 151:902–907, 1994

Marmar CR, Weiss DS, Metzler TJ, et al: Longitudinal course and predictors of continuing distress following critical incident exposure in emergency services personnel. J Nerv Ment Dis 187:15–22, 1999

Morgan III CA, Wang S, Mason J, et al: Hormone profiles in humans experiencing military survival training. Biol Psychiatry 47:891–901, 2000a

Morgan III CA, Wang S, Southwick SM, et al: Plasma neuropeptide-Y in humans exposed to military survival training. Biol Psychiatry 47:902–909, 2000b

Morgan III CA, Hazlett G, Wang S, et al: Symptoms of dissociation in humans experiencing acute uncontrollable stress: a prospective investigation. Am J Psychiatry 158:1239–1247, 2001a

Morgan III CA, Wang S, Rasmusson A, et al: Relationship among plasma cortisol, catecholamines, neuropeptide Y, and human performance during exposure to uncontrollable stress. Psychosom Med 63:412–422, 2001b

Morgan III CA, Rassmusson A, Wang S, et al: Neuropeptide-Y, cortisol and subjective distress in humans exposed to acute stress: replication and extension of a previous report. Biol Psychiatry 52:136–142, 2002

Morgan III CA, Southwick SM, Krystal JH: Toward a pharmacology of acute stress disorders. Biol Psychiatry 53:834–843, 2003

Morgan III CA, Hazlett G, Rasmusson A, et al: Relationships among plasma de-hydroepiandrosterone sulfate and cortisol levels, symptoms of dissociation and objective performance in humans exposed to acute stress. Arch Gen Psychiatry 61:819–825, 2004

Osterrieth PA: Le test de copie d'une figure complex: contribution a l'étude de la perception et de la mémoire. Arch Psychol 30:286–356, 1944

Shalev AY, Peri T, Canetti L, et al: Predictors of PTSD in injured trauma survivors: a prospective study. Am J Psychiatry 153:219–225, 1996

Schnurr PP, Spiro A: Combat exposure, posttraumatic stress disorder symptoms, and health behaviors as predictors of self-reported physical health in older veterans. J Nerv Ment Dis 187:353–359, 1999

Southwick SM, Krystal JH, Morgan CA, et al: Abnormal noradrenergic function in posttraumatic stress disorder. Arch Gen Psychiatry 50:266–274, 1993

Southwick SM, Krystal JH, Bremner JD: Noradrenergic and serotonergic function in posttraumatic stress disorder. Arch Gen Psychiatry 54:749–758, 1997

Spiegel D, Hunt T, Dondershine HE: Dissociation and hypnotizability in posttraumatic stress disorder. Am J Psychiatry 145:301–305, 1988

Vaiva G, Thomas P, Ducrocq F, et al : Low posttrauma GABA plasma levels as a predictive factor in the development of acute posttraumatic stress disorder. Biol Psychiatry 55:250–254, 2004

Zahrt J, Taylor JR, Mathrew RG, et al: Supranormal stimulation of D1 dopamine receptors in the rodent cortex impairs spatial working memory performance. J Neurosci 17:8528–8535, 1997

C H A P T E R   9

PERITRAUMATIC DISSOCIATION

Time Perception and Cerebellar Regulation of
Psychological, Interpersonal, and Biological Processes

ROBERT J. URSANO, M.D.
CAROL S. FULLERTON, PH.D.
DAVID M. BENEDEK, M.D.

Traumatic events place in stark relief the process of behavior change in response to environmental stressors. Behavior changes through experience and learning. It may be changed by positive life experiences, and it certainly changes after traumatic life events. However, the neurobiological processes governing behavior changes are still poorly understood.

PERITRAUMATIC DISSOCIATION

Dissociation at the time of a traumatic event—*peritraumatic dissociation*—is a poor prognostic sign (Shalev et al. 1996; Ursano and Fullerton 1999; Ursano et al. 1999b), increasing the risk of both acute and chronic post-traumatic stress disorder (PTSD; Birnes et al. 2003; Griffin et al. 1997; Marmar et al. 1997; Punamaki et al. 2005; Ursano et al. 1999b). In one study, those experiencing peritraumatic dissociation were 4.12 times more likely to have acute PTSD and 4.86 times more likely to develop chronic PTSD. The risk was independent of risk associated with prior PTSD (i.e., before a motor vehicle accident [MVA]; Ursano et al. 1999a).

A number of studies support the hypothesis that the risk for PTSD associated with peritraumatic dissociation is independent of general dissociative tendencies (Grieger et al. 2003; Marmar et al. 1994) and of the risk attributable to prior PTSD (Fullerton et al. 2000). However, few prospective studies have examined the predictors of peritraumatic dissociation. The relationship of this phenomenon to prior trauma, prior peritraumatic dissociation, prior PTSD, and prior major depression has not been well characterized.

Emergency workers who reported greater levels of peritraumatic dissociation after the 1989 San Francisco earthquake (Marmar et al. 1996) were younger, had a higher level of disaster exposure, perceived greater threat, had poorer general psychological adjustment, and had greater external locus of control. Prior trauma itself has been suggested as a risk factor for later peritraumatic dissociation (Marmar et al. 1996; Shalev et al. 1996); however, this has not been examined empirically. If prior trauma is a risk factor for peritraumatic dissociation, this relationship may be due to the presence of earlier episodes of peritraumatic dissociation or prior PTSD. Depression may also be a factor in peritraumatic dissociation (Ursano et al. 1999b). Individuals with mood disorders report high rates of dissociative symptoms, especially those related to transient sensory, cognitive, and affective phenomena even in intervals between illness episodes.

MVAs are an important cause of PTSD and also of the related but more transient acute stress disorder. In addition to occurring more immediately after a traumatic event, acute stress disorder requires the presence of peritraumatic dissociative symptoms. The rates of PTSD in victims of serious MVAs have ranged from 8% (Malt and Blikra 1993) to 46% (Blanchard et al. 1994). In one study, MVA survivors who reported the dissociative experiences of feeling numb or dazed at the time of the accident were at greater risk of chronic PTSD at 3 months and at 1 year later (Ehlers et al. 1998). Harvey and Bryant (1998) reported that MVA-related dissociative symptoms predicted chronic PTSD and that approximately 78% of MVA survivors with acute stress disorder developed PTSD 6 months after their MVA. Barton et al. (1996) compared a small sample of MVA victims with both acute stress disorder (diagnosed retrospectively) and subsequent PTSD with a sample of MVA victims with only PTSD. Findings suggested prior mood disorder (not major depression), previous Axis I disorders, and previous Axis II disorders predisposed MVA victims to acute stress disorder.

Changes in one's sense of time and place are common symptoms during a traumatic event, as is altered spatial memory, in which individuals describe feelings of "losing track of what is going on around me" and of feeling "detached." Altered sense of time, such as feeling that time either slowed down or sped up, is the most common peritraumatic dissociative

TABLE 9–1. Frequency of peritraumatic dissociative symptoms

Peritraumatic symptom	Frequency, *n* (%)
1. Losing track or blanking out	39 (32)
2. Acting on "automatic pilot"	31 (25)
3. Sense of time changed (slowing or speeding up)	69 (56)
4. Seemed unreal, like in a dream or play	48 (39)
5. Felt as if floating above scene	17 (14)
6. Felt disconnected from body or body distorted	19 (16)
7. Felt as though what happened to someone else was happening to self	1 (0.8)
8. Unaware of things that happened	32 (26)

Note. N=122
Source. Adapted from Ursano et al. 1999b.

symptom reported by individuals during or shortly after a traumatic event (Cardeña and Spiegel 1993; Noyes and Kletti 1997; Shalev et al. 1996; Terr 1984). Ursano et al. (1999b) examined peritraumatic dissociation following MVAs (*N*=122) in people with acute stress disorder. Using the Structured Clinical Interview for DSM-III-R and the Peritraumatic Dissociative Experiences Questionnaire—Rater Version, they found the most common peritraumatic symptom was sense of time change during the event, reported by slightly more than half the participants (*n*=69, 56%; see Table 9–1). Alteration in the perception of time is most often experienced as time slowed down. Peritraumatic dissociative symptoms reported by about one-third of subjects were 1) the event seemed unreal, as though a dream or play (*n*=48, 39%) and 2) moments of losing track or blanking out (*n*=39, 32%). The other four commonly reported peritraumatic dissociative symptoms (as listed in Table 9–1) were endorsed by 14%–26% of the study population. Twenty five percent reported one peritraumatic dissociative symptom, 19% reported two symptoms, 13% reported three symptoms, and 22% reported four or more symptoms. Younger subjects were more likely to experience peritraumatic dissociation, as were white versus nonwhite subjects and single versus married subjects. Younger subjects reported a greater number of peritraumatic dissociative symptoms, as did subjects with an injured passenger. After adjusting for age and passenger injury, prior major depression was significantly related to more peritraumatic dissociative symptoms. An interaction of age and prior major depression indicated that those who were younger and reported a history of major depression had the greatest number of peritraumatic dissociative symptoms (Fullerton et al. 2000; Ursano et al. 1999b).

CEREBELLAR REGULATION OF PERITRAUMATIC DISSOCIATION AND FEAR MEMORIES

Regulators operate to maintain diverse behavioral responses—from body temperature control to sleep-wake cycles. Biological and behavioral regulation is maintained by our neurobiology and interpersonal interactions. For example, the interpersonal environment, including the mother's voice (Hofer 1984, 1987) or the presence of a trusted other for a phobic child approaching a feared object, can operate as a critical regulator of arousal and fear. Like the thermostat on the wall, regulators at the interpersonal or neurobiological levels modulate complex systems and simultaneously explain more than one effect (e.g., heat and cold). Alterations in regulators can result in profound effects or subtle shifts in the level of function (Staab et al. 1999). Two prominent and clearly definable peritraumatic dissociative symptoms that often follow traumatic events are time perception changes (e.g., time seeming to go slower) and spatial memory changes (e.g., inability to recall the location of items or directions). These symptoms both describe alteration or deficits in processes that are usually automatic (or unconsciously accomplished). From the perspective described in the following section, these symptoms may represent altered modulator and regulator functions attributable to the cerebellum.

    The cerebellum—that part of the brain that in the past had been only associated with balance and coordination—may be a fundamental regulator in the response to trauma. The cerebellum is an important regulator of time, space awareness, and fear memory consolidation. Specifically, trauma (fear) related alterations in the perception of sense of time and space may be evidence of cerebellar dysregulation (Ursano and Fullerton 1999).

Sense of Time

Distortion of the sense of time has been examined in laboratory studies. Both the basal ganglia (Harrington et al. 1998) and cerebellum (Ivry and Spencer 2004; Jueptner et al. 1996; Meck 2005) have been linked to a brain timing system. Brain imaging studies have shown both decreased cerebellar blood flow (Mathew et al. 1998) and increased left cerebellar blood flow (Jueptner et al. 1996) associated with an altered sense of time. However, some studies do not support this idea (Harrington et al. 2004b). A recent investigation using event-related functional magnetic resonance imaging showed that timing sensitivity was related to activation of the left cerebellum along with the right caudate nucleus and the right inferior parietal cortex (Harrington et al. 2004a). Tetrahydrocannabinol (THC) receptors in particular may be related to altered time sense (Matthew et al. 1998). Interestingly, the endogenous cannabinoid system (in the amygdala) has also been related to control of fear extinction (Marsicano et al. 2002). For an endogenous time clock, the subjective experience of time speeding up would mean that the time clock regulator had slowed down—that is, each second took longer to pass and vice versa (McCrone 1997).

Spatial Memory

Both clinical and experimental studies suggest that the cerebellum and its network are involved in spatial processing. Three search strategies are generally described for spatial memory (Molinari et al. 1997). A *place strategy* depends on using an allocentric spatial map identifying markers based on their absolute relationships to each other. For example, a place strategy to locate a parked car in a parking lot may be "it is straight ahead, out the door 50 meters, and to the left." A *praxic strategy* is repeating specific sequences of movements covering the same distance and angles. This would be the equivalent of finding one's car in the parking lot by remembering "I turn left, then go 100 feet, turn right, and look to my left." Last, a *taxic strategy* can be used, whereby one approaches specific cues associated with the target, such as "I will remember that my car is parked near the tall tree." Thus spatial localization is a sequencing of cues or actions, much like the sequencing on which muscular movement is dependent. This has been one of the perspectives supporting cerebellar involvement in spatial memory—and more importantly, the experimental findings described in the following discussion.

Animal studies (Petrosini et al. 1996) have shown that hemicerebellectomized rats lose the ability to use praxic and taxic strategies but preserve place strategy for spatial memory tasks in the Morris water maze (Morris 1981). The spatial system appears to continue to operate when other systems of memory are lost. The deficit is in impaired memory acquisition rather than utilization—that is, the animals are fine if they have an already acquired internal "map." (The opposite observation has been made with hippocampal injury—that is, lesioned animals learn cues for location but cannot perform under a place strategy.) Thus, cerebellar- and perhaps basal ganglia–dependent aspects of spatial memory appear to be related to the procedural and performance-based aspects of spatial memory in contrast to the declarative representational-based components. This may be a result of the cerebellar contribution to the timing and ordering of cognitive functions (Ivry and Baldo 1992; Silveri et al. 1994).

Fear Memory Consolidation

Although the basolateral amygdala complex has been hypothesized to play a central role in fear conditioning, cerebellar processes have also been related to the elaboration and storage of emotion-laden memories in the brain in animal models (Thompson et al. 1997). Sacchetti et al. (2002) demonstrated that the interpositus nucleus and the cortex of the cerebellum are part of a wide network of brain regions responsible for associating emotional memory with behavior response. Bao et al. (1998) demonstrated that the absence of a brain-derived neurotrophic factor in cerebellar granule cells massively impaired conditioned response to painful stimuli, and they suggested that brain-derived neurotrophic factor may mediate cerebellar processes important in memory formation.

In summary, recent observations on the cerebellum indicate that 1) the cerebellum may be central to time sense, 2) cerebellar THC receptors may be specifically related to altered time sense, 3) endogenous cannabinoids may play a role in fear extinction, 4) spatial memory depends on cerebellar function, and 5) fear memory consolidation is dependent on specific areas of the cerebellum. Taken together, these findings suggest an important role for the cerebellum in peritraumatic dissociation, in particular the symptom of altered time sense and the development of "fear memories."

CONCLUSION

Disturbances in the regulation of our sense of time and space perception are important peritraumatic dissociation symptoms that predict the onset of posttraumatic stress and subsequent PTSD (*fear memory disorder* or perhaps better termed *impaired fear memory extinction/forgetting disorder*). The cerebellum appears to be a critical neurobiological component of one's sense of time and space and consolidation of fear memories, the disturbances of which are core symptoms and features of PTSD (see Figure 9–1). We know little about the interpersonal and developmental aspects of time and space awareness. The disturbance of sense of time has often been reported during or immediately after a traumatic event. It can be proposed that arousal or anxiety is the initiator of the alterations of time and spatial sense. Alternatively, these time-space alterations may be an indicator of a more general regulator disturbance that affects cognition, arousal, and memory elaboration. Brain imaging studies of cerebellar function in stressful settings may be able to delineate whether this brain region makes substantial contributions to the disturbances seen after traumatic events.

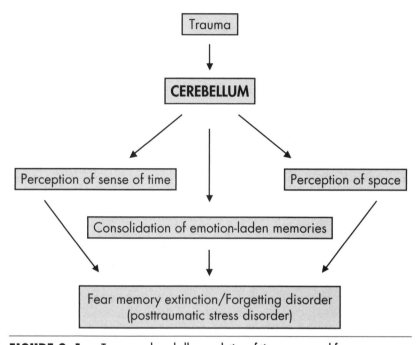

FIGURE 9–1. Trauma and cerebellar regulation of time, space, and fear memory consolidation.

Study of the relationship between onset conditions and the development of PTSD can offer new avenues for research and clinical intervention that studies of the chronic disorder may overlook. The transitory symptoms of loss of time and spatial sense do not appear to persist after the early period of the trauma exposure and therefore may not be evident in studies of chronic PTSD. Studies of chronic PTSD may identify sustaining factors of the illness rather than initiating factors. Prevention of chronic PTSD will require attention to the factors determining early onset symptoms of PTSD. The cerebellum may play a role in peritraumatic dissociation, particularly symptoms of time distortion and spatial memory, and therefore in the initiation of the PTSD process.

REFERENCES

Bao S, Chen L, Qiao X, et al: Impaired eye-blink conditioning in waggler, a mutant mouse with cerebellar BDNF deficiency. Learn Mem 5:355–364, 1998

Barton KA, Blanchard EB, Hickling EJ: Antecedents and consequences of acute stress disorder among motor vehicle accident victims. Behav Res Ther 34:805–813, 1996

Birnes P, Brunet. A, Carreras D et al: The predictive power of peritraumatic dissociation and acute stress symptoms for posttraumatic stress symptoms: a three-month prospective study. Am J Psychiatry 160:1337–1339, 2003

Blanchard EB, Hickling EJ, Taylor AE, et al: The psychological morbidity associated with motor vehicle accidents. Behav Res Ther 31:283–90, 1994

Cardeña E, Speigel D: Dissociative reactions to the San Francisco Bay Area earthquake of 1989. Am J Psychiatry 150:474–478, 1993

Ehlers A, Mayou RA, Bryant B: Psychological predictors of chronic posttraumatic stress disorder after motor vehicle accidents. J Abnorm Psychol 107:508–519, 1998

Fullerton CS, Ursano RJ, Epstein RS, et al: Peritraumatic dissociation following motor vehicle accidents: relationship to prior trauma and prior major depression. J Nerv Ment Dis 188:267–272, 2000

Grieger TA, Fullerton CS, Ursano RJ: Posttraumatic stress disorder, alcohol use, and perceived safety after the terrorist attack on the Pentagon. Psychiatr Serv 54:1380–1382, 2003

Griffin MG, Resick PA, Mechanic MB: Objective assessment of peritraumatic dissociation: psychophysiological indicators. Am J Psychiatry 154:1081–1088, 1997

Harrington DL, Haaland KY, Hermanowicz N: Temporal processing in the basal ganglia. Neuropsychology 12:1–10, 1998

Harrington DL, Boyd LA, Mayer AR, et al: Neural representation of interval encoding and decision making. Brain Res Cogn Brain Res 21:193–205, 2004a

Harrington DL, Lee RR, Boyd LA, et al: Does the representation of time depend on the cerebellum? Effect of cerebellar stroke. Brain 127:561–574, 2004b

Harvey AG, Bryant RA: The relationship between acute stress disorder and posttraumatic stress disorder: a prospective evaluation of motor vehicle accident survivors. J Consult Clin Psychol 66:507–512, 1998

Hofer MA: Relationships as regulators: a psychobiological perspective on bereavement. Psychosom Med 46:183–197, 1984

Hofer MA: Early social relationships: a psychobiologist's view. Child Dev 58:633–647, 1987

Ivry RB, Baldo JV: Is the cerebellum involved in learning and cognition? Curr Opin Neurobiol 2:212–216, 1992

Ivry RB, Spencer RM: The neural representation of time. Curr Opin Neurobiol 14:225–232, 2004

Jueptner M, Fleurich L, Weiller C, et al: The human cerebellum and temporal information processing: results from a PET experiment. Neuroreport 7:2761–2765, 1996

Malt UF, Blikra G: Psychosocial consequences of road accidents. Eur Psychiatry 8:227–28, 1993

Marmar CR, Weiss DS, Schlenger WE, et al: Peritraumatic dissociation and posttraumatic stress in male Vietnam theater veterans. Am J Psychiatry 151:902–907, 1994

Marmar CR, Weiss DS, Metzler TJ, et al: Characteristics of emergency services personnel related to peritraumatic dissociation during critical incident exposure. Am J Psychiatry 153:94–102, 1996

Marmar CR, Weiss DS, Metzler TJ: The Peritraumatic Dissociative Experiences Questionnaire, in Assessing Psychological Trauma and PTSD. Edited by Wilson JP, Keane TM. New York, Guilford, 1997, pp 412–428

Marsicano G, Wotjak CT, Azad SC, et al: The endogenous cannabinoid system controls extinction of aversive memories. Nature 418:530–534, 2002

Mathew RJ, Wilson WH, Turkington TG, et al: Cerebellar activity and disturbed time sense after THC. Brain Res 797:183–189, 1998

McCrone J: When a second lasts forever. New Scientist 156:52–56, 1997

Meck WH: Neuropsychology of timing and time perception. Brain Cogn 58:1–8, 2005

Molinari M, Petrosini L, Grammaldo LG: Spatial event processing, in The Cerebellum and Cognition (International Review of Neurobiology, Vol 14). Edited by Schmahmann JD. New York, Academic Press, 1997, pp 217–230

Morris RGM: Spatial localization does not require the presence of local cues. Learn Motiv 12:239–260, 1981

Noyes R, Kletti R: Depersonalization in response to life-threatening danger. Comp Psychiatry 18:375–384, 1997

Petrosini L, Molinari M, Dell'Anna ME: Cerebellar contribution to spatial event processing: Morris water maze and T-maze. Eur J Neurosci 8:1882–1896, 1996

Punamaki RL, Komproe IH, Quota S, et al: The role of peritraumatic dissociation and gender in the association between trauma and mental health in a Palestinian community sample. Am J Psychiatry 162:545–551, 2005

Sacchetti B, Baldi E, Lorenzi CA, et al: Cerebellar role in fear conditioning consolidation. Proc Natl Acad Sci 99:8406–8411, 2002

Shalev AY, Peri T, Canetti L, et al: Predictions of PTSD in injured trauma survivors: a prospective study. Am J Psychiatry 153:219–225, 1996

Silveri MC, Leggio MG, Molinari M: The cerebellum contributes to linguistic production: a case of agrammatic speech following a right cerebellar lesion. Neurology 44:2047–2050, 1994

Staab J, Fullerton CS, Ursano RJ: A critical look at PTSD: constructs, concepts, epidemiology, and implications, in Response to Disaster: Psychosocial, Community, and Ecological Approaches. Edited by Gist R, Lubin B. Bristol, PA, Taylor & Francis, 1999, pp 101–132

Terr LC: Time and trauma. Psychoanal Study Child 39:633–665, 1984

Thompson RF, Bao S, Chen L, et al: Associative learning, in The Cerebellum and Cognition (International Review of Neurobiology, Vol 14). Edited by Schmahmann JD. New York, Academic Press, 1997, pp 151–189

Ursano RJ, Fullerton CS: Posttraumatic stress disorder: cerebellar regulation of psychological, interpersonal and biological responses to trauma? Psychiatry 62:325–328, 1999

Ursano RJ, Fullerton CS, Epstein RS, et al: Acute and chronic posttraumatic stress disorder in motor vehicle accident victims. Am J Psychiatry 156:589–595, 1999a

Ursano RJ, Fullerton CS, Epstein RS, et al: Peritraumatic dissociation and posttraumatic stress disorder after motor vehicle accidents. Am J Psychiatry 156:1808–1810, 1999b

CHAPTER 10

POSTTRAUMATIC STRESS DISORDER SYMPTOM PROVOCATION AND NEUROIMAGING

Heterogeneity of Response

RUTH A. LANIUS, M.D., PH.D.
ROBYN BLUHM, M.A.
ULRICH LANIUS, PH.D.

Dissociation is commonly observed in individuals who have experienced psychological trauma. Acute dissociative responses to psychological trauma have been found to predict the later development of chronic posttraumatic stress disorder (PTSD) (Bremner and Brett 1997; Bremner et al. 1992; Koopman et al. 1994; Marmar et al. 1994; Shalev et al. 1996). Moreover, individuals who experience acute dissociative responses to psychological trauma have been shown to develop a chronic pattern of dissociation in response to minor stressors or reminders of the original trauma (Bremner 1999). Bremner (1999) hypothesized that there may be two subtypes of acute trauma response, one primarily dissociative and the other predominantly intrusive and hyperaroused, that represent unique pathways to chronic stress-related psychopathology. Neuroimaging studies by Lanius et al. (2001, 2002, 2005) have shown that these two subtypes of response persist, occurring in individuals with chronic PTSD upon exposure to reminders of traumatic events.

This chapter discusses the neuroimaging literature on the heterogeneity of response to traumatic reminders in PTSD. Comparison of dissociative phenomena in PTSD with those observed in other psychiatric conditions, as well as neurological conditions, together with a broader understanding of the nature of dissociation in PTSD itself, may lead to a deeper understanding of the alterations in neural functioning that are associated with PTSD.

DEFINING DISSOCIATION

DSM-IV-TR defines *dissociation* as "a disruption in the usually integrated functions of consciousness, memory, identity, or perception of the environment. The disturbance may be sudden or gradual, transient or chronic" (American Psychiatric Association 2000, p. 477). Dissociation has been shown to be etiologically connected to psychological trauma (Boon and Draijer 1993; Coons 1994; Kluft 1995; Lewis et al. 1997; Nijenhuis et al. 1998). Dissociation in response to psychological trauma promotes a discontinuity between conscious experience and memory. There are two broad components to this discontinuity: detachment from the overwhelming emotional content of the experience and a compartmentalization of the experience (Allen 2001; van der Kolk 1996). As a result, the traumatic experience is not integrated into a unitary whole or into an integrated sense of self. Several authors (e.g., Bremner et al. 1992; Butler et al. 1996; Nijenhuis et al. 2002; Spiegel 1997) have seen this disruption as serving a protective function in response to acute or chronic stress.

Dissociation may include alterations in perception, emotion, cognition, and behavior. For instance, perceptual alterations may occur in the experience of time (e.g., flashback; see Chapter 9 in this volume, "Peritraumatic Dissociation"); in changes in self-experience (e.g., depersonalization), and in the perception of reality (e.g., derealization). Similarly, cognitive abnormalities of dissociation can include amnesia, fugue states, confusional states, and deficits in attention. Somatic or sensory motor and behavioral changes can involve sensory distortions, motor weakness, paralysis, ataxia, tremors, shaking, and convulsions.

Van der Kolk et al. (1996) described primary, secondary, and tertiary types of dissociation in an attempt to classify the wide range of phenomena experienced by traumatized individuals with dissociative experiences. *Primary dissociation* refers to the fragmented nature of traumatic memories, such as observed during flashback experiences. It has been well established that the imprints of traumatic experiences are initially dissociated and retrieved as sensory fragments that have little linguistic component (van der Kolk 1996). *Secondary dissociation* is the subtype of dissociation that most closely resembles the DSM-IV-TR definition cited earlier. It includes alterations in the experience of time, place, and person. Symptoms such as depersonalization, derealization, altered body image, tunnel vision, altered pain perception, and peritraumatic dissociation are included in this category. *Tertiary dissociation* includes the expression of distinct ego states, as observed in dissociative identity disorder.

SYMPTOM PROVOCATION NEUROIMAGING STUDIES IN POSTTRAUMATIC STRESS DISORDER

Heterogeneity of Response

When we first began studying the neural correlates of traumatic memory recall in our laboratory, we realized that patients can have distinctly different responses to recalling memories of their traumatic experiences. The first patient we studied told us that as soon as she tried to recall her traumatic experience, she felt as though she were outside of her body watching herself. She also described herself as feeling completely disconnected from the emotional content of the traumatic memory. Her heart rate showed a small decline from baseline. Our research group was extremely surprised by this response, particularly because the literature on traumatic recall in PTSD patients focused on the experience of intrusive sensory and emotional fragments of the traumatic event. We therefore decided to pursue these pilot findings through a more systematic investigation and divided our subsequent subjects into two groups based on whether their response to script-driven imagery was primarily one of hyperarousal (or reliving the event or aspects of the event) or dissociation.

Some patients have also reported experiencing some symptoms of dissociation despite having a response to script-driven imagery that is primarily characterized by hyperarousal and reliving symptoms. Although extreme dissociative symptoms, like dissociative disorders, have been linked to the experience of severe and chronic abuse, often beginning in childhood, it is not yet clear what characteristics are common to patients who experience these "mixed" responses (see Chapter 4 in this volume, "Relationships Between Dissociation and Posttraumatic Stress Disorder"). The approximately 30% of patients in our studies who respond to trauma reminders by dissociating do tend to report histories of chronic abuse. Further research, however, will be required to tease out the factors that are associated with milder dissociative responses to script-driven imagery. Some of the possible factors may be age, gender, experience of peritraumatic dissociation, time since trauma, type of trauma, presence of comorbid conditions, trait anxiety, and variability in baseline psychophysiological reactivity. In some cases, too, patients may respond in one manner at one time and in the other at a later time, for example, generally responding to trauma reminders with hyperarousal but sometimes dissociating. Because this involves differences in response over time, this type of variation cannot generally be captured in a single neuroimaging session and must therefore be noted in a screening session. The strength of the link between having a phenomenological experience of hyperarousal/flashback/reliving and psychophysiological reactivity also requires further investigation.

Over the past several years, a number of neuroimaging script-driven symptom provocation studies have appeared in the PTSD literature. Most of these studies focus on patients who experience a pattern of response characterized by flashbacks or a hyperarousal response. Patients often report that the memories of the trauma they experience are more vivid and have a stronger sensory character than normal memories. They also tend to experience emotional and autonomic arousal. This pattern of response is similar to what van der Kolk et al. (1996) described as primary dissociation. We have found, however, that approximately 30% of patients with PTSD experience a different response to traumatic cues, one that is characteristic of van der Kolk et al.'s secondary dissociation (Lanius et al. 2002, 2005). In these patients, exposure to trauma-related cues results in feelings of "leaving their body," or of experiencing their traumatic memory "at a distance." In many of these patients, there is no increase in heart rate during traumatic script-driven imagery, and they also exhibit a very different pattern of brain activation than the hyperaroused/flashback/reliving patients.

The Hyperarousal/Flashback/Reliving Response

Compared with control subjects, patients who had a hyperarousal/flashback/reliving response and relived their traumatic experience after being exposed to the traumatic script showed an average increase in heart rate of 12 bpm and reported significantly higher levels of anger, fear, disgust, sadness, guilt, and shame while recalling the traumatic memory (Lanius et al. 2001). This group of PTSD subjects showed significantly less activation of the thalamus, anterior cingulate gyrus (Brodmann's area [BA] 32), medial prefrontal cortex (mPFC; BA 10,11), and inferior frontal gyrus (BA 47) than did healthy control subjects (Lanius et al. 2001) (see Figure 10–1). Altered levels of anterior cingulate activation and medial prefrontal activation are consistent with positron emission tomography (PET) studies of sexual abuse and combat-related

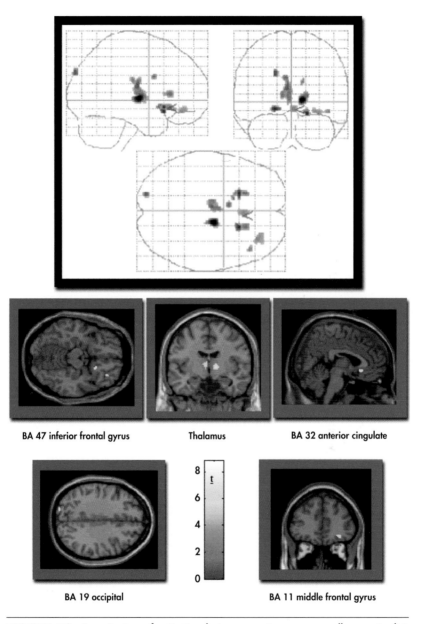

FIGURE 10–1. Regions of activation during traumatic memory recall versus implicit baseline in which the comparison group shows greater activation than the hyperarousal/flashback/reliving posttraumatic stress disorder group.

Corrected for multiple comparisons, $P<0.001$, maximum cluster siz=10 voxels ($2\times2\times2$ mm). Comparison group, $n=10$; posttraumatic stress disorder group, $n=11$. The center gradient bar shows the approximate t value for regions of activation depicted on the figure.

PTSD (Bremner et al. 1999a, 1999b; Lanius et al. 2001, 2002, 2003b; Liberzon et al. 1999; Shin et al. 1997, 1999, 2004).

Functional Connectivity During Hyperarousal/Flashback/Reliving States

More recently, we have conducted an analysis of the connections between different brain regions involved in the response to script-driven imagery seen in PTSD patients with hyperarousal/flashback/reliving responses compared with control subjects (Lanius et al. 2004). The "subtraction analyses" usually used in PTSD neuroimaging studies to date are able to delineate specific brain regions involved in different responses to traumatic script-driven imagery; however, functional connectivity analyses are required to assess interregional brain activity correlations. Abnormal connectivity among regions involved in different responses to the recall of traumatic material may be an important means of studying the neuronal networks underlying hyperarousal/flashback/reliving versus dissociative responses.

Functional connectivity analyses of patients experiencing hyperarousal/flashback/reliving responses to the traumatic script showed markedly different patterns of brain activation. PTSD subjects showed neural networks consistent with a nonverbal pattern of memory recall (i.e., occipital lobes, right parietal lobe, and posterior cingulate gyrus) as compared with control subjects who showed neural networks more consistent with verbal patterns of memory retrieval (i.e., left prefrontal and anterior cingulate) (BA 32) (see Figure 10–2). Cabeza and Nyberg (2000, 2003) suggested that prefrontal activations during episodic memory retrieval have sometimes been shown to be bilateral but show a clear tendency for right lateralization. It has been hypothesized that anterior cingulate activation during memory recall is related to language processes, because activation of this area is more frequent for verbal than nonverbal materials. For nonverbal episodic memory retrieval, however, occipital, right parietal, and posterior cingulate activations have been shown to predominate.

Key Brain Areas Involved in Hyperarousal/Flashback/Reliving Responses

Emerging evidence from the PTSD symptom provocation neuroimaging literature has shown that several key brain areas, including the anterior cingulate gyrus, the mPFC, the amygdala, and the thalamus are involved in the pathophysiology underlying PTSD. Therefore, the functional significance of each of these areas in context with the symptomatology of PTSD is reviewed in the following sections.

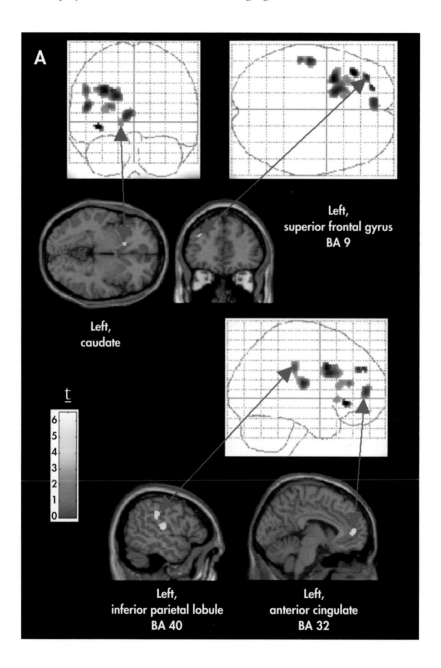

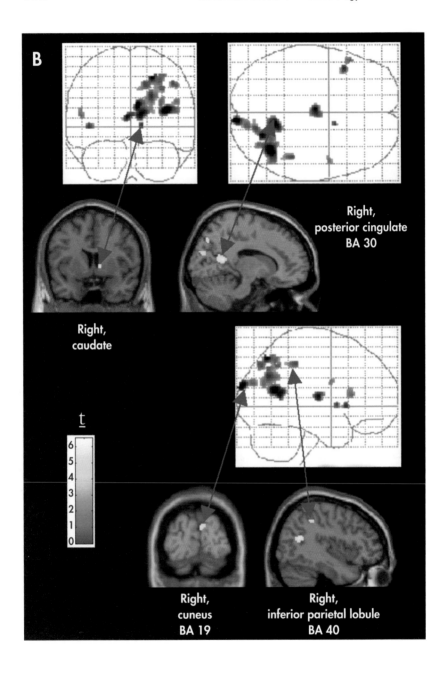

FIGURE 10–2. Analyses of connectivity patterns underlying the response to script-driven imagery in posttraumatic stress disorder (PTSD) subjects with hyperarousal/flashback/reliving responses compared with traumatized subjects without PTSD. *(Pages 197–198)*

(A) Comparison of PTSD and comparison psychophysiological internaction maps between right anterior cingulate gyrus (Talairach coordinates x=2, y=20, z=36) and traumatic script-driven imagery in which comparison subjects (*n*=13) showed greater levels of brain activation than the PTSD subjects (*n*=11). (B) Comparison of PTSD and comparison PPI maps between right anterior cingulate gyrus (Talairach coordinates x=2, y=20, z=36) and traumatic script-driven imagery in which PTSD subjects (*n*=11) showed greater levels of brain activation than comparison subjects (*n*=11). The glass brains show an overlay of all significant activations; the cross-sectional images show areas of interest in which the *t* values are represented by the color of the activation site.

Source. Reprinted from Lanius RA, Williamson PC, Densmore M, et al.: "The Nature of Traumatic Memories: A 4-T fMRI Functional Connectivity Analysis." *American Journal of Psychiatry* 160:1–9, 2004. Copyright 2004, American Psychiatric Association. Used with permission.

Anterior cingulate cortex. The anterior cingulate gyrus is thought to play a key role in a number of functions, including the representation of subjective experience, the integration of bodily responses with behavioral demands (Critchley et al. 2002), and emotion (Lane et al. 1998). Animal research has suggested that the anterior cingulate gyrus has extensive connections with multiple brain structures, including the amygdala, hypothalamus, nucleus accumbens, ventral tegmental area, substantia nigra, raphe, locus coeruleus, periaqueductal grey, and brain stem autonomic nuclei (Carmichael and Price 1995; Frysztak and Neafsey 1994; Neafsey et al. 1993; Sesack and Pickel 1992; Sesack et al. 1989). Thus, the anterior cingulate gyrus appears to be part of a complex system coordinating the autonomic, neuroendocrine, and behavioral aspects of emotional response. It may also play a key role in the visceral aspects of emotion (Vogt and Gabriel 1993). These functions suggest that the altered levels of activity of the anterior cingulate gyrus observed in patients with PTSD on exposure to reminders of trauma may contribute to emotional dysregulation. Emotional dysregulation in these patients includes extremes of reexperiencing and avoiding emotionally distressing memories as well as generalized problems with physiological hyperarousal and emotional numbing.

Medial prefrontal cortex. The mPFC has been hypothesized to play a role in the extinction of conditioned fear responses (Morgan et al. 1993). This region has also been shown to suppress the stress response that is mediated by the hypothalamic-pituitary-adrenal axis (Crane et al. 2003).

PET studies have shown negative correlations between blood flow in the left prefrontal cortex and the amygdala (Davidson and Sutton 1995; Drevets et al. 1992). Moreover, the mPFC may exert inhibitory influences over the limbic system, including the amygdala in PTSD (Shin et al. 2004; but also see Gilboa et al. 2004).

The mPFC has also been shown to play an important role in the retrieval of episodic memory (Tulving et al. 1994) and may be involved in the temporal segregation of memories (Schnider et al. 2000). Moscovitch and Winocur (2002) described this function as ensuring that "currently relevant memories can be differentiated from memories that may have been relevant once but are no longer" (p. 202). Thus, the mPFC may be in part responsible for the "timeless" nature of the traumatic memories experienced by many PTSD patients.

Thalamus. In PTSD patients with a hyperarousal/flashback/reliving response to traumatic script-driven imagery, the thalamus has been shown to be less active than in control subjects (Lanius et al. 2001; Liberzon et al. 1999). Several studies have reported thalamic dysfunction in PTSD (Bremner et al. 1999b; Lanius et al. 2001, 2003b; Liberzon et al. 1996), but this is by no means consistent across all studies. Possible factors that may account for such discrepancies between studies include 1) differences in the response variables measured in different studies (e.g., metabolism, blood oxygenation) and their relative time courses, 2) variability in scanner resolution, and 3) variability in the details of the experimental paradigm (e.g., chronicity of illness of PTSD subjects, comorbidity, type of trauma).

The thalamus relays information from all sensory modalities, except for olfaction, to the cerebral cortex. It has also been suggested that the thalamus is involved in mediating the interaction between attention and arousal (Portas et al. 1998), both of which are clearly relevant to the phenomenology of traumatic stress syndromes. High levels of arousal during traumatic experiences may lead to alterations in sensory processing in the thalamus (Krystal et al. 1995). This in turn disrupts transmission of sensory information to the frontal cortex, cingulate gyrus, amygdala, and hippocampus and is one mechanism that has been hypothesized to underlie dissociative symptoms (Krystal et al. 1998). Alterations in sensory processing may be one of the mechanisms underlying flashbacks in PTSD.

An interesting approach that has been put forward suggests that the inability to integrate memories into the present context may be related to disruptions in thalamus-mediated temporal cognitive binding, "a temporally coherent event that binds, in the time domain, the fractured components of external and internal reality into a single construct...the 'self'"

(Llinas 2002, p. 126; see also Joliot et al. 1994). Such a lack of temporal cognitive binding and the resulting lack of corticothalamic dialogue may be a process underlying flashback experiences or primary dissociation (van der Hart et al. 1998; van der Kolk et al. 1996). This phenomenon has been described as an inability to integrate the totality of what is happening into personal memory and identity. Therefore these memories remain isolated from ordinary consciousness. Such a conceptualization raises the question of whether dynamic state changes in the corticothalamic system may account for the fragmented nature of memory observed in PTSD and whether PTSD is a neuropsychiatric disorder that can be characterized by thalamocortical dysrhythmia (Llinas et al. 1998).

Amygdala. The amygdala is another structure that has been implicated in the pathophysiology of PTSD, with several neuroimaging studies reporting an increase in amygdala activation (Liberzon et al. 1999; Pissiota et al. 2002; Rauch et al. 1996, 2000; Shin et al. 1997). However, we and others have not found altered amygdala activation (Bremner et al. 1999a, 1999b; Lanius et al. 2001, 2002, 2003; Shin et al. 1999). Although we have not found amygdala dysfunction in the studies conducted in our laboratory, this may be due to differences in activation patterns in individual subjects. In a recent case study, we described the response to traumatic script-driven imagery of two subjects (husband and wife), both of whom developed acute PTSD secondary to a motor vehicle accident (Lanius et al. 2003a). Although both subjects experienced the identical stressor, their subjective, psychophysiological, and neurobiological responses to traumatic script-driven imagery were significantly different. The husband exhibited a hyperarousal/flashback/reliving response with concomitant amygdala activation, and the wife showed a numbing response with no concomitant amygdala activation.

One possible explanation for the divergent findings with respect to amygdala activation in PTSD subjects is also suggested by Williams et al. (2001). This group examined the amygdala response to fearful faces in normal adults and demonstrated that two distinct response systems may be implicated in this task, depending on arousal levels. During individual trials in which exposure to these faces was accompanied by arousal, as measured by a change in skin conductance, activation occurred in the amygdala and in the mPFC. In contrast, in trials in which there was no skin conductance response, activity was seen instead in the hippocampus and lateral prefrontal cortex. These authors hypothesized that their data reflect two distinct types of processing of fearful stimuli, which they described as involving networks associated with visceral experience versus declarative fact. If this hypothesis is true, then future studies in PTSD patients may find more consistency in amygdala response by measuring arousal levels. The amygdala has also been shown to play a crucial role in fear conditioning and contextual learning (Le Doux 2002). In addition, the basolateral amygdala appears to play a role in stress-mediated alterations of memory, including postevent memory consolidation (Cahill 2000), which is of particular relevance in PTSD.

Dissociative Responses

Some of the PTSD subjects in our study who experienced dissociative responses to the traumatic script-driven imagery (Lanius et al. 2002, 2005) described their experience during the procedure by saying "I was looking down at myself from above," "I was detached from my body," "I was completely zoned out and floating," or "I was emotionless." All of the PTSD patients had chronic histories of emotional, physical, and/or sexual abuse beginning in childhood and often continuing to the present. They also reported that dissociation was a defense they had used throughout their lives to escape overwhelming experiences. Unlike the group of patients who experienced a hyperarousal/flashback/reliving response to reminders of a traumatic experience, the patients who had a dissociative response did not show a mean increase in heart rate. In fact, there was variability of autonomic response in these patients, with some subjects showing decreases in heart rate, and others showing increases.

In contrast to subjects experiencing a hyperarousal/flashback/reliving response to the traumatic script-driven imagery, patients who responded to the traumatic script with a dissociative response exhibited higher levels of brain activation in the superior and middle temporal gyri (BA 38), the inferior frontal gyrus (BA 47), the occipital lobe (BA 19), the parietal lobe (BA 7), the medial frontal gyrus (BA 10), the mPFC (BA 9), and the anterior cingulate gyrus (BA 24 and BA 32) (see Figure 10–3). The results of increased brain activation in all of these areas in dissociative PTSD patients are consistent with previous findings of increased global cerebral blood flow in the frontal lobes and anterior cingulate gyrus in tetrahydrocannabinol-induced depersonalization (Mathew et al. 1999) and of increased activation of the frontal cortex in patients with depersonalization disorder (Hollander et al. 1992). In addition, changes in metabolism in parietal area BA 7B and occipital area BA 19 during states of depersonalization in DSM-IV-TR depersonalization disorder (Simeon et al. 2000) and in dissociative identity disorder (Reinders et al. 2003; see Chapter 11 in this volume, "Psychobiology of Traumatization and Trauma-Related Structural Dissociation of the Personality," for further discussion) have been reported. In two studies of patients with dis-

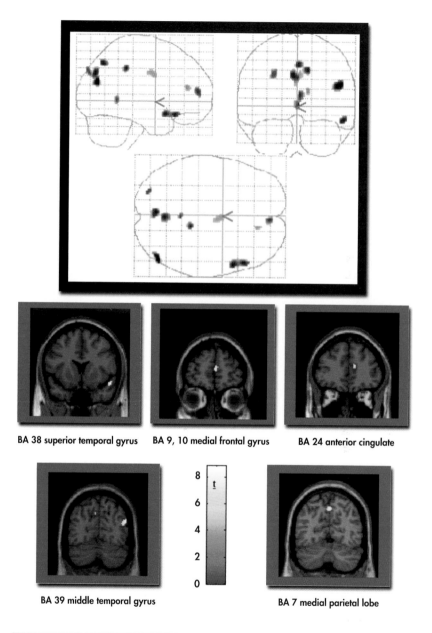

FIGURE 10–3. Regions of activation during traumatic memory recall versus implicit baseline in which the dissociated PTSD group shows greater activation than the comparison group.

Corrected for multiple comparisons, $P<0.001$, maximum cluster size = 10 voxels ($2\times2\times2$ mm). Comparison group, $n=10$; posttraumatic stress disorder (PTSD) group, $n=10$.

sociative identity disorder, increased activation was also reported in the left temporal lobes (Sar et al. 2000; Saxe et al. 1992).

In comparison with studies of the hyperarousal/flashback/reliving response in PTSD, there are few neuroimaging studies of dissociative phenomena, and the majority of these do not use symptom provocation paradigms, as is common in most PTSD research. Care must therefore be taken when generalizing from studies that examine dissociative states in patients with disorders other than PTSD (such as epilepsy or depersonalization disorder). Even in cases in which the patients have a history of trauma, differences in the way in which dissociative symptoms are elicited may be associated with differences in the brain regions involved. For example, the study by Reinders et al. (2003) examining subjects with dissociative identity disorder subsequent to a history of trauma included only subjects who could voluntarily "switch" between personality states and who did not remember the traumatic events presented during the scanning session when in their "apparently normal" personality state. By contrast, the subjects in our studies remembered their traumatic event but dissociated involuntarily when reminded of the event during the script-driven imagery session.

Functional Connectivity During Dissociative States

Analyses of connectivity patterns underlying the response to script-driven imagery seen in PTSD patients with dissociative responses compared with control subjects have also been conducted (Lanius et al. 2005). Differences in connectivity patterns involving the insula were observed, with activation in the right insula in dissociated PTSD subjects, but not in control subjects, correlating with activity in the left ventrolateral thalamus (see Figure 10–4). The insula has been shown to receive signals related to pain states, body temperature, and visceral sensations as well as signals regarding the state of the smooth musculature in blood vessels and other viscera (Craig 2003).

Damasio (1999) emphasized the role of the insula and the somatosensory cortices in processing signals regarding bodily state and suggested that these signals form the basis for emotions. The dissociative PTSD subjects in this study reported that they experienced both changes in their perception of their own bodily states and an inability to feel emotion. In a PET study investigating brain activity during self-generated emotion, Damasio et al. (2000) found insula activation across a range of emotions. Bilateral activation of the insula was seen during recall of memories causing sadness and anger, whereas right hemispheric activation was seen during recall of happiness and fear. In this study, subjects

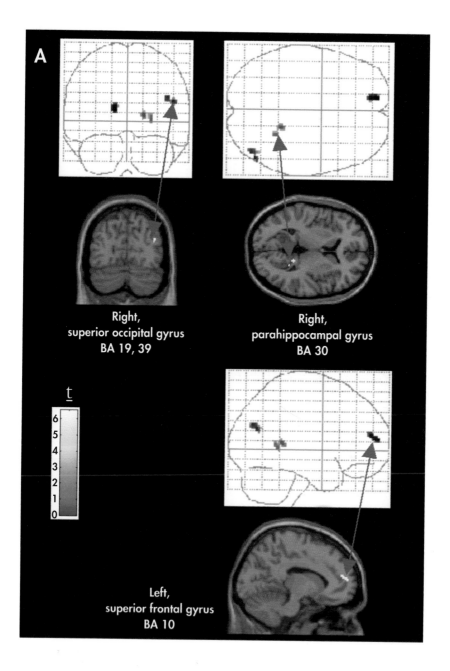

Right,
superior occipital gyrus
BA 19, 39

Right,
parahippocampal gyrus
BA 30

Left,
superior frontal gyrus
BA 10

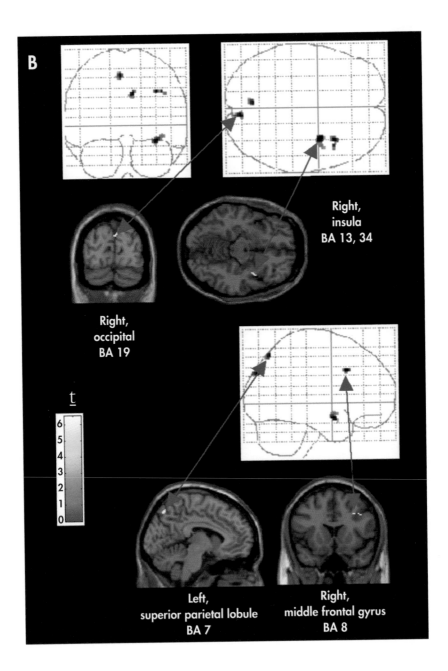

FIGURE 10–4. Analyses of connectivity patterns underlying the response to script-driven imagery in posttraumatic stress disorder (PTSD) subjects with dissociative responses compared with traumatized subjects without PTSD. *(Pages 205–206)*

(A) Brain regions with activation showing significantly greater functional connectivity/covariation with activation in the left thalamus in traumatized subjects without PTSD than in PTSD subjects with dissociative responses during recall of a traumatic event. **(B)** Brain regions with activation showing significantly greater functional connectivity/covariation with activation in the left thalamus in PTSD subjects with dissociative responses than in traumatized subjects without PTSD during recall of a traumatic event.

Areas of functional connectivity/covariation determined by the statistical parametric map of the *t* statistic (SPM[t]) showing the psychophysiological interaction between activity in the left thalamus (Talairach coordinates $x=-14$, $y=-16$, $z=4$) and activity in other brain regions. The grid diagrams show all areas with significantly greater covariation in the subjects without **(A)** or with **(B)** PTSD. The cross-sectional brain images show sites of significant covariation in areas of interest.

Source. Reprinted from Lanius RA, Williamson PC, Bluhm RL, et al.: "Functional Connectivity of Dissociative Responses in Posttraumatic Stress Disorder: A Functional Magnetic Resonance Imaging Investigation," *Biological Psychiatry* 57:873–884, 2005. Copyright 2005, with permission from American Society of Biological Psychiatry.

were healthy volunteers, and care was taken (using both subjective reports and objective measures of psychophysiological arousal) to ensure that subjects were actually experiencing the required emotion during data acquisition. The dissociated PTSD subjects in our study, however, reported difficulties in feeling emotions. Thus the insula activation seen in this study may reflect this altered perception or, possibly, alterations in the "body map" constructed by the insula, which has been hypothesized by Damasio (1999) to contribute to emotional experiences.

Key Brain Areas Involved in Dissociative Processes in Posttraumatic Stress Disorder

Even though the neuroimaging literature on dissociation has been sparse, emerging evidence is beginning to show several important brain areas to be involved in the pathophysiology underlying dissociation, including the prefrontal cortex, the temporal cortex, the parietal cortex, the anterior cingulate gyrus, and the amygdala. The functional significance of each of these areas in context with dissociative symptomatology is reviewed in the following sections.

Insula. Our finding of differences in functional connectivity between the right insula and the left ventrolateral thalamus in dissociative PTSD patients and in healthy control subjects is interesting in light of the insula's role in two processes relevant to the dissociative response: perception of bodily processes (interoception) and perception of emotions. Critchley et al. (2001) also investigated the role of the insula in the perception of internal states. These investigators measured state-dependent regional brain activity in subjects with pure autonomic failure; such patients cannot modulate their bodily state via the autonomic nervous system due to peripheral autonomic degeneration. Subjects with pure autonomic failure showed less activity in the right insula and left somatosensory cortex than did healthy control subjects. These differences occurred consistently across a number of task conditions, indicating that they are due to an alteration in the cortical mapping of bodily states rather than to a task-specific response. Together with Damasio's findings of insula activation in recall of emotional states discussed earlier, it may be that the alterations in bodily state and in emotional response to memories experienced by dissociative PTSD subjects are mediated in part by insula activity.

Temporal cortex. The temporal cortex has multiple functions, including the processing of auditory information as well as aspects of learning, memory, and emotion. In epilepsy, dissociative experiences have been reported to occur during seizures with various foci in either the right or the left hemisphere, including the temporal lobes (Devinsky et al. 1989; Kenna and Sedman 1965). One reported series of 32 cases of patients with temporal lobe epilepsy included 11 individuals who exhibited symptoms of depersonalization—4 with a left-sided focus, 3 with a right-sided focus, and 4 with general dysrhythmia (Kenna and Sedman 1965). Another report of 71 epileptic patients in whom dissociative symptoms were quantified noted that depersonalization was most commonly induced by partial complex seizures, in particular in those with left-sided foci (Devinsky et al. 1989). Scores on the Dissociative Experiences Scale in this patient population were lower than those seen in patients with psychiatric dissociative disorders.

Work by Penfield and Rasmussen (1957) examining the effects of direct stimulation of the temporal lobe during surgery shows depersonalization symptoms associated with stimulation of the superior and middle temporal gyrus. Patients reported "queer sensations of not being present and floating away" and "far off and out of this world" in response to stimulation of the superior and middle temporal gyrus, respectively. Penfield and Rasmussen (1957) suggested that depersonalization involves an "alteration in the usual mechanism of comparison of immediate sensory perception with memory records" (cited in Simeon et al. 2000, p. 1782).

Teicher and others have explored the relationship between early abuse and limbic system dysfunction as measured by the Limbic System Checklist-33 (Teicher et al. 1993). This symptom checklist includes symptoms often experienced by people with temporal lobe epilepsy (Teicher et al. 1993). Changes in brain activation in the superior and middle temporal gyri may therefore contribute to the dissociative responses that patients experience while recalling their traumatic experience.

Parietal and occipital cortex. The parietal and occipital cortices play an important role in the processing of sensory information. Such processing begins in modality-specific primary sensory areas and continues in association areas that may be either unimodal or polymodal and in the prefrontal cortex (Fuster and Joaquin 2003). The alterations in activation in the occipital area BA 19 and the parietal area BA 7 observed in dissociative PTSD patients and subjects with depersonalization disorder (Lanius et al. 2002; Simeon et al. 2000) may underlie the lack of integration of sensory experience that is characteristic of dissociative symptoms.

Corticolimbic Model of Dissociation

Sierra and Berrios (1998) proposed a corticolimbic model of dissociation in which depersonalization is thought to occur due to corticolimbic disconnection. They suggested that left medial prefrontal activation with reciprocal amygdala inhibition results in hypoemotionality and decreased arousal on traumatic reminders. However, it has been proposed that right dorsolateral prefrontal cortex activation with reciprocal anterior cingulate inhibition leads to hypervigilance, attentional difficulties, and emptiness of mental contents. In support of their model, Sierra and Berrios cited evidence for medial prefrontal involvement in both the monitoring and modulation of emotions (Damasio 1994; Reiman et al. 1997). In this model, the mPFC inhibits emotional processing on limbic structures (the amygdala) once a threshold of anxiety is reached. This in turn leads to a dampening of sympathetic output and reduced emotional experiencing.

Several studies have suggested that the prefrontal cortex has inhibitory influences on the emotional limbic system, including PET studies showing a negative correlation between blood flow in the left prefrontal cortex and the amygdala (Davidson and Sutton 1995; Drevets et al. 1992;

TABLE 10–1.   Main subtypes of response to recall of traumatic events

	Phenomenology	Autonomic response	Brain activation in key regions
Hyperarousal/ Flashback/ Reliving response	Subjects experience emotional and attentional hyperarousal as well as reexperiencing aspects of the traumatic event as emotional or sensory fragments.	Tendency toward increased heart rate; may have increased galvanic skin response and/or systolic or diastolic blood pressure	↓Anterior cingulate ↓Medial prefrontal cortex ↑Amygdala ↓Thalamus
Dissociative response	Subjects may report feeling emotionally distant from the event or having no emotions at all. They may also report alterations in their experience of their body, in intensity or quality of visual or auditory stimuli, or in perception of time. Some feel completely disconnected from their body.	Variable heart rate response; rate may increase, decrease, or remain unchanged from baseline Increased heart rate is the least common response observed in these patients and, when it occurs, is a smaller increase than that observed in patients who experience a hyperarousal/flashback/ reliving response.	↑Temporal cortex ↑Parietal/occipital cortex ↑Anterior cingulate ↑Medial prefrontal cortex ↑Insula

Shin et al. 2004). Our findings partially lend support to the above model proposed by Sierra and Berrios (1998). The dissociative PTSD patients showed increased activation in the medial frontal cortex (BA 10). They also did not exhibit increased amygdala activation. Increased activation of the mPFC may underlie the lack of autonomic response observed in these patients (Lanius et al. 2002).

CONCLUSION

In summary, research suggests that PTSD patients can have very different responses to traumatic script-driven imagery, and these differences may shed light on key biological dimensions of the disorder (see Table 10–1). In our functional neuroimaging studies of PTSD, approximately 70% of patients relived their traumatic experience and showed an increase in heart rate while recalling the traumatic memory (Lanius et al. 2001, 2004), whereas the other 30% showed a dissociative response with variable heart rate changes. (Lanius et al. 2002, 2005) Our findings are consistent with Bremner's previous hypothesis describing two subtypes of acute trauma response—one primarily dissociative and the other characterized predominantly by intrusions and hyperarousal—each of which represents unique pathways to chronic stress-related psychopathology (Bremner 1999). Moreover, the results support the suggestion by Foa et al. (1995) that our understanding of posttrauma psychopathology may be hindered when PTSD subjects with different symptom patterns are grouped in the same diagnostic category. The functional neuroimaging findings described in this chapter also suggest that different neuronal mechanisms may generate these two distinct reactions and that the heterogeneity of neurobiological, physiological, and phenomenological responses to traumatic reminders in PTSD needs to be addressed in the designs of functional imaging studies.

Further investigation may also help to elucidate the factors that are associated with differences in response. Although dissociative symptoms and disorders have been historically linked with chronicity of abuse/trauma exposure, we do not yet know why some patients experience a dissociative response to script-driven imagery. Although anecdotally it appears that many of these patients do experience particularly severe or prolonged abuse, it is likely that the complete story is more complex than this. For example, some of our patients who participated in the script-driven imagery protocol twice had a hyperarousal response on one occasion and a dissociative response on the other. Other patients have reported experiencing both reliving sensory or emotional aspects of their traumatic event and dissociative symptoms. Future research may clarify how common these mixed patterns of response are and may also allow us to elucidate the conditions that are more likely to underlie a hyperarousal/flashback/reliving versus a dissociative response in the same patient. In terms of clinical applications of this research, it may also be beneficial to design studies that examine the effects of standard and novel PTSD treatments on both hyperarousal/flashback/reliving as well as dissociative responses in an attempt to refine our treatment strategies for specific symptoms of this complex disorder.

REFERENCES

Allen JG: Traumatic Relationships and Serious Mental Disorders. Chichester, New York, Wiley, 2001

American Psychiatric Association: Diagnostic and Statistical Manual of Mental Disorders, 4th Edition, Text Revision. Washington DC, American Psychiatric Association, 2000

Boon S, Draijer N: Multiple personality disorder in The Netherlands: a clinical investigation of 71 patients. Am J Psychiatry 150:489–494, 1993

Bremner JD: Acute and chronic responses to psychological trauma: where do we go from here? Am J Psychiatry 156:349–351, 1999

Bremner JD, Brett E: Trauma-related dissociative states and long-term psychopathology in posttraumatic stress disorder. J Trauma Stress 10:37–49, 1997

Bremner JD, Southwick S, Brett E, et al: Dissociation and posttraumatic stress disorder in Vietnam combat veterans. Am J Psychiatry 149:328–332, 1992

Bremner JD, Narayan M, Staib LH, et al: Neural correlates of memories of childhood sexual abuse in women with and without posttraumatic stress disorder. Am J Psychiatry 156:1787–1795, 1999a

Bremner JD, Staib LH, Kaloupek D, et al: Neural correlates of exposure to traumatic pictures and sound in Vietnam combat veterans with and without posttraumatic stress disorder: a positron emission tomography study. Biol Psychiatry 45:806–816, 1999b

Butler LD, Duran RE, Jasiukaitis P, et al: Hypnotizability and traumatic experience: a diathesis-stress model of dissociative symptomatology. Am J Psychiatry 153:42–63, 1996

Cabeza R, Nyberg L: Imaging cognition II: an empirical review of 275 PET and fMRI studies. J Cogn Neurosci 12:1–47, 2000

Cabeza R, Nyberg L: Functional neuroimaging of memory. Neuropsychologia 41:241–244, 2003

Cahill L: Modulation of long-term memory in humans by emotional arousal: adrenergic activation and the amygdala, in The Amygdala. Edited by Aggleton J. New York, Oxford University Press, 2000, pp 425–446

Carmichael ST, Price JL: Limbic connections of the orbital and medial prefrontal cortex in macaque monkeys. J Comp Neurol 363:615–641, 1995

Coons PM: Confirmation of childhood abuse in child and adolescent cases of multiple personality disorder and dissociative disorder not otherwise specified. J Nerv Ment Dis 182:461–464, 1994

Craig AD: Interoception: the sense of the physiological condition of the body. Curr Opin Neurobiol 13:500–505, 2003

Crane JW, Ebner K, Day TA: Medial prefrontal cortex suppression of the hypothalamic-pituitary-adrenal axis response to a physical stressor, systemic delivery of interleukin-1beta. Eur J Neurosci 17:1473–1481, 2003

Critchley HD, Mathias CJ, Dolan RJ: Neuroanatomical basis for first- and second-order representations of bodily states. Nat Neurosci 4:207–212, 2001

Critchley HD, Melmed RN, Featherstone E, et al: Volitional control of autonomic arousal: a functional magnetic resonance study. Neuroimage 16:909–919, 2002

Damasio AR: Descartes' Error: Emotion, Reason, and the Human Brain. New York, Putnam, 1994

Damasio AR: The Feeling of What Happens: Body and Emotion in the Making of Consciousness. New York, Harcourt Brace, 1999

Damasio AR, Grabowski TJ, Bechara A, et al: Subcortical and cortical brain activity during the feeling of self-generated emotions. Nat Neurosci 3:1049–1056, 2000

Davidson RJ, Sutton SK: Affective neuroscience: the emergence of a discipline. Curr Opin Neurobiol 5:217–224, 1995

Devinsky O, Putnam F, Grafman J, et al: Dissociative states and epilepsy. Neurol 39:835–840, 1989

Drevets WC, Videen TO, Price JL, et al: A functional anatomical study of unipolar depression. J Neurosci 12:3628–3641, 1992

Foa EB, Riggs DS, Gershuny BS: Arousal, numbing, and intrusion: symptom structure of PTSD following assault. Am J Psychiatry 152:116–120, 1995

Frysztak RJ, Neafsey EJ: The effect of medial frontal cortex lesions on cardiovascular conditioned emotional responses in the rat. Brain Res 643:181–193, 1994

Fuster O, Joaquin M: Cortex and Mind: Unifying Cognition. New York, Oxford University Press, 2003

Gilboa A, Shalev AY, Laor L, et al: Functional connectivity of the prefrontal cortex and the amygdala in posttraumatic stress disorder. Biol Psychiatry 55:263–272, 2004

Hollander E, Carrasco JL, Mullen LS, et al: Left hemispheric activation in depersonalization disorder: a case report. Biol Psychiatry 31:1157–1162, 1992

Joliot M, Ribary U, Llinas R: Human oscillatory brain activity near 40 Hz coexists with cognitive temporal binding. Proc Natl Acad Sci 91:11748–11751, 1994

Kenna JC, Sedman G: Depersonalization in temporal lobe epilepsy and the organic psychoses. Br J Psychiatry 111:293–299, 1965

Kluft RP: The confirmation and disconfirmation of memories of abuse in dissociative identity disorder patients. Dissociation 8:235–258, 1995

Koopman C, Classen C, Spiegel D: Predictors of posttraumatic stress symptoms among survivors of the Oakland/Berkeley, Calif., firestorm. Am J Psychiatry 151:888–894, 1994

Krystal JH, Bennett AL, Bremner JD, et al: Toward a cognitive neuroscience of dissociation and altered memory functions in post-traumatic stress disorder, in Neurobiological and Clinical Consequences of Stress: From Normal Adaptation to PTSD. Edited by Friedman MJ, Charney DS, Deutch AY. New York, Raven, 1995, pp 239–269

Krystal JH, Bremner JD, Southwick SM, et al: The emerging neurobiology of dissociation: implications for the treatment of posttraumatic stress disorder, in Trauma, Memory, and Dissociation. Edited by Bremner JD, Marmar CR. Washington, DC, American Psychiatric Press, 1998, pp 321–363

Lane RD, Reiman EM, Axelrod B, et al: Neural correlates of levels of emotional awareness: evidence of an interaction between emotion and attention in the anterior cingulate cortex. J Cogn Neurosci 10:525–535, 1998

Lanius RA, Williamson PC, Densmore M, et al: Neural correlates of traumatic memories in posttraumatic stress disorder: a functional MRI investigation. Am J Psychiatry 158:1920–1922, 2001

Lanius RA, Williamson PC, Boksman K, et al: Brain activation during script-driven imagery induced dissociative responses in PTSD: a functional magnetic resonance imaging investigation. Biol Psychiatry 52:305–311, 2002

Lanius RA, Hopper JW, Menon RS: Individual differences in a husband and wife who developed PTSD after a motor vehicle accident: a functional MRI case study. Am J Psychiatry 160:667–669, 2003a

Lanius RA, Williamson PC, Hopper J, et al: Recall of emotional states in posttraumatic stress disorder: an fMRI investigation. Biol Psychiatry 53:204–210, 2003b

Lanius RA, Williamson PC, Densmore M, et al: The nature of traumatic memories: a 4-T fMRI functional connectivity analysis. Am J Psychiatry 161:36–44, 2004

Lanius RA, Williamson PC, Bluhm RL, et al: Functional connectivity of dissociative responses in posttraumatic stress disorder: a functional magnetic resonance imaging investigation. Biol Psychiatry 57:873–884, 2005

Le Doux J: Synaptic Self: How Our Brains Become Who We Are. New York, Penguin Putnam, 2002

Lewis DO, Yeager CA, Swica Y, et al: Objective documentation of child abuse and dissociation in 12 murderers with dissociative identity disorder. Am J Psychiatry 154:1703–1710, 1997

Liberzon I, Taylor SF, Fig LM, et al: Alteration of corticothalamic perfusion ratios during a PTSD flashback. Depress Anxiety 4:146–150, 1996

Liberzon I, Taylor SF, Amdur R, et al: Brain activation in PTSD in response to trauma-related stimuli. Biol Psychiatry 45:817–826, 1999

Llinas RR: I of the Vortex: From Neurons to Self. Cambridge, MA, MIT Press, 2002

Llinas R, Ribary U, Contreras D, et al: The neuronal basis for consciousness. Philos Trans R Soc Lond B Biol Sci 353:1841–1849, 1998

Marmar CR, Weiss DS, Schlenger WE, et al: Peritraumatic dissociation and posttraumatic stress in male Vietnam theater veterans. Am J Psychiatry 151:902–907, 1994

Mathew RJ, Wilson WH, Chiu NY, et al: Regional cerebral blood flow and depersonalization after tetrahydrocannabinol administration. Acta Psychiatr Scand 100:67–75, 1999

Morgan MA, Romanski LM, LeDoux JE: Extinction of emotional learning: contribution of medial prefrontal cortex. Neurosci Lett 163:109–113, 1993

Moscovitch M, Winocur G: The frontal cortex and working with memory, in Principles of Frontal Lobe Function. Edited by Stuss DT, Knight RT. New York, Oxford University Press, 2002, pp 188–209

Neafsey EJ, Terreberry RR, Hurley KM, et al: Anterior cingulate cortex in rodents: connections, visceral control functions and implications for emotion, in Neurobiology of Cingulate Cortex and Limbic Thalamus: a Comprehensive Handbook. Edited by Vogt BA, Gabriel M. Boston, MA, Birkhäuser, 1993, pp 206–223

Nijenhuis ER, Spinhoven P, van Dyck R, et al: Degree of somatoform and psychological dissociation in dissociative disorder is correlated with reported trauma. J Trauma Stress 11:711–730, 1998

Nijenhuis ER, van der Hart O, Steele, K: The emerging psychobiology of trauma-related dissociation and dissociative disorders, in Biological Psychiatry. Edited by D'haenen H, den Boer JA, Willner P. Hoboken, NJ, Wiley, 2002, pp 1079–1098

Penfield W, Rasmussen T: The Cerebral Cortex of Man: A Clinical Study of Localization of Function. New York, Macmillan, 1957

Pissiota A, Frans O, Fernandez M, et al: Neurofunctional correlates of posttraumatic stress disorder: a PET symptom provocation study. Eur Arch Psychiatry Clin Neurosci 252:68–75, 2002

Portas CM, Rees G, Howseman AM, et al: A specific role for the thalamus in mediating the interaction of attention and arousal in humans. J Neurosci 18:8979–8989, 1998

Rauch SL, van der Kolk BA, Fisler RE, et al: A symptom provocation study of posttraumatic stress disorder using positron emission tomography and script-driven imagery. Arch Gen Psychiatry 53:380–387, 1996

Rauch SL, Whalen PJ, Shin LM, et al: Exaggerated amygdala response to masked facial stimuli in posttraumatic stress disorder: a functional MRI study. Biol Psychiatry 47:769–776, 2000

Reiman EM, Lane RD, Ahern GL, et al: Neuroanatomical correlates of externally and internally generated human emotion. Am J Psychiatry 154:918–925, 1997

Reinders AA, Nijenhuis ER, Paans AM, et al: One brain, two selves. Neuroimage 20:2119–2125, 2003

Sar V, Kundakci T, Kiziltan E, et al: Differentiating dissociative disorders from other diagnostic groups through somatoform dissociation. J Trauma Dissociation 1:67–80, 2000

Saxe GN, Vasile RG, Hill TC, et al: SPECT imaging and multiple personality disorder. J Nerv Ment Dis 180:662–663, 1992

Schnider A, Ptak R, von Daniken C, et al: Recovery from spontaneous confabulations parallels recovery of temporal confusion in memory. Neurol 55:74–83, 2000

Sesack SR, Pickel VM: Prefrontal cortical efferents in the rat synapse on unlabeled neuronal targets of catecholamine terminals in the nucleus accumbens septi and on dopamine neurons in the ventral tegmental area. J Comp Neurol 320:145–160, 1992

Sesack SR, Deutch AY, Roth RH, et al: Topographical organization of the efferent projections of the medial prefrontal cortex in the rat: an anterograde tract-tracing study with Phaseolus vulgaris leucoagglutinin. J Comp Neurol 290:213–242, 1989

Shalev AY, Peri T, Canetti L, et al: Predictors of PTSD in injured trauma survivors: a prospective study. Am J Psychiatry 153:219–225, 1996

Shin LM, Kosslyn SM, McNally RJ, et al: Visual imagery and perception in posttraumatic stress disorder: a positron emission tomographic investigation. Arch Gen Psychiatry 54:233–241, 1997

Shin LM, McNally RJ, Kosslyn SM, et al: Regional cerebral blood flow during script-driven imagery in childhood sexual abuse-related PTSD: a PET investigation. Am J Psychiatry 156:575–584, 1999

Shin LM, Orr SP, Carson MA, et al: Regional cerebral blood flow in the amygdala and medial prefrontal cortex during traumatic imagery in male and female Vietnam veterans with PTSD. Arch Gen Psychiatry 61:168–176, 2004

Sierra M, Berrios GE: Depersonalization: neurobiological perspectives. Biol Psychiatry 44:898–908, 1998

Simeon D, Guralnik O, Hazlett EA, et al: Feeling unreal: a PET study of depersonalization disorder. Am J Psychiatry 157:1782–1788, 2000

Spiegel D: Trauma, dissociation, and memory, in Psychobiology of Posttraumatic Stress Disorder. Edited by Yehuda R, McFarlane AC. Ann NY Acad Sci 821:225–237, 1997

Teicher MH, Glod CA, Surrey J, et al: Early childhood abuse and limbic system ratings in adult psychiatric outpatients. J Neuropsychiatry Clin Neurosci 5:301–306, 1993

Tulving E, Kapur S, Craik FI, et al: Hemispheric encoding/retrieval asymmetry in episodic memory: positron emission tomography findings. Proc Natl Acad Sci 91:2016–2020, 1994

van der Hart O, van der Kolk BA, Boon S: The treatment of dissociative disorders, in Trauma, Memory, and Dissociation. Edited by Bremner JD, Marmar CR. Washington, DC, American Psychiatric Press, 1998, pp 253–283

van der Kolk BA: Trauma and Memory, in Traumatic Stress: The Effects of Overwhelming Experience on Mind, Body, and Society. Edited by van der Kolk BA, McFarlane AC, Weisaeth L. New York, Guilford, 1996, pp 279–302 van der Kolk BA, van der Hart O, Marmar CR: Dissociation and information processing in posttraumatic stress disorder, in Traumatic Stress: The Effects of Overwhelming Experience on Mind, Body, and Society. Edited by van der Kolk BA, McFarlane AC, Weisaeth L. New York, Guilford, 1996, pp 303–327

Vogt BA, Gabriel M: Neurobiology of Cingulate Cortex and Limbic Thalamus: A Comprehensive Handbook. Boston, MA, Birkhäuser, 1993

Williams LM, Phillips ML, Brammer MJ, et al: Arousal dissociates amygdala and hippocampal fear responses: evidence from simultaneous fMRI and skin conductance recording. Neuroimage 14:1070–1079, 2001

CHAPTER 11

PSYCHOBIOLOGY OF TRAUMATIZATION AND TRAUMA-RELATED STRUCTURAL DISSOCIATION OF THE PERSONALITY

ELLERT R. S. NIJENHUIS, PH.D.
JOHAN A. DEN BOER, M.D., PH.D.

Traumatized individuals tend to alternate between reexperiencing traumatic events and being more or less detached from these painful memories on account of not integrating such experiences into their personality. Moreover, the survivor's sense of self typically changes with these alternations. These essential features of survivors have been insufficiently recognized in psychobiological studies of traumatization. The bulk of the studies to date rests on the implicit assumption that reminders of traumatic experience will typically evoke reaction patterns mediated by the sympathetic nervous system. This perspective may be overly simplistic.

This chapter addresses the complexity of psychobiological reactions to traumatizing events using predictions drawn from the theory of trauma-related structural dissociation of the personality (Nijenhuis et al. 2002; Steele et al. 2005; van der Hart et al. 2004). This theory proposes that survivors' psychobiological reaction patterns to stressors and reminders of stressors depends on the part or parts of the personality structure that are activated during exposure to the stressor.

THE THEORY OF STRUCTURAL DISSOCIATION IN A NUTSHELL

According to the theory of structural dissociation, traumatization involves a division of personality structure into two or more different but more or less intensely interacting prototypical components, each with its own distinct psychobiological underpinnings. The lack of peritraumatic and posttraumatic integration of the personality is primarily due to exposure to highly stressful events, limitations of the integrative capacity, and lack of social support. In its basic form, the personality becomes divided into an *apparently normal part* (ANP) of the personality that is focused on fulfilling functions in daily life and an *emotional part* (EP) of the personality that is largely fixated on physical defense from major threat, in particular, threat to the integrity of the body.

The ANP and EP are guided by insufficiently integrated evolutionary prepared action systems or constellations of such psychobiological systems. In their ANPs, survivors are predominantly mediated by action systems for functioning in daily life, and in their EPs they are mediated by action systems for defense, including attachment cry—that is, the desperate cry for (re)union with a caretaker from which the EP has become separated. (The reaction pattern is more generally known as the "separation cry." However, the separated youngster does not cry for separation from his caretakers, but cries for reunion.) These dissociative parts are each endowed with their own sense of self, which can range from rudimentary (as applies, for example, to EPs that only have a very limited existence, i.e., basic autobiography) to highly complex (as applies to many ANPs that have an extended existence, i.e., an extended autobiography). They may encompass just one psychobiological state (e.g., an EP fixated on flight, implying a rudimentary sense of self) or complex assemblies of different states (implying a more extended sense of self). All dissociative parts are fixated in maladaptive action tendencies that maintain structural dissociation.

The theory of structural dissociation holds that the psychobiological functioning of survivors changes with structural alternations and will be dependent on the part or parts of the personality that are activated at the time of measurement of the dependent psychological or psychobiological variable under study. Some survivors may predominantly display ANPs during measurement, others may display EPs, and still others may alternate among or have parallel activation of the different parts.

These ideas contrast with the dominant, contemporary assumptions that different survivors have in principle similar (abnormal) reactions to natural and experimental threat cues and that their functioning is relatively stable over time. These assumptions are at odds with 150 years of clinical observation and associated theoretical analyses suggesting that survivors' psychobiological reactions to (perceived) threat can be different between individuals and changeable within an individual. Indeed, an increasing number of studies suggest that different survivors can display different, sometimes even opposite, psychobiological features (e.g., Mason et al. 2002), including contrasting cortisol levels and autonomic nervous system reactions as well as different patterns of cerebral blood flow.

POLYVAGAL THEORY AND STRUCTURAL DISSOCIATION

Different psychobiological reaction patterns of different prototypical dissociative parts (i.e., the ANP or the EP engaging in active and/or passive physical defense) to real or perceived threat may relate to mediation by different action systems and different components of the autonomic nervous system.

Porges's (2001, 2003) polyvagal theory details essential neural structures and neurobehavioral systems we share with, or have adapted from, our phylogenetic ancestry. His theory proposes three response systems that relate to different branches of the autonomic nervous system: the 1) ventral vagal and 2) dorsal vagal branches of the parasympathetic nervous system and the 3) sympathetic-catecholaminergic nervous system. In this paradigm, state can be changed in a predictable manner, and specific state changes are associated with potentiating or limiting the range of specific behaviors. Porges maintained that the three systems each have their own adaptive biobehavioral response strategies to different environmental challenges. We agree that these systems involve adaptation but also suggest that integration of the three systems is required for adaptive behavior beyond threat exposure (i.e., for adaptation when threat has passed).

The functions of the ventral vagal system, the phylogenetically most recent system, are social communication, self-soothing and calming (a major component of self-regulation and affect regulation), and inhibition of sympathetic-catecholaminergic influences. This mammalian signaling system for motion, emotion, and communication involves cranial nerve regulation of the striated facial muscles coordinated with a myelinated vagus that inhibits sympathetic activity at the level of the heart. Ventral vagal control involves the vagal brake that regulates the heart and allows the individual to stay calm in safe environments. The ventral vagal system involves pathways that originate in the frontal cortex. Thus there is cortical control of these medullar motor neurons.

The second and phylogenetically older system serves active defense from threat and is dependent on the sympathetic nervous system. The sympathetic system mobilizes energy under prolonged challenge. This adaptive system innervates the heart to provide the energy required to focus on threat cues to run or to fight. The quickest way to achieve mobilization is to release the ventral vagal brake. This action instantly activates the heart and thus provides energy for active defense. Individuals can rapidly calm themselves by reengaging the ventral vagal system that decreases metabolic output.

The third and phylogenetically oldest system is the dorsal vagal system, which serves major immobilization under threat. It provides inhibitory input to the sinoatrial node of the heart (i.e., the heart's pacemaker) via unmyelinated fibers and also provides low tonic influences on the bronchi. Low heart rate in response to severe stress may thus be determined by the unmyelinated dorsal vagal fibers. We hold that this system serves total submission rather than mere immobilization.

Structural dissociation may involve a lack of integration of the three systems. In ANPs and EPs that can engage in attachment behaviors, play, and some exploration when they feel safe, survivors would be predominantly guided by the ventral vagal complex. However, ANPs also encompass the sympathetic system to the degree that they engage in defensive actions when they feel threatened (e.g., by threatening internal experiences such as intrusions of traumatic memories from EPs). ANPs can engage in detachment as well (i.e., detachment from the traumatic past and reminders of this past), which may involve a degree of dorsal vagal hypoarousal. The EPs' active defensive actions (e.g., flight, freeze) would be mediated by the sympathetic-catecholaminergic system and their passive defensive actions (e.g., submission) by the dorsal vagal complex. Many authors refer to (predominantly parasympathetic) states of hypoarousal as dissociative but exclude sympathetic hyperarousal states from this category (Perry et al. 1995; Schore 2003).

In EPs that engage in active (sympathetically mediated) defenses when they feel threatened, survivors have increased heart rates and blood pressure and decreased skin conductance response compared with their ANPs. However, in totally submissive (parasympathetically mediated) EPs, survivors have decreased heart rates and blood pressure when exposed to (perceived) threat. Furthermore, sympathetically mediated EPs, parasympathetically mediated EPs, and ANPs would all have different patterns of cerebral metabolism. For example, in sympathetically mediated EPs, survivors would have more activity in the amygdala, insula, and somatosensory cortex. ANPs would have more activity in the anterior cingulate and the medial prefrontal cortex (mPFC) when exposed to major reminders of traumatizing events (i.e., brain structures that exert inhibitory influences on the "emotional brain"). Many ANPs display efforts to evade reminders of traumatizing events and other trauma-related stimuli. Their mental efforts to escape prominently include the narrowing of attention to concerns of daily life, which we speculate may include conscious or unconscious efforts to keep the ventral vagal system online. We now explore some recent findings in light of these hypotheses.

DIFFERENT REACTION PATTERNS IN DIFFERENT SURVIVORS

Neuroendocrinological Features

Different survivors can have different cortisol levels (Bourne et al. 1967; Mason et al. 2001). For example, Vietnam veterans with posttraumatic stress disorder (PTSD) who felt guilt about their military actions in Vietnam (i.e., were emotionally engaged in their traumatic history at the time of measurement) had elevated cortisol, whereas veterans with PTSD who were emotionally numb, avoidant, and generally disengaged had low cortisol levels (Mason et al. 2001).

Mason et al. (2001) suggested that emotional engagement and disengagement may represent primary (i.e., immediate) and secondary (i.e., subsequent avoidant) emotional responses to traumatizing events, respectively. In our terms, the immediate reactions could denote an EP engaging in flight, freeze, or fight, and the avoidant reactions could denote ANP or EPs under dorsal vagal control. We are not aware of direct studies of cortisol levels in ANPs and EPs.

Psychophysiological Features

Several studies have found that survivors tend to have elevated heart rates and blood pressure in the acute stage of PTSD (Bryant et al. 2000) and when exposed to perceived threat cues such as script-driven imagery (Kinzie et al. 1998; Orr et al. 1997). These effects could be due to sympathetic control or to the release of the ventral vagal brake. Some preliminary findings indeed suggest that elevated sympathetic tone in survivors in response to mild cognitive challenge can relate to a dysfunctional parasympathetic system (Sahar et al. 2001).

Kinzie et al. (1998) and Osuch et al. (2001) found that only a small proportion of survivors had increased psychophysiological responses to general emotional challenge and to trauma cue exposure. These subgroups have been labeled "physiologic responders" and "nonresponders." Lack of heart rate increases in resonse to challenge in a substantial proportion of PTSD patients may suggest not a flight or fight but rather a giving-up response that involves inhibition (i.e., total submission). This inhibition could be related to dorsal vagal parasympathetic control in these survivors. In our terms, heart rate decreases in response to emotional challenge mark EPs that engage in total submission, whereas lack of heart rate changes in response to such challenge would be characteristic of ANPs. Flight, freeze, and fight EPs would have increased heart rates.

Lack of heart rate changes in response to emotional challenge may relate to negative dissociative symptoms, suggesting parasympathetic dominance. Thus, adult rape victims with high degrees of negative dissociative symptoms had lower heart rates when talking about their rapes compared with survivors with low degrees of negative dissociation (Griffin et al. 1997). In this study there was a general suppression of autonomic physiological responses in the high dissociation group. Delinquent, traumatized adolescents with many negative dissociative symptoms also had lower heart rates compared with those with few negative dissociative symptoms (Koopman et al. 2000). However, higher mean heart rates were found among youths reporting greater frequency and intensity of adverse childhood experiences.

Different survivors of childhood abuse can also have different subjective psychological and physiological reactions to trauma scripts (Schmahl et al. 2002). A woman with PTSD and a woman with histrionic personality disorder had elevated heart rates and blood pressures during the experiment. However, a woman with borderline personality disorder who experienced a negative dissociative reaction in response to an abandonment script had an extreme decline in physiological reactivity.

Neural Activity

Utilizing functional magnetic resonance imaging to study the neural circuitry underlying the response patterns of sexual abuse–related PTSD patients to trauma scripts, Lanius et al. (2002) found that reactivity depended on whether the patients tended to reexperience the traumatizing event or to become detached. In terms of the theory of structural dissociation, reexperiencing constitutes a positive dissociative response and probably an EP engaging in active defense. Detachment pertains to negative dissociative symptoms (and perhaps also some alterations in consciousness) and possibly a detached ANP or EP. Compared with control subjects, the "detached" PTSD patients showed more activation in the superior and middle temporal gyri (Brodmann's area [BA] 38), the inferior frontal gyrus (BA 47), the occipital lobe (BA 19), the medial frontal gyrus (BA 10), the parietal lobe (BA 7), the medial cortex (BA 9), and the anterior cingulate gyrus (BA 24 and 32). However, the PTSD patients who reexperienced traumatizing events showed significantly less activation of the thalamus, the anterior cingulate gyrus (BA 32), and the medial frontal gyrus (BA 10 and 11) than did comparison subjects (see Chapter 10 in this volume, "Posttraumatic Stress Disorder Symptom Provocation and Neuroimaging," for further discussion).

Similarly, Lanius et al. (2003) described a husband and wife who had developed PTSD in the context of a serious motor vehicle accident. Whereas both reported peritraumatic dissociative symptoms, they exhibited different subjective, psychophysiological, and neurobiological responses to trauma script-driven imagery (see Chapter 10). During the accident, the husband became extremely aroused and rescued himself and his wife by breaking the windshield. His wife could hardly move because she, in her words, was "frozen." When reexperiencing the accident during testing, he was psychologically and physically aroused, and she felt "numb and frozen." They thus reengaged in their original response patterns. The woman's description and her high peritraumatic dissociation score suggests that she may not have been frozen (i.e., sympathetically aroused) but rather paralyzed, thus dominated by dorsal vagal influences. His heart rate increased from baseline, and he had increased activity in his anterior frontal, anterior cingulate, superior and medial temporal, thalamic, parietal, and occipital brain regions. She had no heart rate change from baseline and had only increased activity in occipital regions. Lanius et al. (2003) concluded that their "results demonstrate that PTSD patients can have very different responses, both subjectively and biologically, while re-experiencing traumatic events" (p. 668).

DIFFERENT PSYCHOBIOLOGICAL REACTIONS FOR DIFFERENT DISSOCIATIVE PARTS

In addition to the suggestion that different individuals with PTSD have very different psychobiological profiles, the theory of structural dissociation suggests that these profiles can also shift *within* patients depending on which part of them has executive control. Several studies using dissociative identity disorder (DID) patients have indeed suggested that different dissociative parts of the personality can have different psychobiological profiles that are not reproduced by DID-simulating controls (see Nijenhuis et al. 2002). Further advances in the field critically depend on theoretical predictions as to the *kinds* of differences that exist among different *types* of dissociative parts of the personality. The theory of structural dissociation offers such predictions.

Psychophysiological Reactivity

Reinders and colleagues studied the psychophysiological reactions of DID patients to auditory scripts while functioning as their ANP and as a clinically fearful, hyperaroused EP (Reinders et al. 2006). Each participant listened to two scripts. One involved a neutral personal memory that the ANPs and the fearful and thus emotionally engaged EPs experienced as a personal narrative memory. The other script described a traumatic experience that the EPs but not the ANPs regarded as a personal experience. Consistent with the hypotheses, the ANPs and the EPs did not have increased heart rates and blood pressures in response to neutral memories. However, the EPs but not the ANPs had highly significant increases in heart rates and systolic blood pressures compared with baseline and with neutral script exposure when listening to the trauma scripts, and they also responded to these scripts with stronger subjective emotional and sensorimotor reactions. The EPs had significantly less heart rate variability compared with the ANPs when these dissociative personalities listened to the trauma scripts. Only the EPs reported a spectrum of primary emotions, including fear, anger, and disgust, and experienced many positive and negative somatoform dissociative symptoms such as being physically touched, having visual images and olfactory reminders of the traumatic experience, and bodily paralysis.

To examine potential demand characteristics, preliminary analysis has explored whether DID-simulating controls (i.e., low and high fantasy–prone healthy individuals) would replicate the findings in DID patients (Reinders et al. 2006). It is difficult for patients without PTSD to simulate the physiological responses marking traumatized patients (Orr and Pitman 1993). Moreover, simulating controls generally are not able to produce psychophysiological state changes equivalent to those in DID patients (Putnam 1997). Initial findings suggest that low and high fantasy–prone healthy individuals had similar levels of heart rate and blood pressure regardless of whether they simulated an ANP or an EP and of whether they listened to audiotapes with descriptions of neutral personal memories or of painful personal memories (Nijenhuis 2004). Therefore, it seems doubtful that the performance of authentic ANPs and EPs in DID can be explained as effects of suggestion and fantasy proneness.

ANP- and EP-Dependent Neural Activity

Supraliminal Exposure to Perceived Threat

The script-driven study in which psychophysiological reactions of the ANP and the EP in DID patients were examined (Reinders et al. 2006) also assessed regional cerebral blood flow (rCBF) patterns using positron emission tomography (Reinders et al. 2003). Exposure to memories that both the ANP and EP deemed as neutral and personal did not yield differences in rCBF patterns. However, major differences in psychobiological responses emerged between the ANP and the EP when listening to trauma scripts that only the EP regarded as a personal memory.

Compared with the patients' ANPs, the EPs had more activity in the amygdala, the insular cortex, the somatosensory areas I and II of the parietal cortex, and the basal ganglia. This activity may reflect that EPs receive major somatosensory information that they interpret in alarming and painful ways (via amygdala and insular cortex activation) and that urge them to generate defensive motor plans (via basal ganglia activation). The EPs also reported disgust when listening to the trauma scripts. This disgust may relate to increased activation in the insula and caudate.

Compared with the EPs, the ANPs had more brain metabolism in the occipital cortex (BA 19: visual perception), the parietal cortex (BA 7 and 40: somatosensory integration), the anterior cingulate (BA 24 and 32: inhibition of emotional reactions), and other frontal areas, including BA 10 (planning, self-awareness). Many of these areas were also activated in the PTSD patients displaying a detached response in Lanius et al.'s (2002) study.

The ANPs' higher degree of activation in BA 7, BA 40, and BA 19 may be linked with depersonalization. Depersonalization is related to several negative somatoform dissociative symptoms (e.g., experiencing the body as a foreign object). Simeon et al. (2000) reported that the disorder was associated with functional abnormalities along sequential hierarchical areas, secondary and cross-modal areas of the sensory cortex (visual, auditory, and somatosensory), and areas responsible for an integrated body schema. More specifically, they found less blood flow in the right temporal cortex (auditory association area) and more metabolism in the parietal somatosensory association area and the multimodal association area (see Chapter 4 in this volume, "Relationships Between Dissociation and Posttraumatic Stress Disorder"). Dissociation and depersonalization scores among the sample were strongly correlated with activation patterns in the posterior parietal association area (BA 7).

It thus seems that integrative failure with respect to bodily cues— which may be at the heart of basic forms of consciousness (Damasio 1999)—is related to dysfunctioning of temporal, parietal, and occipital association areas. Indeed, "[t]here is a hierarchy of sensory processing in the brain, from primary sensory areas to unimodal and then polymodal association areas and finally to the [prefrontal cortex]" (Simeon et al. 2000, p. 1786). Depersonalization and negative somatoform dissociative symptoms may thus relate to dysfunction of the posterior association areas that negatively affects the input into the prefrontal cortex. Patients in their ANPs indeed report low body awareness and feel generally more or less detached from their body.

Reduced activity in prefrontal areas for EPs (Reinders et al. 2006) suggests lack of inhibition regarding emotional reactivity. Stress hormone–related interference of the mPFC presents a major problem for affect regulation in that hippocampal (McCormick and Thompson 1982) and mPFC (Armony and LeDoux 1997) information processing are crucially involved in inhibiting the amygdala. Bremner et al. (1999) documented mPFC and anterior cingulate dysfunction in women with and without PTSD who reported childhood sexual abuse. Their participants were exposed to neutral personal memories and to descriptions of personalized childhood sexual abuse events. Abuse scripts were associated with greater increases in rCBF in portions of the prefrontal cortex, posterior cingulate, and motor cortex in women with PTSD compared with women without PTSD. These scripts also induced alterations in rCBF in the mPFC (i.e., decreased blood flow in the subcallosal gyrus and the anterior cingulate). Compared with women who had not developed PTSD, those with PTSD also had decreased blood flow in the right hippocampus, fusiform/inferior temporal gyrus, supramarginal gyrus, and visual association cortex. In sum, Reinders and colleagues showed that the subjective, psychophysiological, and neurobiological reactions to trauma scripts of DID patients depend on which dissociative part of the personality (i.e., the ANP or the EP) is activated during testing (Reinders et al. 2006).

Subliminal Exposure to Perceived Threat

Preconscious information processing plays a key role in responding to unconditioned and conditioned threat cues and in fear-related learning (Dolan 2000). The theory of structural dissociation considers that in an ANP survivors aim to avoid this threat and that in an EP they selectively attend to these cues. In line with such predictions, the patients in ANPs named the color of a mask that immediately followed the subliminal presentation of experimental stimuli more quickly when this stimulus involved angry facial expressions compared with neutral facial expressions (Hermans et al. 2006). Those in EPs did not show differential responses to these cues. DID-simulating controls showed the reverse pattern: a tendency toward longer response latencies after exposure to angry faces when enacting ANPs and a tendency toward shorter reaction times after exposure to angry faces when enacting EPs. This pattern of responding was specific to cues that signaled an increased possibility of attack rather than to fear cues in general. These results are consistent with the interpretation that ANPs avoid subliminal threat cues by means of gaze aversion and that EPs particularly attend to bodily threat from a person with increased sympathetic tone.

If ANPs can preconsciously avoid externally presented unconditioned and conditioned threat cues, they may also preconsciously avoid internal unconditioned and conditioned threatening stimuli. If so, it seems possible that the ANP preconsciously avoids the EP and its memories, as the theory of structural dissociation holds. Some neurobiological data are consistent with the interpretation that dissociative amnesia involves inhibited access to episodic memory that involves major conditioned stimuli for the patient (Markowitsch et al. 2000).

Reactions to Perceived Threat in a Clinical Setting

The first author of this chapter (E.R.S.N.) assessed heart rates and bodily movements in response to perceived threat cues in the ANPs and EPs of patients with complex dissociative disorders. This work constituted a clinical exercise designed to help patients develop assertive reactions to real or perceived threat (e.g., to stop ongoing abuse or respond more effectively to threats of further traumatization). A small, insignificant object was moved in the direction of the patient's face. In their ANPs, the patients looked composed, showed no heart rate changes, and reported feeling at ease during the exposure. In their EPs, which engaged in freezing or in inclinations to ward off the threat cue, the patients had profound increases in heart rate with fearful facial expressions, were fixated on the moving object, and reported intense fear and an inability to move (freeze) or a strong impulse to run (flight). Sometimes fight EPs became activated during exposure. Finally, in EPs that engaged in total submission, patients had decreasing heart rates, averted their gaze, were immobile, and reported that they mentally left their body. Some reported amnesia for the experience after exposure.

Emotional support during such exposure in the form of a hand of a trusted person on the participant's back prevented extreme increases and decreases of psychophysiological activity. This support likely activates the ventral vagal nervous system, specifically the attachment action system, which inhibits dominance of defensive systems in response to reminders of traumatic experience. These clinical observations suggest that emotional support raises the survivors' integrative capacity.

Other Psychobiological Studies of ANPs and EPs

In two studies of DID, electroencephalographic (EEG) coherence (Hopper et al. 2002) and quantitative EEG activity (Kowal 2005) were explored for the "host"(ANP); several childlike, trauma-fixated parts of the personality (EP); and healthy control subjects. Differences for the ANP and the EP on these variables were found. Compared with the ANP, EPs had less EEG coherence, suggesting lower neuronal cortical connectivity (Hopper et al. 2002). These patterns—consistent with the theory of structural dissociation—were not reproduced by professional actors emulating these dissociative parts.

POSITIVE FEEDFORWARD EXCITATION AND NEGATIVE FEEDBACK INHIBITION

Based on the findings just described, we offer an overview of how EPs and ANPs seem to have different psychobiological reactions to the stimuli that they consciously and unconsciously perceive as threats.

EP-Dependent Responsivity to Threat

Exposure to major external threat causes rapid activation of the defensive system by the amygdala and related structures. This is mandatory for survival, as is learning and memorizing (through classical conditioning) signals that indicate threat. The range of threat-related responses orchestrated by the amygdala includes activation of the sympathetic nervous system and the hypothalamic-pituitary-adrenal axis, defensive behavior (through the central grey), startle response, and stress-induced hypoalgesia (Aggleton 2000). The lateral amygdala receives sensory inputs directly from the sensory thalamus and indirectly from the sensory cortex. The lateral amygdala projects to the central nucleus of the amygdala, which projects to structures controlling defensive behavior (flight, freeze, fight, total submission), autonomic arousal, hypoalgesia, stress hormones, and potentiated startle. Thus, the amygdala will be hyperactivated in the face of threat (unconditioned stimuli), will encode and store associations between conditioned and unconditioned stimuli, and will modulate memories of traumatizing events more generally. When conditioned stimuli reappear, the amygdala and other aspects of the emotional brain as well as the defensive system tend to become reactivated.

Hyperactivation of the defensive system during traumatic stress may produce hypermnesia through mediation of the basolateral nucleus of the amygdala. The basolateral amygdala has a major role in stress-mediated neuromodulatory influences on memory storage (Cahill 2000). Postevent memory consolidation for emotional experiences involves not only the basolateral amygdala but also the stria terminalis. This is a major afferent/efferent amygdala pathway that interacts with peripheral stress hormone feedback locally in the amygdala and with emotional memory storage elsewhere in the brain (Cahill 2000).

Reactivated traumatic memories represent internal threat and aversion (disgust) in that these memories are not narratives but somatosensory and emotionally charged experiences. Findings of Reiman et al. (2000) suggest that internal threat cues (including body signals) are associated with activity of the insula. We have already noted a correlation between activation of the insula and disgust. Because the insula have afferent/efferent connections with the amygdala, internal threat cues may activate the amygdala through this path.

Hyperactivation of the amygdala in EPs exposed to threat cues may be related to failed inhibition of the amygdala and insula by the hippocampus and the mPFC due to excessive release of stress hormones: uninhibited positive feedforward loops would seem to stabilize the defensive system and impede the integration of the EP and the ANP. In this context, reactivation of traumatic memories and the defensive system (the EP) by conditioned stimuli implies sensitization rather than modulation of associations between conditioned and unconditioned stimuli. Thus it seems that exposure of the EP to (perceived) threat cues (re)activates defensive responses with concomitant lack of contextual information processing, uninhibited conditioned emotional responding within limits of homeostasis, and hampered integration of traumatic memories.

ANP-Dependent Responsivity to Threat

Because ANPs displayed reactivity to masked angry faces, it seems unlikely that the amygdala and related brain structures are completely inactive when ANPs are exposed to threat cues. However, in the EP, the survivors' emotional brain is strongly activated. While in the EP they attend to threat cues, but in the ANP their gaze is averted from threat, and attention is directed to cues that matter to daily life functioning. It seems possible that there is transient activation of the lateral amygdala by means of input from the sensory thalamus when the ANP is exposed to threat. However, due to the ANP's mental avoidance of threat cues and retraction of the field of consciousness to matters of daily life, the lateral amygdala could become readily subject to a form of negative feedback inhibition. When emotional systems that regulate daily life are in executive control, the amygdala—which has a role in attention (Gallagher 2000)—and related structures may operate in a mode that is different from the mode associated with the defensive system.

Activation of the prefrontal cortex inhibits the amygdala. Therefore, another (not incompatible) explanation could be that because the ANP has to rely more on executive functions to operate in daily life, more frontal networks are activated (Fuster 2003), which could involve ventral vagal control. Thus the ANP recruits more neural networks that include the dorsolateral prefrontal cortex and other related areas, thus leading to inhibition of the amygdala.

Because ANPs are often depersonalized, studies of DID could help understand ANP reactivity to threat in various trauma-related disorders. Depersonalization is related to several negative somatoform dissociative symptoms and involves functional abnormalities along sequential hierarchical areas and secondary and cross-modal areas of the sensory cortex (visual, auditory, and somatosensory) as well as areas responsible for an integrated body schema (Simeon et al. 2000). Perhaps the ANP's lack of sensory perception, including bodily and peripheral stress hormone feedback, could be instrumental in inhibiting the defensive system, and hence the insula and amygdala, and the responsivity it orchestrates. One way to study the presumed negative feedback and positive feedforward loops would be to apply functional magnetic resonance imaging while patients' ANPs and EPs are exposed to (perceived) threat cues.

CONCLUSION

Emerging clinical and experimental evidence supports the idea that structural dissociation of the personality reflects a lack of integration among specific psychobiological action systems and among different components of the human central nervous system: the ventral vagal system for social engagement and functioning in daily life, the sympathetic nervous system for active physical defense, and the dorsal vagal parasympathetic system for passive physical defense.

The primary form of this structural dissociation involves failed integration between systems dedicated to daily life (and survival of the species) and systems dedicated to the survival of the individual in the face of severe threat. The evidence to date suggests that in PTSD and the dissociative disorders, (re)activation of active physical defense by trauma-related cues is associated with increased activation of the amygdala, insula, and related structures and decreased activation of the hippocampus, anterior cingulate gyrus, mPFC, and perhaps other prefrontal areas as well. The amygdala orchestrates a range of unconditioned and conditioned reactions to threat, including sympathetic and dorsal vagal activity, analgesia, defensive motor reaction patterns, subjective emotional feelings such as fear, and retraction of the field of consciousness to threat cues in the immediate, subjective present. These reactions seem to lack modulation by the prefrontal cortex.

However, in their ANPs, survivors avoid threat cues (gaze aversion, mental avoidance) and direct their attention to cues that have a bearing on daily life. The depersonalization and negative somatoform dissociative symptoms that characterize the ANP may be related to disturbed metabolism in the somatosensory association areas. Although structural dissociation may be adaptive when the integrative level is not sufficient to integrate action systems for defense (serving to avoid aversive stimuli) and daily life (dedicated to seeking attractive stimuli), continued structural dissociation is maladaptive when integration of traumatic experiences would be feasible.

To date, psychobiological research on PTSD and the dissociative disorders has largely overlooked that findings may depend on the type of dissociative part of the personality that dominates the functioning of the patient at the time of measurement. In this regard, the theory of structural dissociation can serve as a heuristic for future research of trauma-related dissociation. More specifically, the theory may be of help in 1) selecting minimal sets of variables needed to assess the different types of dissociative parts that patients with trauma-related dissociative disorders encompass; 2) conceptualizing and studying the features of these different types of parts in terms of these essential variables; and 3) conceptualizing the dynamics of transition between the parts that, as interacting but insufficiently integrated clusters, constitute these patients' personality (see Vaitl et al. 2005).

REFERENCES

Aggleton JP (ed): The Amygdala: A Functional Analysis. New York, Oxford University Press, 2000

Armony JG, LeDoux JE: How the brain processes emotional information. Ann NY Acad Sci 821:259–270, 1997

Bourne PG, Rose RM, Mason JW: 17-OHCS levels in combat: Special Forces "A" Team under threat of attack. Arch Gen Psychiatry 19:135–140, 1967

Bremner JD, Narayan M, Staib LH, et al: Neural correlates of memories of childhood sexual abuse in women with and without posttraumatic stress disorder. Am J Psychiatry 156:1787–1795, 1999

Bryant RA, Harvey AG, Guthrie RM, et al: A prospective study of psychophysiological arousal, acute stress disorder, and posttraumatic stress disorder. J Abnorm Psychol 109:341–344, 2000

Cahill L: Modulation of long-term memory in humans by emotional arousal: adrenergic activation and the amygdala, in The Amygdala: A Functional Analysis. Edited by Aggleton JP. New York, Oxford University Press, 2000, pp 425–446

Damasio AR: The Feeling of What Happens: Body and Emotion in the Making of Consciousness. New York, Harcourt Brace, 1999

Dolan RJ: Functional neuroimaging of the amygdala during emotional processing and learning, in The Amygdala: A Functional Analysis. Edited by Aggleton JP. New York, Oxford University Press, 2000, pp 631–655

Fuster JM: Cortex and Mind: Unifying Cognition. New York, Oxford University Press, 2003

Gallagher M: The amygdala and associative learning, in The Amygdala: A Functional Analysis. Edited by Aggleton JP. New York, Oxford University Press, 2000, pp 311–329

Griffin MG, Resick PA, Mechanic MB: Objective assessment of peritraumatic dissociation: psychophysiological indicators. Am J Psychiatry 154:1081–1088, 1997

Hermans EJ, Nijenhuis ER, van Honk J, et al: State-dependent attentional bias for facial threat in dissociative identity disorder. Psychiatry Res 141:233–236, 2006

Hopper A, Ciorciari J, Johnson G, et al: EEG coherence and dissociative identity disorder: comparing EEG coherence in DID hosts, alters, controls and acted alters. J Trauma Dissociation 1:75–88, 2002

Kinzie JD, Denney D, Riley C, et al: A cross-cultural study of reactivation of posttraumatic stress disorder symptoms: American and Cambodian psychophysiological response to viewing traumatic video scenes. J Nerv Ment Dis 186:670–676, 1998

Koopman C, Carion V, Sudhakar S, et al: Dissociation, childhood abuse and heart rate during a stressful speech. Poster presented at the 16th Conference of the International Society for Traumatic Stress Studies, San Antonio, TX, November 2000

Kowal J: QEEG comparisons of persons with and without DID. Proceedings of the 22nd Fall Conference of the International Society for the Study of Dissociation. Toronto, ON, Canada, November 2005

Lanius RA, Williamson PC, Boksman K, et al: Brain activation during script-driven imagery induced dissociative responses in PTSD: a functional magnetic resonance imaging investigation. Biol Psychiatry 52:305–311, 2002

Lanius RA, Hopper JW, Menon RS: Individual differences in a husband and wife who developed PTSD after a motor vehicle accident: a functional MRI case study. Am J Psychiatry 160:667–669, 2003

Markowitsch HJ, Kessler J, Weber-Luxenburger G, et al: Neuroimaging and behavioral correlates of recovery from amnestic block syndrome and other cognitive deteriorations. Neuropsychiatry Neuropsychol Behav Neurol 13:60–66, 2000

Mason JW, Wang S, Yehuda R, et al: Psychogenic lowering of urinary cortisol levels linked to increased emotional numbing and a shame-depressive syndrome in combat-related posttraumatic stress disorder. Psychosom Med 63:387–401, 2001

Mason JW, Wang S, Yehuda R, et al: Marked lability in urinary cortisol levels in subgroups of combat veterans with posttraumatic stress disorder during an intensive exposure treatment program. Psychosom Med 64:238–246, 2002

McCormick DD, Thompson RF: Locus coeruleus lesions and resistance to extinction of a classically conditioned response: involvement of the neocortex and hippocampus. Brain Res 245:239–249, 1982

Nijenhuis ER: Structural dissociation of the personality: phenomena, theory, and psychobiological research. Keynote presented at the Fifth European EMDR Conference, Stockholm, Sweden, June 2004

Nijenhuis ER, van der Hart O, Steele K: The emerging psychobiology of trauma-related dissociation and dissociative disorders, in Biological Psychiatry. Edited by D'haenen H, den Boer JA, Willner P. Hoboken, NJ, Wiley, 2002, pp 1079–1098

Orr SP, Pitman RK: Psychophysiologic assessment of attempts to simulate posttraumatic stress disorder. Biol Psychiatry 33:127–129, 1993

Orr SP, Lasko NB, Metzger LJ, et al: Psychophysiologic assessment of PTSD in adult females sexually abused during childhood. Ann NY Acad Sci 821:491–493, 1997

Osuch EA, Benson B, Geraci M, et al: Regional cerebral blood flow correlated with flashback intensity in patients with posttraumatic stress disorder. Biol Psychiatry 50:246–253, 2001

Perry BD, Pollard RA, Blakely TL, et al: Childhood trauma, the neurobiology of adaptation, and "use dependent" development of the brain: how "states" become "traits." Infant Ment Health J 16:271–291, 1995

Porges SW: The polyvagal theory: phylogenetic substrates of a social nervous system. Int J Psychophysiol 42:123–146, 2001

Porges SW: The polyvagal theory: phylogenetic contributions to social behavior. Physiol Behav 79:503–513, 2003

Putnam FW: Dissociation in Children and Adolescents. New York, Guilford, 1997

Reiman EM, Lane RD, Ahern GL, et al: Positron emission tomography in the study of emotion, anxiety, and anxiety disorders, in Cognitive Neuroscience of Emotion. Edited by Lane RD, Nadel I. New York, Oxford University Press, 2000, pp 389–406

Reinders AA, Nijenhuis ER, Paans AM, et al: One brain, two selves. Neuroimage 20:2119–2125, 2003

Reinders AATS, Nijenhuis ERS, Quak J, et al: Psychobiological characteristics of dissociative identity disorder: a symptom provocation study. Biol Psychiatry 60:730–740, 2006

Sahar T, Shalev AY, Porges SW: Vagal modulation of responses to mental challenge in posttraumatic stress disorder. Biol Psychiatry 49:637–643, 2001

Schmahl CG, Elzinga BM, Bremner JD: Individual differences in psychophysiological reactivity in adults with childhood abuse. Clin Psychol Psychother
9:271–276, 2002

Schore AN: Affect Dysregulation and Disorders of the Self. New York, Norton, 2003

Simeon D, Guralnik O, Hazlett EA, et al: Feeling unreal: a PET study of depersonalization disorder. Am J Psychiatry 157:1782–1788, 2000

Steele K, van der Hart O, Nijenhuis ERS: Phase-oriented treatment of structural
dissociation in complex traumatization: overcoming trauma-related pho-
bias. J Trauma Dissociation 6:11–53, 2005

Vaitl D, Birbaumer N, Gruzelier J, et al: Psychobiology of altered states of consciousness. Psychol Bull 131:98–127, 2005

van der Hart O, Nijenhuis ER, Steele K, et al: Trauma-related dissociation: conceptual clarity lost and found. Aust N Z J Psychiatry 38:906–914, 2004

Part III

CONTEMPORARY IMPLICATIONS FOR ASSESSMENT AND TREATMENT

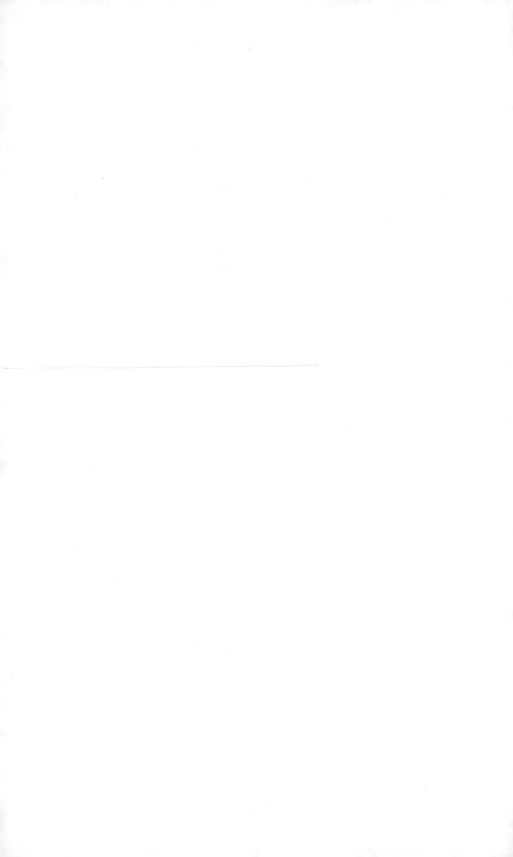

CHAPTER 12

PSYCHIATRIC APPROACHES TO DISSOCIATION

Integrating History, Biology, and Clinical Assessment

J. DOUGLAS BREMNER, M.D.
ERIC VERMETTEN, M.D., PH.D.

The simple notion that psychological trauma can have lasting effects on the individual has led to an abundance of research studies into the effects of trauma on health and disease. Besides the effect of trauma itself, both peritraumatic dissociation and trauma-related persistent dissociation have been shown to be markers for long-term psychopathology (Bremner and Brett 1997; Bremner et al. 1993b; Briere 2006; Irwin 1994; Marmar et al. 1994). The underlying systems involved in the manifestation of trauma-related symptom such as flashbacks, sleep problems, emotional numbing, avoidance, hyperarousal, and irritability have become known through a prolific amount of research since the mid-1990s. Traumatic stress and traumatic dissociation are now known to be associated with a range of symptoms and conditions, including posttraumatic stress disorder (PTSD), dissociation, depression, somatization, substance abuse, and eating disorders. The overlapping nature of this range of symptoms, and their common etiology in psychological trauma, has led to the term *trauma spectrum disorders* (Bremner 2002). This chapter reviews studies in the area of PTSD and dissociation against the context of the current psychiatric classification system. Included in this review are the long-term effects of traumatic stress on the brain and neurobiology in humans (Vermetten and Bremner 2002a, 2002b), which show changes in areas including the hippocampus and frontal cortex as well as alterations in stress hormones (cortisol and norepinephrine). The common neurobiological links between PTSD and dissociative symptoms are also discussed.

BACKGROUND TO THE DIAGNOSTIC DEVELOPMENT OF THE DISSOCIATIVE DISORDERS

The diagnostic development of the dissociative disorders has evolved in a strange fashion parallel to that of PTSD. In the First World War, the diagnosis of shell shock was close to a pure dissociative disorder. Soldiers were described as forgetting their names or who they were and wandering off the battlefield with no memory of what had happened to them. Because of the close proximity of exploding shells, this disorder was originally conceived of as being secondary to the physical impact of the explosions, although this idea was later revised.

The psychiatric approach to the dissociative disorders, however, failed to acknowledge any relationship to psychological trauma. In the early part of the twentieth century American psychiatrists published case reports of individuals who wandered away from their homes, forgot about their past identities, and developed new lives in another city. This became known as *fugue states*. *Depersonalization disorder* (DPD) was similarly developed with a focus on the symptoms rather than the etiology (see Chapter 1 in this volume, "Relationship Between Trauma and Dissociation," for related discussion). *Dissociative amnesia* (originally psychogenic amnesia) had a psychoanalytical bent that emphasized repressed conflicts in the etiology; in the mid-twentieth century it was grouped with the old remnant of hysteria, conversion disorder, and called *dissociative hysteria*. As a result the dissociative disorders had difficulty shaking the suspicion that they were not true disorders or that they were a disguise for secondary gain, malingering, or criminality. Also, a psychoanalytic emphasis on unconscious conflicts in the etiology of psychiatric disorders led to a de-emphasis on the pathogenic role of psychological trauma. When *dissociative identity disorder* (DID; originally multiple personality disorder) emerged from the dissociative disorders spectrum, it was initially fueled by interest in the fascinating phenomena of seemingly multiple personalities emanating out of the same individual. In all of this, there was no appreciation for the critical role that psychological trauma routinely played in these disorders.

Psychological trauma was co-opted by clinicians who originally were advocates for Holocaust survivors and later for Vietnam veterans. An alliance between these groups led to the formulation of PTSD in DSM-III in 1980 (American Psychiatric Association 1980). PTSD then became the sine qua non of a trauma-related psychiatric disorder. In 1980 the dissociative disorders were separated from hysterical neurosis and gained independent status. Since then, PTSD and the dissociative disorders have developed in a parallel fashion, with two separate scientific/clinical societies, the International Society for Traumatic Stress Studies (for PTSD) and the International Society for the Study of Dissociation (for the dissociative disorders). Two groups of researchers developed in each society, focused on their own particular disorders. These two separate groups have only gradually started to realize that they have something in common.

DISSOCIATION IN POSTTRAUMATIC STRESS DISORDER

Despite PTSD's existence in DSM since 1980, remarkably little is known about the relationship between PTSD and dissociation. Several studies, however, have demonstrated a strong relationship between dissociative disorders and psychological trauma (Bremner et al. 1992, 1993b; Cardeña and Spiegel 1993; Chu and Dill 1990; Lewis and Putnam 1996; Loewenstein and Putnam 1998; Marmar et al. 1994; Putnam et al. 1986; Sanders and Giolas 1991; Spiegel 1984, 1994; Spiegel and Cardeña 1991; Spiegel et al. 1988; Stutman and Bliss 1985; see Chapter 4 in this volume, "Relationships Between Dissociation and Posttraumatic Stress Disorder," for further discussion). Furthermore, dissociative symptoms always cluster together. In our own studies, we were not able to find any evidence for the distinctness of amnesia, depersonalization, derealization, and identity diffusion as separate constructs (Bremner et al. 1993b, 1998). In fact, these symptoms are highly correlated.

Yet there appears to be no consistency in DSM in the conceptualization of dissociative symptoms relative to PTSD. For example, reexperiencing trauma is not described as a dissociative symptom, but flashback episodes are unquestionably dissociative. It is unclear what the difference, if any, would be between these positive (i.e., reexperiencing) symptoms. Inability to recall an important aspect of the trauma is not listed as a (negative) dissociative symptom under PTSD but is listed as a dissociative symptom under acute stress disorder (see Chapter 4). Similar confusion exists regarding numbing and detachment, which are identified as dissociative symptoms under acute stress disorder but not under PTSD. Confusion also exists in DSM for the overlap between dissociative symptoms in PTSD and dissociative disorders. For instance, after a car accident, many individuals who go on to develop PTSD report looking down on the scene from above (depersonalization); however, when they are exposed to stressors, things look strange or unreal (derealization), and they may have gaps of memory for the event (amnesia). The identity disturbance of DID is really related to a series of amnesic episodes that, when extreme, can lead the patient to feel as though there are multiple unconnected facets of themselves that are imperfectly connected with one another. Again, the different personality states are almost invariably experienced in a dreamy, dissociative state.

The inconsistency regarding the conceptualization of dissociation also affects which disorders are regarded as dissociative throughout DSM-IV-TR (American Psychiatric Association 2000). This confusion involves not only PTSD but also other conditions, including borderline personality disorder, which is also commonly associated with trauma and is conceptualized as related to aberrations in child development.

PERITRAUMATIC DISSOCIATION AS A PREDICTOR TO POSTTRAUMATIC STRESS DISORDER

Since the late 1990s, there has been an expansion of research in the field of dissociation. The development of instruments including the Dissociative Experiences Scale (Bernstein and Putnam 1986), the Structured Clinical Interview for DSM-III-R Dissociative Disorders (Steinberg et al. 1990), the Dissociative Disorders Interview Schedule (Ross et al. 1990), the Peritraumatic Dissociative Experiences Questionnaire (Marmar et al. 1994), and the Clinician-Administered Dissociative States Scale (CADSS; Bremner et al. 1998) have facilitated research in this field (see Chapter 13 in this volume, "Psychological Assessment of Posttraumatic Dissociation," for review).

There has been some controversy about whether dissociation is a normal psychological response or a pathological symptom seen only in trauma survivors (Bremner and Marmar 1998; Kluft 1985; Lewis and Putnam 1996). Part of this controversy relates to the overlap of dissociation with other constructs, such as hypnotizability and absorption. Both hypnotizability and absorption (e.g., the capacity to become intensely absorbed in a movie) are normal personality features that vary in the general population. *Absorption* is described as a tendency to become fully involved in a perceptual imaginative or ideational experience. Individuals prone to this type of experience are more highly hypnotizable (Tellegen and Atkinson 1974). Absorption and hypnosis share a kind of imaginative involvement (Vermetten et al. 1998). Some of the questions asked on scales to measure dissociation include absorption-type questions, which may identify a normal personality trait instead of a pathological response. In our opinion, dissociative symptoms—such as repeatedly seeing things as though you were in a tunnel—are indicators of psychopathology and are primarily found in patients with pathological responses to trauma. The distinction may involve control over the change in mental state, with absorption being a more controlled, adaptive ability to enter such states, whereas dissociation is more often experienced as unbidden (Barrett 1992).

We asked Vietnam veterans about dissociative symptoms at the time of combat trauma and found that those who dissociated at the time of combat trauma were more likely to later develop PTSD and continued to have dissociative responses to subsequent stressors (Bremner and Brett 1997; Bremner et al. 1992). We found that Vietnam combat veterans with PTSD had increased dissociative symptom levels compared with combat veterans without PTSD (Bremner et al. 1992, 1993b). These studies showed a close relationship between the diagnosis of PTSD and dissociative disorders. For example, 86% of a PTSD sample met criteria for a comorbid dissociative disorder (Bremner and Brett 1997), whereas essentially 100% of patients with DID met criteria for PTSD (Vermetten et al. 2006a). Marmar et al. (1994) found that dissociative responses to trauma predicted long-term PTSD in emergency personnel, and prospective studies have documented the association between dissociative states at the time of trauma and the development of chronic PTSD (Koopman et al. 1994; Shalev et al. 1996). According to Marmar et al. (2006), the strongest predictor as seen in their study after the attacks on the World Trade Center was the immediate response to trauma. From their study it appeared that unmanageable terror and horror at the time of a traumatic event represent the single best predictor of PTSD, and prolonged panic has large, long effects that swamp all pre- and posttrauma predictors. More specifically, as another study showed, it was not dissociative symptoms in the first 24 hours after a trauma that was predictive of chronic PTSD but rather dissociative symptoms about 1 week after trauma that was predictive of long-term outcome (McFarlane 2000). It may be that immediate dissociative responses are nonspecific responses to trauma and that continued dissociation in a situation of chronic stress is the best predictor of pathology.

In order to conduct studies of treatment and neurobiology of dissociation, we developed the CADSS as a scale for use as a repeated measure of dissociative states (Bremner et al. 1998). The CADSS is a 27-item scale with 19 subject-rated items and 8 items scored by an observer. The 19 subjective items are administered by a clinician who begins each question with the phrase "at this time" and then reads the item to the subject.

The subject then endorses one of a range of possible responses: 0 not at all, 1 slightly, 2 moderately, 3 considerably, 4 extremely. Some of the dissociative symptoms measured with the CADSS that were most commonly endorsed in traumatized patients included "Did things seem to be moving in slow motion?"; "Did sounds change, so that that they became very soft or very loud?"; and "Did it seem as if you were looking at things as an observer or a spectator?" We found that these symptoms increased when PTSD patients were reexposed to reminders of their original trauma during a traumatic memories group conducted at the inpatient PTSD program at the Atlanta Veterans Affairs hospital. Moreover, PTSD patients with high dissociative disorder comorbidity showed significantly higher CADSS scores compared with patients with schizophrenia or depression, Vietnam combat veterans without PTSD, and healthy individuals (Bremner et al. 1998). A group of patients with PTSD were assessed before and after exposure to a traumatic memories group. They showed a significant increase in dissociative symptomatology, in comparison with baseline, during exposure to a traumatic memories group.

TRANSLATING ANIMAL MODELS OF STRESS TO HUMAN TRAUMA AND POSTTRAUMATIC STRESS DISORDER

The introduction of PTSD as a psychiatric disorder in DSM-III represented the recognition that psychological trauma can cause changes in brain and physiological responding (Saigh and Bremner 1999). It was another decade, however, before research into the neurobiology of PTSD began in earnest. Initial studies applied findings on the effects of stress in animals to the study of the neurobiology of PTSD. Studies in animals exposed to stress showed deficits in memory function (Luine et al. 1994) and damage to the hippocampus, which mediates this memory function (Sapolsky et al. 1990; Uno et al. 1989). Stress interfered with hippocampal-based mechanisms of memory function, including long-term potentiation (Diamond et al. 1996; Luine et al. 1994). A variety of mechanisms have been proposed for these findings, including elevated levels of glucocorticoids released during stress (Lawrence and Sapolsky 1994; Sapolsky 1996), stress-related inhibition of brain-derived neurotrophic factor (Nibuya et al. 1995; Smith et al. 1995), or changes in serotonergic function (McEwen et al. 1992), although mechanisms continue to be debated (Leverenz et al. 1999). Studies have shown that stress is associated with an inhibition of neurogenesis (the growth of new neurons) in the hippocampus (Fowler et al. 2001; Gould et al. 1997) and that these effects are reversible with antidepressant selective serotonin reuptake inhibitor (SSRI) medications (Duman et al. 2001; Lee et al. 2001; Malberg et al. 2000) as well as other medications, including tianeptine (Czeh et al. 2001) and phenytoin (Watanabe et al. 1992). Antidepressant-induced promotion of neurogenesis may underlie the behavioral effects of these medications (Santarelli et al. 2003), although this question continues to be a matter of debate (Vollmayr et al. 2003).

HIPPOCAMPAL DYSFUNCTION IN POSTTRAUMATIC STRESS DISORDER AND DISSOCIATIVE DISORDERS

The role of the hippocampus in learning and memory and the wide range of memory alterations seen in PTSD patients led to the hypothesis of hippocampal dysfunction in PTSD (Bremner 2003; Bremner et al. 1995a). Initial studies demonstrated deficits in hippocampal-based learning and memory in PTSD (Bremner et al. 1993a, 1995b). The first neuroimaging study in PTSD (Bremner et al. 1995c), using magnetic resonance imaging (MRI), showed an 8% decrease in right hippocampal volume in patients with combat-related PTSD ($n=26$) in comparison with matched control subjects ($n=22$) ($P<0.05$). Decreases in right hippocampal volume in the PTSD patients were associated with deficits in short-term memory (Bremner et al. 1995c). Findings of smaller hippocampal volume and/or a reduction in N-acetylaspartate in the hippocampus (a marker of neuronal integrity) in adults with chronic, long-standing PTSD have been replicated several times in the published literature (Bremner et al. 1997c; Freeman et al. 1998; Gurvits et al. 1996; Schuff et al. 2001; Stein et al. 1997; Villareale et al. 2002). One study used a specific cognitive task to probe hippocampal function and demonstrated a failure of left hippocampal activation with a memory task in women with abuse-related PTSD (Bremner et al. 2003b). This was significant after controlling for differences in hippocampal volume measured on MRI in the same subjects. Women with PTSD had smaller hippocampal volume than both abused and nonabused women without PTSD. We also recently demonstrated that women with DID had both significantly smaller hippocampal (19.2%) and amygdalar volume (31.6%) when compared with healthy female control subjects (Vermetten et al. 2006a). All patients with DID in this study also had a diagnosis of PTSD according to DSM-IV-TR. Studies in children have not shown smaller hippocampal volume in PTSD (Carrion et al. 2001; De Bellis et al. 1999, 2001). Other studies provoked symptoms of PTSD by showing traumatic pictures, reading back personalized scripts of trauma, or other methods. These studies most consistently showed a failure of activation in the frontal cortex (Bremner et al. 1999a, 1999b; Shin et al. 1999), the part of the brain involved in shutting off the fear response by inhibiting the amygdala, which mediates the fear response.

Based on findings related to the effects of antidepressants on neurogenesis, we assessed the effects of the SSRI paroxetine on outcomes related to function of the hippocampus. We studied 28 patients with PTSD and treated them for up to 1 year with variable dosages of paroxetine (Vermetten et al. 2003). Twenty-three patients completed the course of treatment, and MRIs were obtained after treatment in 20 patients. Those who did not complete treatment stopped because of substance abuse relapse or were lost to follow-up (possibly because of a treatment nonresponse). The Wechsler Memory Scale–Revised and the Selective Reminding Test were used to assess hippocampal-based declarative memory function. MRI was used to assess hippocampal volume before and after treatment. Patients with PTSD showed a significant improvement in PTSD symptoms with treatment and altered reactivity to a stress challenge paradigm (Vermetten et al. 2006b). Treatment resulted in significant improvements in verbal declarative memory and a 4.6% increase in mean hippocampal volume. These findings suggested that long-term treatment with paroxetine is associated with improvement of verbal declarative memory deficits and an increase in hippocampal volume in PTSD.

STRESS HORMONES

Norepinephrine

Hormones (including norepinephrine and cortisol) play a critical role in the stress response. Norepinephrine (commonly known as adrenaline) is released in both the brain and the body and has several functions that are critical for survival. It sharpens the senses, focuses attention, raises the level of fear, quickens the heart rate and blood pressure, and in general prepares us for the worst. The norepinephrine system is like a fire alarm that alerts all areas of the brain simultaneously. This system sacrifices the ability to convey specific information to specific parts of the brain in order to obtain more speed. Norepinephrine focuses the senses by activating the neurons that collect sensory information to rapidly and efficiently identify danger in the environment. At the same time, norepinephrine stimulates the heart to beat more rapidly and blood pressure to increase. This effects an emergency transfer of oxygen and nutrients needed for survival to all the cells of the body. The beauty of the system is that the same chemical messenger that "turns on" the brain also stimulates the heart (as well as other bodily organs) in order to facilitate survival. Chronic stress in animals leads to increased levels of norepinephrine (Bremner et al. 1996a).

A variety of studies have shown long-term dysregulation of the noradrenergic system in PTSD (Bremner et al. 1996b). Psychophysiology studies have demonstrated an increase in sympathetic responses (heart rate, blood pressure, and galvanic skin response) to traumatic reminders, such as traumatic slides and sounds or traumatic scripts, in PTSD (Pitman et al. 1987). Studies of norepinephrine in plasma and urine have shown increased levels at baseline, while traumatic reminders resulted in a potentiated release of norepinephrine in PTSD (McFall et al. 1990). Administration of the α_2 antagonist yohimbine, which results in increased release of norepinephrine in the brain, increased PTSD-specific symptomatology (Southwick et al. 1993). A greater release of norepinephrine metabolites in plasma in PTSD patients was also found. Alterations in central metabolic responses to yohimbine were found in PTSD patients using positron emission tomography (PET; Bremner et al. 1997a). Animal studies have shown that increasing norepinephrine release up to a certain level improves cognition and attention, but beyond that point there is a reduction in performance. Using PET, which allows measurement of brain activity while norepinephrine release in the brain is stimulated with medication (yohimbine), we found that lower levels of norepinephrine stimulate brain activity in the prefrontal cortex, but at very high levels (as seen in PTSD) the brain shuts off. These findings are consistent with an inverted U-curve for norepinephrine in which lower levels of norepinephrine stimulation increase the efficiency of the brain, whereas very high levels make it more inefficient. The experience of "choking" during an examination that one is prepared to take reflects the release of too much norepinephrine in the brain. This concept lies behind the common practice of taking propranolol (which blocks the effects of norepinephrine in the brain) to improve performance during public speaking.

Cortisol

The cortisol system also plays an important role in the stress response. Like norepinephrine, cortisol is released during times of threat and is critical to survival. Cortisol redistributes the energy of the body when under attack in order to help survival. This includes suppressing functions not necessary for immediate survival, such as reproduction, the body's immune response, digestion, and the feeling of pain. Cortisol also promotes necessary survival functions, such as increasing heart rate and blood pressure, and shunts energy to the brain and muscles to assist thinking and escape. Although cortisol has actions that are beneficial for short-term survival, it may perform these functions at the expense of long-term viability of the body. For instance, chronically high cortisol levels cause gastric ulcers, thinning of the bones, and possibly even brain damage. Evolution may have preferred the caveman who could survive attacks by woolly mammoths long enough to pass his genes to the next generation, even if it meant that he could not remember where he left his favorite spear when he was old. In other words, evolution prefers short-term survival at the expense of long-term function.

The corticotropin-releasing factor (CRF)/hypothalamic-pituitary-adrenal (HPA) axis system plays an important role in the stress response. Exposure to stressful situations is associated with a marked increase in cortisol release from the adrenal. Glucocorticoid release from the adrenal is regulated by adrenocorticotropic hormone secreted from the pituitary, which in turn is primarily regulated by CRF release from the paraventricular nucleus of the hypothalamus. Intraventricular injection of CRF results in stress-related behaviors (e.g., fearfulness). Stressors early in life may have long-term effects on the CRF/HPA axis, including increased glucocorticoid response to subsequent stressors (Heim et al. 1998, 2000).

PTSD has been associated with long-term dysregulation of the HPA axis. Baseline levels of urinary cortisol were either decreased or unchanged in chronic PTSD, whereas decreased levels were found in 24-hour samples of plasma cortisol levels (Yehuda et al. 1994). However, exposure to a stressor (Bremner et al. 2003a) or a traumatic reminder (Elzinga et al. 2003) was associated with a potentiated release of cortisol in PTSD. Cortisol may also be elevated in the more acute phase of PTSD, although further research is needed in this area. A replicated finding has been a super-suppression of the cortisol response to lower doses of dexamethasone suppression test (DST; 0.5 mg), a finding which is the opposite of patients with major depression who are nonsuppressors with the standard 1 mg DST test (Yehuda et al. 1993; see also review by de Kloet et al. 2005). PTSD patients had elevated levels of CRF in the cerebrospinal fluid (CSF; Baker et al. 1999; Bremner et al. 1997b). One possible explanation of findings to date is an increase in neuronal CRF release, increased central glucocorticoid receptor responsiveness, and resultant low levels of peripheral cortisol due to enhanced negative feedback.

NEUROBIOLOGICAL STUDIES IN DISSOCIATION

Because of the delay in achieving a consensus regarding the diagnostic formulation of the dissociative disorders, there have been few neurobiological studies of these conditions. In one early study, patients with DID were found to have changes in autonomic indices and reactions times when voluntarily moving between alter personality states (Putnam et al. 1990). Hypnotizability, which has been associated with dissociation, was found to correlate with CSF levels of the dopamine metabolite homovanillic acid in a mixed group of psychiatric patients (Spiegel and King 1992). κ Opioid receptor agonists can induce depersonalization, derealization, and perceptual alterations (Pfeiffer et al. 1986). In patients with eating disorders, dissociative symptoms as measured by the Dissociative Experiences Scale were positively correlated with CSF homovanillic acid and negatively correlated with CSF β-endorphin (Demitrack et al. 1993).

The HPA axis is known to play a central role in the stress response, which is critical in the development of dissociative disorders. The role of the HPA axis in mediating dissociation is still unclear. Cortisol levels were found to fall during hypnosis (Sachar et al. 1966). One study in DPD found nonsignificantly lower basal salivary cortisol in DPD patients compared with healthy control subjects (Stanton et al. 2001), whereas another study showed a tendency for elevated basal urinary and plasma cortisol and a resistance to low-dose dexamethasone suppression in DPD compared with control subjects (Simeon et al. 2001).

Apart from single case reports, brain imaging studies of dissociative disorders published in the literature are few. In one study, patients with DPD had higher activity in somatosensory association areas (Simeon et al. 2000). One brain imaging study used functional MRI in PTSD patients who were in a dissociative state while reexperiencing traumatic memories and found they showed more activation in the temporal, inferior and medial frontal, occipital, parietal, anterior cingulate, and medial prefrontal cortical regions (Lanius et al. 2002; see Chapter 10 in this volume, "Posttraumatic Stress Disorder Symptom Provocation and Neuroimaging"). Recently the script-driven paradigm has been applied using PET in DID patients (Reinders et al. 2003, 2006; see Chapter 11 in this volume, "Psychobiology of Traumatization and Trauma-Related Structural Dissociation of the Personality").

Brain regions such as the hippocampus that are sensitive to stress may mediate symptoms of dissociation. Two studies have found a negative correlation between dissociative symptom level as measured by the Dissociative Experiences Scale and hippocampal volume as measured with MRI in women with early childhood sexual abuse–related PTSD (Bremner et al. 2003b; Stein et al. 1997). Electrical stimulation of the hippocampus and adjacent regions in patients with epilepsy resulted in a number of dissociative-like symptoms, including feelings of déjà vu, depersonalization, derealization, and memory alterations (Halgren et al. 1978; Penfield and

Perot 1963). Administration of the N-methyl-D-aspartate (NMDA) receptor antagonist ketamine resulted in dissociative symptoms in healthy subjects, including feeling out of body, time standing still, body distortions, and amnesia (Krystal et al. 1994). NMDA receptors are highly concentrated in the hippocampus and play a role in memory on a molecular level. Stress inhibits long-term potentiation, which is the molecular model for memory (Diamond et al. 1995, 1996). Based on these findings, we have hypothesized that stress, acting through the NMDA receptor in the hippocampus, may mediate symptoms of dissociation (Bremner 2002; Bremner and Marmar 1998). Because of trance-like states seen in some individuals with thalamic lesions, and given the role of the thalamus as a gateway of sensory information from the outside world to the brain, we have also hypothesized that thalamic dysfunction may play a role in dissociation (Krystal et al. 1996).

Medication trials in dissociative disorders have been similarly limited (see Chapter 17 in this volume, "Treatment of Traumatic Dissociation"). The SSRI fluoxetine was shown to reduce symptoms of depersonalization (Fichtner et al. 1992; Hollander et al. 1990; Ratliff and Kerski 1995). The anticonvulsant lamotrigine, which inhibits glutamate release, was found to attenuate ketamine-induced dissociation in healthy subjects (Anand et al. 2000). It has been hypothesized that NMDA antagonists such as ketamine may induce depersonalization via increased glutamate neurotransmission at non-NMDA glutamate receptors. Along these lines, there was a promising preliminary open-label trial of lamotrigine in chronic depersonalization (Sierra et al. 2001). Opioid receptor antagonists have been reported to reduce dissociation, including naltrexone in patients with borderline personality disorder (Bohus et al. 1999) and intravenous naloxone in chronic depersonalization (Nuller et al. 2001).

CONCLUSION

In this chapter we reviewed how traumatic stress results in an activation of brain areas that play a critical role in the stress response. We mentioned the neurohormonal systems cortisol and norepinephrine. These systems help the organism escape from stressors. Brain areas involved in memory and the stress response, including the hippocampus, frontal cortex, and amygdala, also play a critical role in survival in the face of a life-threatening stressor. With chronic stress these systems may become dysfunctional. Research in patients with PTSD shows long-term alterations in stress-responsive systems (e.g., cortisol and norepinephrine) as well as alterations in structure and/or function in brain regions involved in the stress response (e.g., the hippocampus, amygdala, and frontal cortex). These brain areas may also mediate dissociative symptoms that overlap with PTSD symptoms, particularly the hippocampus, which appears to play a key role in dissociation.

The current diagnostic schema does not appropriately address the experiences of clinicians who care daily for patients with stress-related psychiatric disorders. In our opinion, this is an artifact of the continuing drive to create categories and classifications of psychiatric diagnoses that contain discrete disorders that are unrelated to one another and not based on any particular theoretical foundation or view of etiology. This is largely a by-product of the domination of psychiatric diagnosis by the field of psychoanalysis for the better part of the twentieth century and the subsequent reaction to this domination. For psychoanalysis, theories of etiology were central to diagnosis; for example, anxiety neurosis was related to repressed conflicts that were made manifest only in symptoms in which the relationship to the disorder was not immediately obvious. The development of DSM represented a gradual removal of psychiatric diagnosis from the psychoanalysts under the mantle of "science" and "objective diagnosis." A major objective of the move to make psychiatric diagnosis empirical was to remove any etiological underpinning for these diagnoses. However, what is not appreciated is that there often was little or no empirical basis for these new psychiatric diagnoses.

Based on the close relationship among dissociation, PTSD, and trauma, we would argue for a reorganization of the current diagnostic criteria for the anxiety disorders (which currently includes PTSD) and dissociative disorders (Bremner 1999). In the current American Psychiatric Association diagnostic criteria there is the diagnosis of acute stress disorder, which describes dissociative and PTSD symptoms in the first month after psychological trauma. Recent research has indicated that acute stress disorder and PTSD are closely related (Brewin et al. 1999). Their criteria should therefore be made consistent with one another.

There is increasing interest in dissociative disorders and their link with trauma. It appears that traumatic dissociation covers both the etiological concept as well as the so-called response (i.e., peritraumatic dissociation). Future studies may learn that this second factor is more important then we currently believe it to be (Briere 2006). From a phenomenological perspective, dissociative disorders as currently defined have good internal consistency. The interface with symptomatically similar or related disorders needs to be further developed and the validity of the research findings embedded into mainstream medicine. Studies related to the neurobiology of trauma-related disorders will play an important role in this process.

REFERENCES

American Psychiatric Association: Diagnostic and Statistical Manual of Mental Disorder, 3rd Edition. Washington, DC, American Psychiatric Association, 1980

American Psychiatric Association: Diagnostic and Statistical Manual of Mental Disorders, 4th Edition, Text Revision. Washington, DC, American Psychiatric Association, 2000

Anand A, Charney D, Oren DA, et al: Attenuation of the neuropsychiatric effects of ketamine with lamotrigine: support for hyperglutamatergic effects of N-methyl-D-aspartate receptor antagonists. Arch Gen Psychiatry 57:270–276, 2000

Baker DB, West SA, Nicholson WE, et al: Serial CSF corticotropin-releasing hormone levels and adrenocortical activity in combat veterans with posttraumatic stress disorder. Am J Psychiatry 156:585–588, 1999

Barrett D: Fantasizers and dissociaters: data on two distinct subgroups of deep trance subjects. Psychol Rep 71:1011–1014, 1992

Bernstein E, Putnam F: Development, reliability, and validity of a dissociation scale. J Nerv Ment Dis 174:727–735, 1986

Bohus MJ, Landwehrmeyer GB, Stiglmayr CE, et al: Naltrexone in the treatment of dissociative symptoms in patients with borderline personality disorder: an open-label trial. J Clin Psychiatry 60:598–603, 1999

Bremner JD: Acute and chronic responses to psychological trauma: where do we go from here? (editorial). Am J Psychiatry 156:349–351, 1999

Bremner JD: Does Stress Damage the Brain? Understanding Trauma-Related Disorders From a Mind-Body Perspective. New York, WW Norton, 2002

Bremner JD: Functional neuroanatomical correlates of traumatic stress revisited 7 years later, this time with data. Psychopharmacol Bull 37:6–25, 2003

Bremner JD, Brett E: Trauma-related dissociative states and long-term psychopathology in posttraumatic stress disorder. J Trauma Stress 10:37–49, 1997

Bremner JD, Marmar CR (eds): Trauma, Memory, and Dissociation. Washington, DC, American Psychiatric Press, 1998

Bremner JD, Southwick SM, Brett E, et al: Dissociation and posttraumatic stress disorder in Vietnam combat veterans. Am J Psychiatry 149:328–332, 1992

Bremner JD, Scott TM, Delaney RC, et al: Deficits in short-term memory in posttraumatic stress disorder. Am J Psychiatry 150:1015–1019, 1993a

Bremner JD, Steinberg M, Southwick SM, et al: Use of the Structured Clinical Interview for DSM-IV Dissociative Disorders for systematic assessment of dissociative symptoms in posttraumatic stress disorder. Am J Psychiatry 150:1011–1014, 1993b

Bremner JD, Krystal JH, Southwick SM, et al: Functional neuroanatomical correlates of the effects of stress on memory. J Trauma Stress 8:527–554, 1995a

Bremner JD, Randall PR, Capelli S, et al: Deficits in short-term memory in adult survivors of childhood abuse. Psychiatry Res 59:97–107, 1995b

Bremner JD, Randall PR, Scott TM. et al: MRI-based measurement of hippocampal volume in patients with combat-related posttraumatic stress disorder. Am J Psychiatry 152:973–981, 1995c

Bremner JD, Krystal JH, Southwick SM, et al: Noradrenergic mechanisms in stress and anxiety, I: preclinical studies. Synapse 23:28–38, 1996a

Bremner JD, Krystal JH, Southwick SM, et al: Noradrenergic mechanisms in stress and anxiety, II: clinical studies. Synapse 23:39–51, 1996b

Bremner JD, Innis RB, Ng CK, et al: PET measurement of cerebral metabolic correlates of yohimbine administration in posttraumatic stress disorder. Arch Gen Psychiatry 54:246–256, 1997a

Bremner JD, Licinio J, Darnell A, et al: Elevated CSF corticotropin-releasing factor concentrations in posttraumatic stress disorder. Am J Psychiatry 154:624–629, 1997b

Bremner JD, Randall PR, Vermetten E, et al: MRI-based measurement of hippocampal volume in posttraumatic stress disorder related to childhood physical and sexual abuse: a preliminary report. Biol Psychiatry 41:23–32, 1997c

Bremner JD, Krystal JH, Putnam FW, et al: Measurement of dissociative states with the Clinician-Administered Dissociative States Scale (CADSS). J Trauma Stress 11:125–136, 1998

Bremner JD, Narayan M, Staib LH, et al: Neural correlates of memories of childhood sexual abuse in women with and without posttraumatic stress disorder. Am J Psychiatry 156:1787–1795, 1999a

Bremner JD, Staib LH, Kaloupek D, et al: Neural correlates of exposure to traumatic pictures and sound in Vietnam combat veterans with and without posttraumatic stress disorder: a positron emission tomography study. Biol Psychiatry 45:806–816, 1999b

Bremner JD, Vythilingam M, Vermetten E, et al: Cortisol response to a cognitive stress challenge in posttraumatic stress disorder (PTSD) related to childhood abuse. Psychoneuroendocrinology 28:733–750, 2003a

Bremner JD, Vythilingam M, Vermetten E, et al: MRI and PET study of deficits in hippocampal structure and function in women with childhood sexual abuse and posttraumatic stress disorder (PTSD). Am J Psychiatry 160:924–932, 2003b

Briere J: Dissociative symptoms and trauma exposure: specificity, affect dysregulation, and posttraumatic stress. J Nerv Ment Dis 194:78–82, 2006

Brewin CR, Andrews B, Rose S, et al: Acute stress disorder and posttraumatic stress disorder in victims of violent crime. Am J Psychiatry 156:360–366, 1999

Cardeña E, Spiegel D: Dissociative reactions to the San Francisco Bay area earthquake of 1989. Am J Psychiatry 150:474–478, 1993

Carrion VG, Weems CF, Eliez S, et al: Attenuation of frontal asymmetry in pediatric posttraumatic stress disorder. Biol Psychiatry 50:943–951, 2001

Chu JA, Dill DL: Dissociative symptoms in relation to childhood physical and sexual abuse. Am J Psychiatry 147:887–892, 1990

Czeh B, Michaelis T, Watanabe T, et al: Stress-induced changes in cerebral metabolites, hippocampal volume, and cell proliferation are prevented by antidepressant treatment with tianeptine. Proc Natl Acad Sci USA 98:12796–12801, 2001

De Bellis MD, Keshavan MS, Clark DB, et al: A.E. Bennett Research Award. Developmental traumatology, part II: brain development. Biol Psychiatry 45:1271–1284, 1999

De Bellis MD, Hall J, Boring AM, et al: A pilot longitudinal study of hippocampal volumes in pediatric maltreatment-related posttraumatic stress disorder. Biol Psychiatry 50:305–309, 2001

de Kloet CS, Vermetten E, Geuze E, et al: Assessment of HPA axis function in posttraumatic stress disorder: pharmacological and non-pharmacological challenge tests, a review. J Psychiatr Res 40:550–567, 2006

Demitrack MA, Putnam FW, Rubinow DR, et al: Relationship of dissociative phenomena to levels of cerebrospinal fluid monoamine metabolites and beta-endorphin in patients with eating disorders: a pilot study. Psychiatry Res 49:1–10, 1993

Diamond DM, Branch BJ, Fleshner M, et al: Effects of dehydroepiandrosterone and stress on hippocampal electrophysiological plasticity. Ann NY Acad Sci 774:304–307, 1995

Diamond DM, Fleshner M, Ingersoll N, et al: Psychological stress impairs spatial working memory: relevance to electrophysiological studies of hippocampal function. Behav Neurosci 110:661–672, 1996

Duman RS, Malberg JE, Nakagawa S: Regulation of adult neurogenesis by psychotropic drugs and stress. J Pharmacol Exp Ther 299:401–407, 2001

Elzinga BM, Schmahl CS, Vermetten E, et al: Higher cortisol levels following exposure to traumatic reminders in abuse-related PTSD. Neuropsychopharmacology 28:1656–1665, 2003

Fichtner CG, Horevitz RP, Braun BG: Fluoxetine in depersonalization disorder. Am J Psychiatry 149:1750–1751, 1992

Fowler CD, Liu Y, Ouimet C, et al: The effects of social environment on adult neurogenesis in the female prairie vole. J Neurobiol 51:115–128, 2001

Freeman TW, Cardwell D, Karson CN, et al: In vivo proton magnetic resonance spectroscopy of the medial temporal lobes of subjects with combat-related posttraumatic stress disorder. Magn Reson Med 40:66–71, 1998

Gould E, McEwen BS, Tanapat P, et al: Neurogenesis in the dentate gyrus of the adult tree shrew is regulated by psychosocial stress and NMDA receptor activation. J Neurosci 17:2492–2498, 1997

Gurvits TG, Shenton MR, Hokama H, et al: Magnetic resonance imaging study of hippocampal volume in chronic combat-related posttraumatic stress disorder. Biol Psychiatry 40:192–199, 1996

Halgren E, Walter RD, Cherlow DG, et al: Mental phenomena evoked by electrical stimulation of the hippocampal formation and amygdala. Brain 101:83–117, 1978

Heim C, Ehlert U, Hanker JP, et al: Abuse-related posttraumatic stress disorder and alterations of the hypothalamic-pituitary-adrenal axis in women with chronic pelvic pain. Psychosom Med 60:309–318, 1998

Heim C, Newport DJ, Heit S, et al: Pituitary-adrenal and autonomic responses to stress in women after sexual and physical abuse in childhood. JAMA 284:592–597, 2000

Hollander E, Liebowitz MR, DeCaria CM, et al: Treatment of depersonalization with serotonin reuptake blockers. J Clin Psychopharmacol 10:200–203, 1990

Irwin HJ: Proneness to dissociation and traumatic childhood events. J Nerv Ment Dis 182:456–460, 1994

Kluft RP: Childhood Antecedents of Multiple Personality Disorder. Washington, DC, American Psychiatric Press, 1985

Koopman C, Classen C, Spiegel D: Predictors of posttraumatic stress symptoms among survivors of the Oakland/Berkeley, Calif., firestorm. Am J Psychiatry 151:888–894, 1994

Krystal JH, Karper LP, Seibyl JP, et al: Subanesthetic effects of the non-competitive NMDA antagonist, ketamine, in humans: psychotomimetic, perceptual, cognitive, and neuroendocrine responses. Arch Gen Psychiatry 51:199–214, 1994

Krystal JH, Bennett A, Bremner JD, et al: Recent developments in the neurobiology of dissociation: implications for posttraumatic stress disorder, in Handbook of Dissociation: Theoretical, Empirical, and Clinical Perspectives. Edited by Michelson LK, Ray WJ. New York, Plenum, 1996, pp 163–190

Lanius RA, Williamson PC, Boksman K, et al: Brain activation during script-driven imagery induced dissociative responses in PTSD: a functional magnetic resonance imaging investigation. Biol Psychiatry 52:305–311, 2002

Lawrence MS, Sapolsky RM: Glucocorticoids accelerate ATP loss following metabolic insults in cultured hippocampal neurons. Brain Res 646:303–306, 1994

Lee H, Kim JW, Yim SV, et al: Fluoxetine enhances cell proliferation and prevents apoptosis in dentate gyrus of maternally separated rats. Mol Psychiatry 6:725–728, 2001

Leverenz JB, Wilkinson CW, Wamble M, et al: Effect of chronic high-dose exogenous cortisol on hippocampal neuronal number in aged nonhuman primate. J Neurosci 19:2356–2361, 1999

Lewis DO, Putnam FW (eds): Child and Adolescent Psychiatric Clinics: Dissociative Identity/Multiple Personality Disorder. Philadelphia, PA, WB Saunders, 1996

Loewenstein RJ, Putnam FW: A comparison study of dissociative symptoms in patients with complex partial seizures, MPD, and posttraumatic stress disorder. Dissociation 1:17–23, 1998

Luine V, Villages M, Martinez C, et al: Repeated stress causes reversible impairments of spatial memory performance. Brain Res 639:167–170, 1994

Malberg JE, Eisch AJ, Nestler EJ, et al: Chronic antidepressant treatment increases neurogenesis in adult rat hippocampus. J Neurosci 20:9104–9110, 2000

Marmar CR, Weiss DS, Schlenger DS, et al: Peritraumatic dissociation and posttraumatic stress in male Vietnam theater veterans. Am J Psychiatry 151:902–907, 1994

Marmar CR, McCaslin SE, Metzler TJ, et al: Predictors of posttraumatic stress in police and other first responders. Ann N Y Acad Sci 1071:1–18, 2006

McEwen BS, Angulo J, Cameron H, et al: Paradoxical effects of adrenal steroids on the brain: protection versus degeneration. Biol Psychiatry 31:177–199, 1992

McFall ME, Murburg MM, Ko GN, et al: Autonomic responses to stress in Vietnam combat veterans with posttraumatic stress disorder. Biol Psychiatry 27:1165–1175, 1990

McFarlane AC: Posttraumatic stress disorder: a model of the longitudinal course and the role of risk factors. J Clin Psychiatry 61:15–20, 2000

Nibuya M, Morinobu S, Duman RS: Regulation of BDNF and trkB mRNA in rat brain by chronic electroconvulsive seizure and antidepressant drug treatments. J Neurosci 15:7539–7547, 1995

Nuller YL, Morozova MG, Kushnir ON, et al: Effect of naloxone therapy on depersonalization. J Psychopharmacol 15:93–95, 2001

Penfield W, Perot P: The brain's record of auditory and visual experience: a final summary and discussion. Brain 86:595–696, 1963

Pfeiffer A, Brantl V, Herz A, et al: Psychotomimesis mediated by opiate receptors. Science 233:774–776, 1986

Pitman RK, Orr SP, Forgus DF, et al: Psychophysiologic assessment of posttraumatic stress disorder imagery in Vietnam combat veterans. Arch Gen Psychiatry 44:970–975, 1987

Putnam FW, Guroff JJ, Silberman EK, et al: The clinical phenomenology of multiple personality disorder: a review of 100 recent cases. J Clin Psychiatry 47:285–293, 1986

Putnam FW, Zahn TP, Post RM: Differential autonomic nervous system activity in multiple personality disorder. Psychiatry Res 31:251–260, 1990

Ratliff NB, Kerski D: Depersonalization treated with fluoxetine. Am J Psychiatry 152:1689–1690, 1995

Reinders AA, Nijenhuis ER, Paans AM, et al: One brain, two selves. Neuroimage 20:2119–2125, 2003

Reinders AA, Nijenhuis ER, Quak J, et al: Psychobiological characteristics of dissociative identity disorder: a symptom provocation study. Biol Psychiatry 60:730–740, 2006

Ross CA, Joshi S, Currie R: Dissociative experiences in the general population. Am J Psychiatry 147:1547–1552, 1990

Sachar EJ, Cobb JC, Shor RE: Plasma cortisol changes during hypnotic trance. Arch Gen Psychiatry 14:482–490, 1966

Saigh PA, Bremner JD: The history of posttraumatic stress disorder, in Posttraumatic Stress Disorder: A Comprehensive Text. Edited by Saigh PA, Bremner JD. Needham Heights, MA, Allyn & Bacon, 1999, pp 1–17

Sanders B, Giolas MH: Dissociation and childhood trauma in psychologically disturbed adolescents. Am J Psychiatry 148:50–54, 1991

Santarelli L, Saxe M, Gross C, et al: Requirement of hippocampal neurogenesis for the behavioral effects of antidepressants. Science 301:805–809, 2003

Sapolsky RM: Why stress is bad for your brain. Science 273:749–750, 1996

Sapolsky RM, Uno H, Rebert CS, et al: Hippocampal damage associated with prolonged glucocorticoid exposure in primates. J Neurosci 10:2897–2902, 1990

Schuff N, Neylan TC, Lenoci MA, et al: Decreased hippocampal N-acetylaspartate in the absence of atrophy in posttraumatic stress disorder. Biol Psychiatry 50:952–959, 2001

Shalev AY, Peri T, Canetti L, et al: Predictors of PTSD in injured trauma survivors: a prospective study. Am J Psychiatry 153:219–225, 1996

Shin LM, McNally RJ, Kosslyn SM, et al: Regional cerebral blood flow during script-driven imagery in childhood sexual abuse-related PTSD: a PET investigation. Am J Psychiatry 156:575–584, 1999

Sierra M, Phillips ML, Lambert MV, et al: Lamotrigine in the treatment of depersonalization disorder. J Clin Psychiatry 62:826–827, 2001

Simeon D, Guralnik O, Hazlett S, et al: Feeling unreal: a PET study of depersonalization disorder. Am J Psychiatry 157:1782–1788, 2000

Simeon D, Guralnik O, Knutelska M, et al: Hypothalamic-pituitary-adrenal axis dysregulation in depersonalization disorder. Neuropsychopharmacology 25:793–795, 2001

Smith MA, Makino S, Kvetnansky R, et al: Stress and glucocorticoids affect the expression of brain-derived neurotrophic factor and neurotrophin-3 mRNA in the hippocampus. J Neurosci 15:1768–1777, 1995

Southwick SM, Krystal JH, Morgan CA, et al: Abnormal noradrenergic function in posttraumatic stress disorder. Arch Gen Psychiatry 50:266–274, 1993

Spiegel D: Multiple personality as a posttraumatic stress disorder. Psychiatr Clin North Am 7:101–110, 1984

Spiegel D (ed): Dissociation: Culture, Mind, and Body. Washington, DC, American Psychiatric Press, 1994

Spiegel D, Cardeña E: Disintegrated experience: the dissociative disorders revisited. J Abnorm Psychol 100:366–378, 1991

Spiegel D, King R: Hypnotizability and CSF HVA levels among psychiatric patients. Biol Psychiatry 31:95–98, 1992

Spiegel D, Hunt T, Dondershine HE: Dissociation and hypnotizability in posttraumatic stress disorder. Am J Psychiatry 145:301–305, 1988

Stanton BR, David AS, Cleare AJ, et al: Basal activity of the hypothalamic-pituitary-adrenal axis in patients with depersonalization disorder. Psychiatry Res 104:85–89, 2001

Stein MB, Koverola C, Hanna C, et al: Hippocampal volume in women victimized by childhood sexual abuse. Psychol Med 27:951–959, 1997

Steinberg M, Rounsaville B, Cicchetti DV: The Structured Clinical Interview for DSM-III-R Dissociative Disorders: preliminary report on a new diagnostic instrument. Am J Psychiatry 147:76–82, 1990

Stutman RK, Bliss EL: Posttraumatic stress disorder, hypnotizability, and imagery. Am J Psychiatry 142:741–743, 1985

Tellegen A, Atkinson G: Openness to absorbing and self-altering experiences ("absorption"), a trait related to hypnotic susceptibility. J Abnorm Psychol 83:268–277, 1974

Uno H, Tarara R, Else JG, et al: Hippocampal damage associated with prolonged and fatal stress in primates. J Neurosci 9:1705–1711, 1989

Vermetten E, Bremner JD: Circuits and systems in stress, I: preclinical studies. Depress Anxiety 15:126–147, 2002a

Vermetten E, Bremner JD: Circuits and systems in stress, II: applications to neurobiology and treatment of PTSD. Depress Anxiety 16:14–38, 2002b

Vermetten E, Bremner JD, Spiegel D: Dissociation and hypnotizability: a conceptual and methodological perspective on two distinct concepts, in Trauma, Memory, and Dissociation. Edited by Bremner JD, Marmar CR. Washington, DC, American Psychiatric Press, 1998, pp 107–161

Vermetten E, Vythilingam M, Southwick SM, et al: Long-term treatment with paroxetine increases verbal declarative memory and hippocampal volume in posttraumatic stress disorder. Biol Psychiatry 54:693–702, 2003

Vermetten E, Schmahl C, Lindner S, et al: Hippocampal and amygdalar volumes in dissociative identity disorder. Am J Psychiatry 163:630–636, 2006a

Vermetten E, Vythilingam M, Schmahl C, et al: Alterations in stress reactivity after long-term treatment with paroxetine in women with posttraumatic stress disorder. Ann NY Acad Sci 1071:184–202, 2006b

Villareale G, Hamilton DA, Petropoulos H, et al: Reduced hippocampal volume and total white matter in posttraumatic stress disorder. Biol Psychiatry 15:119–125, 2002

Vollmayr B, Simonis C, Weber S, et al: Reduced cell proliferation in the dentate gyrus is not correlated with the development of learned helplessness. Biol Psychiatry 54:1035–1040, 2003

Watanabe Y, Gould E, Daniels DC, et al: Tianeptine attenuates stress-induced morphological changes in the hippocampus. Euro J Pharmacol 222:157–162, 1992

Yehuda R, Southwick SM, Krystal JH, et al: Enhanced suppression of cortisol following dexamethasone administration in posttraumatic stress disorder. Am J Psychiatry 150:83–86, 1993

Yehuda R, Teicher MH, Levengood RA, et al: Circadian regulation of basal cortisol levels in posttraumatic stress disorder. Ann NY Acad Sci 746:378–380, 1994

CHAPTER 13

PSYCHOLOGICAL ASSESSMENT OF POSTTRAUMATIC DISSOCIATION

JOHN BRIERE, PH.D.
JUDITH ARMSTRONG, PH.D.

Dissociation can vary dramatically in form and severity, ranging from mild depersonalization to extreme and debilitating splits in self-awareness and identity. Dissociative symptoms can also mimic the manifestations of other psychological disturbance, from the mood swings of bipolar disorders to the relational variations of personality disorders, the cognitive slippage of schizophrenia, and the loss of focus of attention-deficit disorders. For these reasons, standardized psychological assessment of dissociation can play a particularly important role in clarifying the traumatized client's diagnosis and his or her treatment needs.

We begin this discussion by highlighting some important issues in dissociation that have practical implications for the assessment process. We then discuss specific empirically supported standardized measures for examining dissociation. We suggest here that traumatic dissociation is a complex, multifactorial phenomenon that is best assessed with a battery of psychometrically sound, multidimensional instruments administered by a clinician who is attuned to the behavioral manifestations of dissociation as they are evoked in the client by the testing.

It should be noted at the outset that some of the difficulties in assessing dissociation do not lie within the client but rather with our incomplete understanding of the effects of dissociation on consciousness, memory, and the development of the self. *Dissociation* has been defined in a variety of ways that emphasize varying approaches to this problem. For example,

Putnam (1997) focused on the initial, often developmentally based, integration failures of mental and behavioral states. Nemiah (1993) emphasized the inaccessibility of voluntary recall, whereas the American Psychiatric Association (2000) especially noted variation in identity. Despite these differences in emphasis, most definitions refer to (or imply) significant, but often temporary, changes in normal consciousness or awareness that arise from reduced or altered access to one's thoughts, feelings, perceptions, and/or memories. These changes involve a context that is not noteworthy for dementia, traumatic brain injury, epilepsy, or other organic disturbance.

Intrinsic to most conceptualizations of dissociation is psychological defense; dissociative symptoms are often viewed as a form of emotional avoidance, evoked by the individual to reduce the emotional effects of traumatic events (e.g., Putnam 1993). However, research suggests that the relationship between trauma and dissociation may be less than straightforward. For example, Briere et al. (2005b) found that trauma exposure accounted for only 4.4% of variance in dissociative symptoms, after taking gender and age into account. Similar results are reported by van IJzendoorn and Schuengel (1996), who, in a meta-analysis of 26 Dissociative Experiences Scale (DES; Bernstein and Putnam 1986) studies, found that trauma exposure accounted for 4% ($r=0.21$) to 8% ($r=0.28$) of the variance in dissociative symptoms. In a further evaluation of the trauma-dissociation relationship, Briere (2006) reported that although clinically significant dissociative symptoms were present in only 8% of trauma-exposed individuals in the Multiscale Dissociation Inventory (MDI; Briere 2002) normative sample, most (90%) of those with clinical levels of dissociation on the MDI reported having experienced a traumatic event. Two variables especially increased the likelihood that trauma would be associated with dissociative symptoms: greater levels of posttraumatic stress and reduced affect regulation capacities. These results suggest that although the presence of dissociation may be a marker for trauma, trauma exposure itself is an insufficient condition for dissociation—in much the same way that trauma exposure, in the absence of additional risk factors, is an insufficient condition for the development of posttraumatic stress disorder (PTSD; Yehuda and McFarlane 1995).

A further complexity has been introduced by research indicating that an insecure (especially "disorganized") parent–child attachment in the early years predicts dissociative symptoms later in life (e.g., Main and Morgan 1996; see Chapter 2 in this volume, "Attachment, Disorganization, and Dissociation," for review). Although on one hand this calls into question the inevitability of trauma exposure in the etiology of dissociative symptomatology, developmental studies have also found that insecure attachment style is frequently associated with early child abuse and neglect (e.g., Ogawa et al. 1997). Moreover, depending on what one considers to be a traumatic event—especially if profound caretaker insensitivity and fear-provoking, disorganized parental behavior during childhood is included—attachment-related dissociative phenomena ultimately may be posttraumatic in nature (Cassidy and Mohr 2001).

One implication of attachment-related issues in the relationship between trauma and dissociation is that the client may have very little access to etiologically relevant (i.e., very early) memories (Reviere 1996). As a result, the most careful and thorough of dissociation assessments may not uncover a trauma history in a client who clearly dissociates; an outcome that obscures the potentially posttraumatic etiology of such symptoms and in some cases also increases the likelihood that the assessor will incorrectly hypothesize dissociative amnesia. Another implication is that an evaluation of dissociation in those with early trauma—or those with seemingly trauma-related symptoms but no known trauma history—may be assisted by the addition of a measure that examines very early negative experiences, such as Westen's (1991) Social Cognition and Object Relations Scale.

ISSUES IN DISSOCIATION ASSESSMENT

Taken together, the available literature suggests that dissociation is both an important clinical issue and a surprisingly complex, if not multidetermined, phenomenon. As a result, clinical intervention in this area typically benefits from a detailed assessment of the psychological context and specific phenomenology of dissociative presentations. Several issues warrant consideration when planning an assessment strategy.

Problems With Nonstructured Assessment

Although the need to assess dissociation is relatively clear, clinicians vary in the methodology they use to accomplish this task. To the extent that these approaches do not involve standardized, normed- or diagnostic criterion–referenced procedures, however, they may be incomplete or even misleading.

In many cases, symptom assessment occurs informally, in the context of a general clinical interview. Typically, the client is asked about various dissociative experiences, and his or her behavior is monitored for evidence of disengagement, reduced responsivity, or altered cognitive-emotional states. Although such interviews can yield a considerable amount of helpful information, they inevitably have the same risks as any informal or ad hoc evaluation procedure, including inadequate query of the full range of dissociative symptoms, variability among clinicians in their ability to elicit information on dissociative symptoms from the client, and the intrinsic subjectivity entailed in the clinician's perceptions of the client's internal state. For these reasons, the validity of informal assessments rests heavily on the background, experience, and competence of evaluators and their ability to motivate clients to self-disclose, a situation that potentially compromises the meaningfulness and objectivity (if not portability) of any given clinical evaluation.

The Importance of Norms

Of equal importance, many tests of dissociative symptomatology have not been normed on individuals in the general population. Without normative data, it is difficult to determine what a given score on a dissociation measure actually means. For example, without knowing the average score on test X in the general population, and its standard deviation, a client's score on X will be hard to interpret in terms of its statistical extremity and, thus, its clinical significance. The importance of normative data is well appreciated in the general clinical assessment literature. Unfortunately, until recently, most measures of dissociative symptomatology have not met this requirement.

In some instances, this problem is partially addressed through the use of cutoff scores. In this approach, clinicians use research data on the utility of scores above a certain value in predicting the presence of a dissociative disorder. For example, in a large sample of psychiatric patients a score of 30 or higher on the DES correctly identified 74% of those with dissociative identity disorder (DID) and 80% of those without DID (Carlson et al. 1993). Assessors often use this value as an indication of whether a dissociative disorder is present in a given client, overlooking the fact that the DES was developed as a brief screening measure for further, more in-depth assessment. In fact, a significant number of people who do not have DID nevertheless score above 30 on the DES, others with DID are known to score below that value, and a score above 30 does not necessarily predict the presence of a non-DID dissociative disorder (Armstrong 1995). In addition, the specific cutoff for a dissociation diagnosis may vary from sample to sample, and this approach does not allow for interpretation of the entire range of scores below (or even above) the cutoff point.

Multidimensionality

Beyond normative and standardization issues, the apparent complexity of dissociative symptoms is relevant to assessment. When a single-score (i.e., unidimensional) measure such as the DES is used clinically, it is not clear whether a client's elevated score is due to high levels of depersonalization, fugue phenomena, and/or multiplicity, for example, or greater endorsement of other symptoms such as derealization or dissociative amnesia. As long as dissociation is thought to refer to a single dimension or continuum, differential symptom endorsement is not a major issue: the primary concern is whether the client dissociates or whether scores of a given magnitude indicate a dissociative disorder. Current research, however, casts doubt on the unidimensionality of dissociation. Several published factor analyses of the DES, for example, have revealed multiple distinct sources of variance in dissociative symptomatology. These statistically independent factors vary from study to study but often include some version of absorption, depersonalization-derealization, and amnesia (e.g., Amdur and Liberzon 1996; Ross et al. 1991). More recently, Briere et al. (2005b) examined dissociative symptoms in a combined sample of general population, clinical, and university participants who completed the MDI. Factor analysis identified five symptom clusters, any two of which had, on average, only 15% of variance in common. Such results suggest that "dissociation" may refer to a variety of separate symptom clusters whose ultimate commonality is more theoretical than empirical. As a result, assessment approaches that evaluate different forms of dissociation are likely to be more helpful than those that provide a single score.

Multidimensional instruments also offer an opportunity for more focused clinical intervention. Treatment for a depersonalization disorder, for example, will differ from treatment for DID. In addition, by quantifying the specific level of various dissociative symptom clusters, multidimensional assessment can assist in tracking differential symptom improvement (or the lack thereof) during treatment.

MEASUREMENT OF DISSOCIATIVE SYMPTOMS

There are a number of measures available for the assessment of dissociative symptoms and disorders. Aside from the two semistructured interviews discussed in the next section, these measures are either self-report instruments or projective tests. Self-report tests can be further divided into generic instruments, broadband trauma measures, and stand-alone dissociative scales.

Semistructured Interviews

The Structured Clinical Interview for DSM-IV Dissociative Disorders

The Structured Clinical Interview for DSM-IV Dissociative Disorders—Revised (SCID-D-R; Steinberg 1994) is a semistructured standardized interview that evaluates the existence and severity of five core dissociative symptom clusters: amnesia, depersonalization, derealization, identity confusion, and identity alteration. Ratings are based on symptom frequency, duration, distress, and level of impairment. In agreement with the multidimensionality of dissociative symptomatology, the SCID-D-R generates diagnoses for each of the five DSM-IV-TR (American Psychiatric Association 2000) dissociative disorders. Acute stress disorder can also be diagnosed with the SCID-D-R, although probably with less accuracy than for the dissociative disorders (Briere 2004).

The reliability and validity of the SCID-D has been assessed in several studies (M. Steinberg, D.V. Cicchetti, J. Buchanan, et al., "NIMH Field Trials of the Structured Clinical Interview for DSM-IV Dissociative Disorders [SCID-D]," unpublished manuscript, Yale University School of Medicine, 1989–1993; Steinberg et al. 1990). However, few data are available on the diagnostic utility (including sensitivity and specificity) of the SCID-D in relation to actual dissociative disorder diagnoses, a situation that is potentially problematic given the absence of validity scales to measure defensiveness or malingering. Nevertheless, the SCID-D has high interrater reliability, and individuals with dissociative disorders have been shown to score significantly higher than those without a dissociative disorder (Steinberg et al. 1990). An added benefit of this interview is that it contains a section for rating dissociative behaviors seen during the interview.

The Dissociative Disorders Interview Schedule

The Dissociative Disorders Interview Schedule (DDIS; Ross et al. 1989) consists of 131 items, each of which is coded as "yes," "no," or "unsure." This interview provides diagnoses for all DSM-IV-TR dissociative disorders and a range of other, often comorbid diagnoses and symptoms, including major depression and borderline personality disorder. Although the DDIS has been used in a number of studies (e.g., Dorahy et al. 2004) and is widely available, there are limited diagnostic utility data (i.e., sensitivity and specificity) available on this measure other than for DID (Ross et al. 1991, 2002) and dissociative disorder not otherwise specified (Ross et al. 2002). Given its semistructured format, the DDIS is probably best employed by those with expertise in assessing dissociative symptomatology.

Generic Measures

Although there are a number of generic psychological tests, two are especially noteworthy for both their broad acceptance and the availability of post hoc scoring systems for dissociation.

Minnesota Multiphasic Personality Inventory–2

Encouraged by the partial success of the post hoc PTSD scale (Keane et al. 1984), and the significant correlation between scale 8 (schizophrenia) and measures of dissociation (e.g., Elhai et al. 2001), clinical researchers have attempted to create dissociation scales from the items of the Minnesota Multiphasic Personality Inventory–2 (MMPI-2; Butcher et al. 1989). Unfortunately, dissociation was not a focus of MMPI item writers. As a result, although several MMPI or MMPI-2 dissociation scales have been devised (e.g., Leavitt 2001; Mann 1995; Phillips 1994), none have been shown to have sufficient sensitivity or specificity (or evidence of cross-validation in other samples) to justify their general clinical use.

That said, a broadband measure of psychopathology such as the MMPI-2 can be useful in making treatment decisions for dissociating clients. Information on symptoms other than dissociation allows both the determination of comorbidity and the evaluation of the client's broader psychological context. Consider, for example, two clients with equally elevated depersonalization and amnesia scores on a stand-alone dissociation measure. One client obtains high scores on MMPI scale 1, a measure of somatization, and scale 3, a measure of denial. This pattern suggests a tendency to mask or displace psychological pain—a defense that may make it considerably harder to identify dissociation and its trauma-related triggers during the treatment process. In this case, intervention may be required to address cognitive and somatic avoidance mechanisms before dissociation, per se, can be fully addressed. In contrast, the second client may have elevations on scale 2, a measure of depression, and scale 9, a measure of hypomania. This client may especially experience dissociative symptoms in the context of mood swings. Although this obviously raises the possibility of a coexisting bipolar disorder, it also may signal the affect regulation difficulties often found among those with dissociative symptoms (e.g., Briere 2006; Schore 2003). In such cases, the client may need to develop a more effective affect regulation repertory (e.g., through approaches delineated by Cloitre et al. 2002 and Linehan 1993) or begin a regimen of mood-stabilizing medication before traumatic material can receive significant attention in therapy.

Rorschach

Considerable research has been done on indicators of dissociation in clients' Rorschach responses (Armstrong 1995; Exner 1986; Luxenberg and Levin 2004). Many correlates of dissociation appear to parallel those of posttraumatic avoidance. This includes the avoidance of feelings associated with low Affective Ratio scores (Levin 1993), emotional distancing associated with high Form Dimension scores (Armstrong and Loewenstein 1991), and escape from the nuances through either high fantasy production (yielding high introversive/super-introversive Experience Balance scores [Armstrong and Loewenstein 1991; Scroppo et al. 1998]) or "tunnel vision" (reflected by high Lambda scores [Hartman et al. 1990]). It should be noted that a number of these signs of dissociation also are potential strengths that can be used in therapy. For example, emotional distancing suggests an ability to self-reflect, whereas high fantasy production may reflect an underlying ability to think before acting (Armstrong 2002).

Several studies also suggest that the actual content of clients' Rorschach responses can indicate dissociative symptomatology associated with traumatic flooding. For example, Armstrong and Loewenstein (1991) documented especially frequent sex, blood, anatomy, morbidity, and aggression content scores among those with DID, which can be enumerated to yield a Trauma Content Index. Since its creation, this scale has been shown to discriminate traumatized from nontraumatized individuals in several studies (e.g., Kamphuis et al. 2000; Nordström and Carlsson 1997), suggesting that it may relate as much to the traumatic etiology of dissociation as to dissociative symptomatology, per se. One important clinical implication for clients who obtain high Trauma Content scores is the possibility that the Rorschach has ceased to be a test and has become, instead, a traumatic trigger. Thus, the typical interpretations of scores cannot always be utilized because the respondent no longer has the appropriate test set (Carlson and Armstrong 1995). Such trauma responses are often associated with significant Thought Disorder Index scores that reflect the client's failure to resolve, or even recognize, contradictory ideas, which is a characteristic of dissociative compartmentalization (Armstrong and Kaser-Boyd 2003; Levin and Reis 1996). Thus, much as some dissociating clients may not understand the contradiction inherent in leaving their own children with parents who abused them as children or in declaring that although their parents fought and hit each other they were not violent, so they may describe on the Rorschach a "crippled butterfly with no body" or a "friendly bomber." For this reason, Holaday (2000) has suggested that the presence of a high Trauma Content score should discourage a premature diagnosis of psychosis in clients with seemingly thought-disordered protocols, because traumatic dissociation may be an alternative explanation. The most recent revision of the Exner Comprehensive Scoring system, which has replaced the Schizophrenia Index with the Perception and Thinking Index, reflects this change in viewpoint (Exner 2000).

In an approach similar to Armstrong and Loewenstein's, Leavitt and Labott (1996) also suggested three Rorschach indicators of dissociation: 1) "reference to forms seen through obscuring media," 2) "reference to unusual responses in which distance appears exaggerated," and 3) "reference to a sense of disorientation in which Rorschach stimuli are experienced as unstable, shifting, moving, or rapidly changing" (p. 488). It should be noted, however, that the reliability and predictive validity of these indicators for dissociation have yet to be fully established.

Standardized Scales Within Broadband Trauma Measures

There are currently two standardized trauma inventories that include specific dissociation scales. Although they offer the advantage of assessing dissociation in the context of a range of other posttraumatic symptoms, the dissociation scales used in these tests are, by necessity, relatively brief and more appropriate for screening than detailed assessment.

Trauma Symptom Inventory Dissociation Scale

The Trauma Symptom Inventory (TSI; Briere 1995) contains 100 symptom items rated according to their frequency of occurrence on a four-point scale ranging from 0 ("never") to 3 ("often") over the prior 6 months. Among the 3 validity and 10 clinical scales of the TSI is the Dissociation scale, which taps "a variety of dissociative experiences, including cognitive disengagement, depersonalization and derealization, out-of-body experiences, and emotional numbing" (Briere 1995, p. 14). Although the Dissociation scale is internally consistent and correlates with trauma and posttraumatic stress (Briere 1995), the underlying unidimensional structure of this scale constrains, to some extent, its interpretive specificity. In addition, as opposed to some other measures, this scale does not tap symptoms of fugue or DID.

Detailed Assessment of Posttraumatic Stress Trauma-Specific Dissociation Scale

The Detailed Assessment of Posttraumatic Stress (DAPS; Briere 2001) is a 104-item inventory that provides information on a client's history of trauma exposure; immediate cognitive, emotional, and dissociative reactions to an index trauma; subsequent posttraumatic reexperiencing, avoidance, and hyperarousal; likelihood of acute stress disorder or PTSD; experienced disability associated with the index traumatic event; and evidence of suicidality, substance abuse, and dissociation.

In addition to the Peritraumatic Dissociation scale, which measures dissociation that occurred during or immediately after a traumatic event, the DAPS Trauma-Specific Dissociation scale evaluates derealization, depersonalization, and detachment symptoms that arise directly from a specific trauma (Briere 2001). It is the only standardized measure of posttraumatic dissociation associated with an index trauma available to clinicians. The other instruments described in this chapter measure the overall level of dissociative symptoms reported by the client at the time of evaluation and thus, probably index dissociative responses to multiple traumatic events (as well as possible early attachment disturbance) in the client's history (Briere et al. 2005a). Like other single-score dissociation scales, however, the Trauma-Specific Dissociation scale does not discriminate between different types of dissociative phenomena.

Stand-Alone Tests of Dissociative Symptomatology

Given the incidence of trauma in clinical populations (e.g., Bryer et al. 1987) and the need for more complete assessment of dissociative symptomatology, stand-alone dissociation measures are often used as part of a general assessment battery. They are also a valuable resource when, during treatment, dissociation emerges as an issue.

Dissociative Experiences Scale

The DES is the best-known dissociation measure (Carlson and Putnam 1993). It taps "disturbance in identity, memory, awareness, and cognitions and feelings of derealization or depersonalization or associated phenomena such as déjà vu and absorption" (Bernstein and Putnam 1986, p. 729). The DES has been shown to be psychometrically reliable and to discriminate trauma victims and those with dissociative disorders in a wide variety of studies (for review see Carlson and Armstrong 1995 or van IJzendoorn and Schuengel 1996).

Because the DES is a popular and well-validated dissociation measure, trauma clinicians sometimes administer it in the context of a psychological test battery, despite its absence of normative data. If the 30-point cutoff is used to assess for possible DID, the clinician should note in his or her report the only moderate sensitivity and specificity of that cutoff (Armstrong 1995). More generally, as is true of the TSI Dissociation scale and other similar scales, the single "dissociation" score yielded by the DES can obscure differential patterns of dissociative symptomatology among clients. Although this might potentially be addressed by extrapolating DES factor scores from dimensionality studies (e.g., Ross et al. 1991), DES factor scores vary in composition from study to study, lack normative data, and do not provide clinical cutoff values (Briere 2004). There is also a post hoc subset of DES items thought to measure pathological (as opposed to normal) dissociation (Waller et al. 1996), although the sum of these items also may obscure multidimensionality.

Beyond its psychometric application, Armstrong (1995) has suggested that the DES can be used as an informal interview tool to facilitate discussion of dissociation. After the DES is completed, the clinician can ask the client for a concrete example of each highly endorsed item, framing the request as an inquiry about skills (e.g., "When do you remember first doing this?"; "How did it help?"), to stimulate the client's nonshameful curiosity about an automatic reaction that he or she may have used since early childhood. This tactic also can help to clarify whether a high score reflects misunderstanding, malingering, or other nondissociative phenomena, such as depressive withdrawal. Importantly, this technique reflects the art of assessment and should be followed by a more objective measure to confirm and extend findings.

Multiscale Dissociation Inventory

The MDI (Briere 2002) is a 30-item, standardized, self-report test of dissociative symptomatology. It is normed on 444 trauma-exposed individuals from the general population and has scales measuring six different types of dissociative response: Disengagement, Depersonalization, Derealization, Emotional Constriction, Memory Disturbance, and Identity Dissociation (Briere 2002). Raw scale scores on the MDI can be converted to normative T-scores that allow for empirically based clinical interpretation of clients' level of dissociative disturbance in each area. Forms are available to graph MDI scale T-scores, yielding a dissociation profile for the client.

MDI scales are reliable and demonstrate multiple indices of validity (Briere 2002). Scales of the MDI have been shown to have differential and specific relationships to child abuse history, adult trauma exposure, clinical status, PTSD, scores on other dissociation measures, and criminal behavior (Briere 2002; Briere et al. 2005a, 2005b; Dietrich 2003). A raw score of 15 or higher on the Identity Dissociation scale had a sensitivity of 0.93 and specificity of 0.92 for DID in a combined clinical/community sample (Briere 2002).

Multidimensional Inventory of Dissociation

The Multidimensional Inventory of Dissociation (P.F. Dell, "MID: Multidimensional Inventory of Dissociation," unpublished assessment battery, 2004) consists of 218 items that yield "14 major facets of dissociation, 23 symptoms of dissociation,…and 5 validity scales" (Dell and

Somers 2005, p. 31). It is available in English (Dell 2002) and Hebrew (Dell and Somers 2005) versions. A study of the English version suggests that individuals with DID score higher than others on many of the scales and items. Somewhat surprisingly, given its multidimensional orientation, both the English and Hebrew versions are described as tapping a single underlying dissociation factor. The Hebrew version has been shown to be reliable and to demonstrate convergent, discriminant, and construct validity. Although norms are not available for this measure, and there are limited published psychometric data for the English version, research is ongoing and future psychometric publications are anticipated.

CONCLUSION

In many ways, the development of psychological tests for dissociation has paralleled and interacted with the development of theory and treatment of dissociation, with each process informing the other and highlighting areas for future investigation. Although the psychometric research at present alerts us to the unknowns and complexities of the relationship between trauma, attachment, and dissociation in general, it also serves to clarify the role these factors play in the individual case by extending the objectivity and thoroughness of the diagnostic assessment. We have emphasized that the complexity and variability of dissociative presentations seen in the treatment context are paralleled by the low correlations between different dissociative processes. This means that testing, especially if it includes a multidimensional measure of dissociation, helps to clarify not only the question of *whether* clients dissociate but also *how* they dissociate. We also have described how inclusion of generic measures of psychopathology—although they do not contain validated dissociation scales—helps to clarify the personality context in which the client's dissociation occurs and thus can guide treatment decisions.

We conclude with a modest caveat. Testing, like diagnostic interviewing, is never infallible, no matter how well standardized, informed, and researched. As with any defensive process, dissociation becomes more visible, and therefore more measurable, when it begins to fail. As a result, clinicians should be aware that a nonfinding of dissociation at one point in treatment can transition into a finding at another point. The fact that this occurs does not necessarily indicate a lack of sensitivity on the part of the test but, rather, is likely to be a natural by-product of the ever-changing interaction between the client's personality, his or her life context, and the effects of treatment. In this regard, the boundary be-

tween diagnostic assessment and treatment is not as compartmentalized as is often presented (Finn and Tonsager 1997). Whatever tests are
chosen to assess dissociation, the results can be brought into treatment
to stimulate the client's metacognitive appreciation of these largely nonverbal responses, the situations that provoke them, and the costs and
benefits of such adaptations in his or her ongoing life.

REFERENCES

Amdur R, Liberzon I: Dimensionality of dissociation in subjects with PTSD. Dissociation 9:118–124, 1996

American Psychiatric Association: Diagnostic and Statistical Manual of Mental Disorders, 4th Edition. Washington, DC, American Psychiatric Association, 1994

American Psychiatric Association: Diagnostic and Statistical Manual of Mental
Disorders, 4th Edition, Text Revision. Washington, DC, American Psychiatric Association, 2000

Armstrong J: Psychological assessment, in Treating Dissociative Identity Disorder. Edited by Spira JL. San Francisco, CA, Jossey-Bass, 1995, pp 3–37

Armstrong J: Deciphering the broken narrative of trauma: signs of traumatic
dissociation on the Rorschach. Rorschachiana 25:11–27, 2002

Armstrong J, Kaser-Boyd N: Projective assessment of psychological trauma, in
The Comprehensive Handbook of Psychological Assessment: Personality
Assessment, Vol 2. Edited by Segal DL, Hilsenroth MD. New York, Wiley,
2003, pp 500–512

Armstrong J, Loewenstein RJ: The psychological organization of multiple personality disordered patients as revealed in psychological testing. Psychiatr
Clin North Am 14:533–546, 1991

Bernstein EM, Putnam FW: Development, reliability, and validity of a dissociation scale. J Nerv Ment Dis 174:727–734, 1986

Briere J: Trauma Symptom Inventory (TSI). Odessa, FL, Psychological Assessment Resources, 1995

Briere J: Detailed Assessment of Posttraumatic Stress (DAPS). Odessa, FL, Psychological Assessment Resources, 2001

Briere J: Multiscale Dissociation Inventory. Odessa, FL, Psychological Assessment Resources, 2002

Briere J: Psychological Assessment of Adult Posttraumatic States: Phenomenology, Diagnosis, and Measurement, 2nd Edition. Washington, DC, American
Psychological Association, 2004

Briere J: Dissociative symptoms and trauma exposure: specificity, affect dysregulation, and posttraumatic stress. J Nerv Ment Dis 194:78–82, 2006

Briere J, Scott C, Weathers FW: Peritraumatic and persistent dissociation in the
presumed etiology of PTSD. Am J Psychiatry 162:2295–2301, 2005a

Briere J, Weathers FW, Runtz M: Is dissociation a multidimensional construct? Data from the Multiscale Dissociation Inventory. J Trauma Stress 18:221–231, 2005b

Bryer JB, Nelson BA, Miller JB, et al: Childhood sexual and physical abuse as factors in adult psychiatric illness. Am J Psychiatry 144:1426–1430, 1987

Butcher JN, Dahlstrom WG, Graham JR, et al: MMPI-2: Minnesota Multiphasic Personality Inventory-2: Manual for Administration and Scoring. Minneapolis, MN, University of Minnesota Press, 1989

Carlson EB, Armstrong J: Diagnosis and assessment of dissociative disorders, in Dissociation: Theoretical, Clinical, and Research Perspectives. Edited by Lynn SJ, Rhue JL. New York, Guilford, 1995, pp 159–174

Carlson EB, Putnam W: An update on the Dissociative Experiences Scale. Dissociation 6:16–27, 1993

Carlson EB, Putnam FW, Ross CA, et al: Validity of the Dissociative Experiences Scale in screening for multiple personality disorder: a multicenter study. Am J Psychiatry 150:1030–1036, 1993

Cassidy J, Mohr JJ: Unsolvable fear, trauma, and psychopathology. Clin Psychol Sci Pract 8:275–298, 2001

Cloitre M, Koenen KC, Cohen LR, et al: Skills training in affective and interpersonal regulation followed by exposure: a phase-based treatment for PTSD related to childhood abuse. J Consult Clin Psychol 70:1067–1074, 2002

Dell PF: Dissociative phenomenology of dissociative identity disorder. J Nerv Ment Dis 190:10–15, 2002

Dell PF, Somers E: Development of the Hebrew-Multidimensional Inventory of Dissociation (H-MID): a valid and reliable measure of pathological dissociation. J Trauma Dissociation 6:31–53, 2005

Dietrich AM: Characteristics of child maltreatment, psychological dissociation, and somatoform dissociation of Canadian inmates. J Trauma Dissociation 4:81–100, 2003

Dorahy MJ, Middleton W, Irwin HJ: Investigating cognitive inhibition in dissociative identity disorder compared to depression, posttraumatic stress disorder and psychosis. J Trauma Dissociation 5:93–110, 2004

Elhai JD, Gold SN, Mateus LF, et al: Scale 8 elevations on the MMPI-2 among women survivors of childhood sexual abuse: evaluating posttraumatic stress, depression, and dissociation as predictors. J Fam Violence 16:47–57, 2001

Exner JE Jr: The Rorschach: A Comprehensive System. Basic Foundations, Vol 1, 2nd Edition. New York, Wiley, 1986

Exner JE Jr: A Primer for Rorschach Interpretation. Asheville, NC, Rorschach Workshops, 2000

Finn SE, Tonsager MD: Information-gathering and therapeutic models of assessment: complementary paradigms. Psychol Assess 9:374–385, 1997

Hartman WR, Clark ME, Morgan MK, et al: Rorschach structure of a hospitalized sample of Vietnam veterans with PTSD. J Pers Assess 54:146–159, 1990

Holaday M: Rorschach protocols from children and adolescents diagnosed with posttraumatic stress disorder. J Pers Assess 75:143–157, 2000

Kamphuis JH, Kugeares SL, Finn SE: Rorschach correlates of sexual abuse: trauma content and aggression indexes. J Pers Assess 75:212–224, 2000

Keane TM, Malloy PF, Fairbank JA: Empirical development of an MMPI subscale for the assessment of combat-related posttraumatic stress disorder. J Consult Clin Psychol 52:888–891, 1984

Leavitt F: The development of the Somatoform Dissociation Index (SDI): a screening measure of dissociation using MMPI-2 items. J Trauma Dissociation 2:69–80, 2001

Leavitt F, Labott SM: Authenticity of recovered sexual abuse memories: a Rorschach study. J Trauma Stress 9:483–496, 1996

Levin P: Assessing PTSD with the Rorschach projective technique, in The International Handbook of Traumatic Stress Syndromes. Edited by Wilson J, Raphael B. New York, Plenum, 1993, pp 189–200

Levin P, Reis B: Use of the Rorschach in assessing trauma, in Assessing Psychological Trauma and PTSD. Edited by Wilson JP, Keane T. New York, Guilford, 1996, pp 529–543

Linehan MM: Cognitive-behavioral treatment of borderline personality disorder. New York, Guilford, 1993

Luxenberg T, Levin P: The utility of the Rorschach in the assessment and treatment of trauma, in Assessing Psychological Trauma and PTSD, 2nd Edition. Edited by Wilson J, Keane T. New York, Guilford, 2004, pp 190–225

Main M, Morgan HJ: Disorganization and disorientation in infant strange situation behavior: phenotypic resemblance to dissociative states, in Handbook of Dissociation: Theoretical, Empirical, and Clinical Perspectives. Edited by Michelson LK, Ray WJ. New York, Plenum, 1996, pp 107–138

Mann BJ: The North Carolina Dissociation Index: a measure of dissociation using items from the MMPI-2. J Pers Assess 64:349–359, 1995

Nemiah JC: Dissociation, conversion, and somatization, in Dissociative Disorders: A Clinical Review. Edited by Spiegel D. Lutherville, MD, Sidran, 1993

Nordström K, Carlsson AM: Rorschach comparison of borderline patients with and without a history of childhood sexual abuse. Paper presented at the annual meeting of the Society for Personality Assessment, San Diego, CA, March 1997

Ogawa JR, Sroufe LA, Weinfield NS, et al: Development and the fragmented self: longitudinal study of dissociative symptomatology in a nonclinical sample. Dev Psychopathol 9:855–879, 1997

Phillips DW: Initial development and validation of the Phillips Dissociation Scale (PDS) of the MMPI. Dissociation 7:92–100, 1994

Putnam FW: Dissociative phenomena, in Dissociative Disorders: A Clinical Review. Edited by Spiegel D. Lutherville, MD, Sidran, 1993, pp 1–16

Putnam FW: Dissociation in Children and Adolescents: A Developmental Perspective. New York, Guilford, 1997

Reviere SL: Memory of Childhood Trauma: A Clinician's Guide to the Literature. New York, Guilford, 1996

Ross CA, Heber S, Norton GR, et al: The Dissociative Disorders Interview Schedule: a structured interview. Dissociation 2:169–189, 1989

Ross CA, Joshi S, Currie R: Dissociative experiences in the general population: a factor analysis. Hosp Community Psychiatry 42:297–301, 1991

Ross CA, Duffy CMM, Ellason JW: Prevalence, reliability and validity of dissociative disorders in an inpatient setting. J Trauma Dissociation 3:7–17, 2002

Schore AN: Affect Dysregulation and Disorders of the Self. New York, WW Norton, 2003

Scroppo JC, Weinberger JL, Drob SL, et al: Identifying dissociative identity disorder: a self-report and projective study. J Abnorm Psychol 107:272–284, 1998

Steinberg M: Structured Clinical Interview for DSM-IV Dissociative Disorders–Revised (SCID-D-R). Washington, DC, American Psychiatric Press, 1994

Steinberg M, Rounsaville B, Cicchetti DV: The Structured Clinical Interview for DSM-III-R Dissociative Disorders: preliminary report on a new diagnostic instrument. Am J Psychiatry 147:76–82, 1990

van IJzendoorn M, Schuengel C: The measurement of dissociation in normal and clinical populations: meta analytic validation of the Dissociative Experiences Scale (DES). Clin Psychol Rev 16:365–382, 1996

Waller NG, Putnam FW, Carlson EB: Types of dissociation and dissociative types: a taxometric analysis of dissociative experiences. Psychol Methods 1:300–321, 1996

Westen D: Social cognition and object relations. Psychol Bull 109:429–455, 1991

Yehuda R, McFarlane A: Conflict between current knowledge about posttraumatic stress disorder and its original conceptual basis. Am J Psychiatry 152:1705–1713, 1995

CHAPTER 14

DISSOCIATIVE IDENTITY DISORDER

Issues in the Iatrogenesis Controversy

RICHARD J. LOEWENSTEIN, M.D.

Controversies about what we now call dissociative disorders existed throughout much of the past two centuries, when the study of hysteria was a major focus of psychology, psychiatry, and neurology (Ellenberger 1970; Guillain 1959). Just as today, debates included the importance of trauma in the etiology of hysteria; the impact of disordered sexuality, either sexual frustration or sexual indulgence, on the etiology of hysterical disorders; whether constitutional or environmental factors were most central to understanding hysteria; and the authenticity of hysterical symptoms altogether (Breuer and Freud 1893/2001; Briquet 1859; Janet 1889; Mai and Merskey 1980; Roy 1979). In addition, at those early times the role of suggestion and suggestibility in producing hypnotic states and the symptoms of hysteria was a major focus of debate (Ellenberger 1970; Guillain 1959). These debates prefigured modern disputes between the special state theorists and the sociocognitive theorists of hypnosis and, by extension, the dissociative disorders. Fugue, amnesia, hypnosis, and multiple personality were topics of many popular plays and fiction during the latter part of the nineteenth century, just as they are today.

It has been hypothesized that the development of a trauma model for dissociative identity disorder (DID) was congruent with a number of historical forces in the latter part of the twentieth century (Loewenstein and Putnam 2004). These twentieth-century dynamics included an increased awareness of the prevalence of domestic violence and childhood sexual and physical abuse, systematic research into these topics, and the rise of mandated reporting (D. W. Brown et al. 1998; Kempe et al. 1962). Feminist psychological theories also were important, because they countered classical psychoanalytic formulations that incest reports were mostly based on oedipal fantasies (J. Goodwin 1989; Herman 1981). These feminist scholars also challenged the more general societal view that children or women who reported sexual maltreatment and/or assaults were mendacious or had brought the sexual assaults on themselves (Chesler 1972). The increase in serious, scientific study of hypnosis and dissociation also led to more systematic understanding of these factors in the diagnosis and treatment of a variety of disorders (Barber 2000; Hilgard 1986; Orne 1959; H. Spiegel and Spiegel 2004). The popularization of the trauma-based etiology of DID based on biographical/autobiographical accounts such as that of Sybil (Schreiber 1976), among others, led to renewed media and societal interest in dissociative disorders that paralleled an interest in personal accounts of childhood abuse. Finally, there was the influence of DSM-III (American Psychiatric Association 1980), which eliminated the term *hysteria* from the diagnostic system. The DSM system separated dissociative disorders from the somatoform disorders and provided diagnostic criteria for the dissociative disorders (previously subsumed under "hysterical neurosis" in DSM-II [American Psychiatric Association 1968]). Disorders in the DSM system that are derived from the classical concept of hysteria are listed in Table 14–1.

EXPLANATORY MODELS FOR DISSOCIATIVE IDENTITY DISORDER

There are now two major explanatory models for multiple personality disorder/DID: the iatrogenesis/suggestibility model (D. W. Brown et al. 1998; McHugh 1992, 1995a, 1995b, 1995c; Merskey 1994; Piper 1994; Piper and Merskey 2004a, 2004b) and the trauma model (Kluft 1991; Loewenstein and Putnam 2004; Putnam 1989, 1997; D. Spiegel 1984). Recently, the iatrogenesis/suggestibility model has been renamed the sociocognitive model to emphasize the affinity of this model to the sociocognitive model of hypnosis (Lilienfeld et al. 1999; Spanos 1996; Spanos and Burgess 1994). The sociocognitive model for hypnosis attempts to counter the notion that hypnotic responsiveness results from discontinuities in experience caused by dissociation or altered states of consciousness (Bowers 1976; Evans 2000; Hilgard 1986). This model posits that the hypnotized subject is solely reacting to a variety of cognitions, motivations, expectancies, and role enactments, resulting in behavior as though he or she were being hypnotized (Spanos 1996). Others have

TABLE 14–1. DSM-IV-TR disorders that devolve from the classical hysteria concept

- Dissociative disorders
- Somatoform disorders
- Posttraumatic stress disorder
- Acute stress disorder
- Personality disorders
  Borderline personality disorder
  Histrionic personality disorder
- Anorexia nervosa

Source. Adapted from Guillain 1959; Loewenstein and Putnam 2004.

suggested a more integrated model of hypnotic responding (Banyai 1991; Barber 2000; D. Brown and Fromm 1986). In the integrated model, it is proposed that hypnosis involves both an altered state as well as sociocognitive factors.

The sociocognitive model for DID basically claims that DID derives from a learned social role usually, but not exclusively, generated iatrogenically in a psychotherapeutic situation, when highly suggestible patients, usually those with borderline personality disorder (BPD), are influenced by implicit or explicit cues or demand characteristics from naïve therapists who believe in the existence of DID and who have overly simplistic notions of memory and psychopathology (Brenneis 1996; Ganaway 1994; Lilienfeld et al. 1999; Yapko 1994). The postulated result is that these therapists oversimplify complex clinical problems as only resulting from a posttraumatic etiology. In addition, according to some proponents of the sociocognitive model, the development of DID taps into "universal capacities for multiple role enactments" found in many cultures. According to Spanos (1996),

> The sociocognitive perspective suggests that patients learn to construe themselves as possessing multiple selves, learn to present themselves in terms of this construal, and learn to recognize and elaborate a personal biography so as to make it congruent with their understanding of what it means to be a multiple. ...I argue that (a) multiple identities are usefully conceptualized as rule-governed social constructions; (b) neither childhood trauma nor a history of severe psychopathology is necessary for the maintenance of multiple identities; and (c) multiple identities are established, legitimated, maintained, and altered through social interaction. (p. 3–4)

Until recently, research that attempted to test this model on clinical samples of presumptive dissociative patients has been lacking. To the extent that it is empirically based, the sociocognitive model for DID relies primarily on extrapolation from studies with nonclinical samples of individuals in experiments on hypnosis, memory, suggestibility, and fantasy proneness as well as a critique of a small subsample of the many clinical and research studies on DID and dissociation as a dimensional construct (D.W. Brown et al. 1998, 1999; Gleaves 1996; Gleaves et al. 2001; Kluft 1989; Lilienfeld et al. 1999; Putnam 1995a, 1995b; Ross 1997). Basic postulates of the sociocognitive model are found in Table 14–2.

Primarily since the 1970s, a second explanatory model—the trauma model—has been promulgated with the central tenet that DID is a "posttraumatic developmental disorder" (Loewenstein 1993) based on a child's experience of overwhelming or traumatic experiences during early development (Armstrong 1995; Kluft 1985, 1988a, 2005; Loewenstein and Putnam 2004; Putnam 1989, 1997; Ross 1997; D. Spiegel 1984, 1986, 1991; D. Spiegel and Cardeña 1991; D. Spiegel et al. 1988). The trauma model posits that severe dissociative disorders occur in children subjected to a variety of overwhelming early life experiences, primarily repetitive, multiple types of maltreatment in environments that are neglectful or damaging to the child in several crucial developmental dimensions (Courtois 2004). In addition, the child is provided little soothing or comfort after being hurt and is left to comfort him- or herself (Kluft 1984a). The child then fails to consolidate a normal sense of self across different experiences and contexts. Alternative senses of self develop, with different affects and memory subsystems that may increase in complexity and stability over time. The consolidation of self states may be shaped by a variety of developmental needs and pressures, including normal developmental substrates, additional overwhelming experiences, object relational needs, and attachment issues and cultural mores, among others (Kluft 1984a; Putnam 1997), especially related to betrayal by parents and other close caretakers (Becker-Blease and Freyd 2005; Freyd 1996; Freyd et al. 2005).

Once this process is in place, additional self states may be created to cope with a variety of issues across the life cycle, including additional traumas, more prosaic distressing life experiences and conflicts, losses of important others, the need to provide concrete symbolism to life problems, and even the stress of psychotherapy, among many others (Kluft 1984a). In addition, secondary structuring of the self states may occur in many ways, leading to the creation of a subjectively personified inner world, or "third reality" (Kluft 2005). This secondary structuring may be shaped by a variety of developmental, intrapsychic, symbolic, social, and cultural factors leading to the subjective experience of personified multiplicity and the outward presentational characteristics that the DID self states exhibit or claim when they emerge in treatment (Kluft

TABLE 14–2. Sociocognitive model of dissociative identity disorder

- Produced through social learning of a role
- Not an authentic form of psychopathology (although may be reliably diagnosed)
- Multiple identities are usefully conceptualized as rule-governed social constructions
- Neither childhood trauma nor a history of severe psychopathology is necessary
- Taps into universal capacities for "multiple role enactments" found in many cultures
- Multiple identities are established, legitimated, maintained, and altered through social interaction

Patient factors

High suggestibility

High hypnotizability

High fantasy proneness

Hysteria

Borderline personality disorder as etiological substrate

Can be explained by other disorders: personality disorders, somatization disorder, bipolar disorder, psychosis, etc.

Primarily North American

Social influences: movies, biographies/autobiographies, television, recovery movement, self-help books, the Internet

Clinician factors

Naïve beliefs about hypnosis, memory, etc.

Therapist believes in multiple personalities and cues patient implicitly and explicitly to enact multiple personalities (demand characteristics)

Belief in repressed/recovered memories

Etiological importance of these for psychopathology

Therapy techniques contain instructions as to how to construe history, role, and behavior

Note. See Lillienfeld et al. 1999 for a review.

1989). In short, the trauma model, as described earlier, posits that DID involves the development of alternate self states due to overwhelming early developmental experiences. However, in addition, the trauma model posits that many aspects of the structuring of this process can be shaped by a variety of psychological, social, and cultural factors, including psychotherapy (Kluft 1988b, 1989).

DID can be conceptualized as an understandable adaptation of the child to unpredictable and malevolent environments (Armstrong 1995). The development of DID allows the child to develop, preserve, and consolidate normal cognitive resources, ego functions, and healthy adaptive resources by using dissociation to compartmentalize memory, cognitions, and affects related to traumatic and neglectful experiences. By doing so the child can protect the development of these normal capacities from the destructive impact of repeated traumatization and neglect. These include artistic and intellectual abilities, an ability to connect and bond with others, empathy, cognitive complexity and imagination, good reality testing under nonstressful conditions, excellent self-observing abilities, a sense of humor, and hope. Characteristics of the trauma model are found in Table 14–3.

THE CONCEPT OF IATROGENESIS

Despite claims of iatrogenesis of DID by sociocognitive model proponents and impassioned rebuttals by trauma model advocates, it is surprising that little attempt has been made to define the term itself. Proponents of the sociocognitive model as well as the trauma model seem to accept *iatrogenesis* as though it were a well-accepted, carefully defined, lucid term.

The term *iatrogenic* derives from the Greek words for *doctor* (*iatros*) and *cause* (*genesis*), literally meaning a problem "caused by a doctor." In clinical medicine, iatrogenesis is neutrally defined primarily as unwanted medical conditions that arise as a result of the diagnosis or treatment of illness: "a symptom or illness brought on unintentionally by something a doctor says or does" (Soukhanov 1999). The term *iatrogenic* is used most commonly to signify errors of commission (e.g., inaccurate diagnosis or incorrect treatment); less commonly it is used to signify errors of omission. In this view, iatrogenic problems are very common and most are relatively minor. On the other hand, studies have shown that "adverse events" occur in almost 4% of hospitalizations in some large studies. About one-third to one-half of adverse events were thought to be due to "negligence or preventable causes." Deaths resulted from as many as 13.6% of these adverse events (Brennan et al. 1991; Leape et al. 1991; Localio et al. 1991).

Despite this, the term *iatrogenic* is rarely applied to side effects of medications or surgical complications in the medical literature or in formal clinical discussions (Fleming 1996). It is most commonly used in informal discussions among physicians, often accompanied by a rueful or shameful tone, when discussing problematic outcomes in one's own patients. On the other hand, the term is used contemptuously and pejoratively when discussing the adverse outcomes produced by colleagues who are not thought to have been following the best practices.

In terms of research to study the sociocognitive model in DID, it is important to clarify the boundaries between the terms *misdiagnosis* and

TABLE 14–3. Trauma model of dissociative identity disorder (DID)

- Developmentally based posttraumatic disorder
- Severe early trauma/Overwhelming situations disrupt normal development of sense of self across different behavioral states
- Disordered early attachments (type D, disorganized) associated with higher dissociation (see Lyons-Ruth et al. 2006)
- Reliable and valid measures of both dissociation as dimensional construct and dissociative disorders
- In studies, diagnostic instruments (e.g., Structured Clinical Interview for DSM-IV Dissociative Disorders) discriminate dissociative disorders from patients with other DSM Axis I and II disorders
- Studies show differences on assessment measures between Cluster B personality disorder patients and multiple personality disorder/DID patients
- Described in case studies, clinical case series, structured interview series in children, adolescents, and adults, and studies in North America, Europe, Latin America, Turkey, Japan
- High rates of reported early trauma, maltreatment, neglect in every study that has examined occurence in association with DID
- Documented trauma in all studies that have attempted to do so (e.g., child studies)
- Construct related to that of complex posttraumatic stress disorder (PTSD): multiple developmental deficits related to multiple traumas across several developmental epochs
- Polysymptomatic clinical picture
  Complex dissociative amnesias
  DID process symptoms (switching, passive influence, pseudohallucinations)
  Depersonalization, derealization
  Autohypnotic symptoms
  Somatoform symptoms
  Mood symptoms
  PTSD symptoms
- Dissociation as a dimensional trait widely studied in clinical and non-clinical samples
- Levels of fantasy proneness, suggestibility, etc. are open, researchable questions

Note. See Loewenstein and Putnam 2004 for a review. DID=dissociative identity disorder; PTSD=posttraumatic stress disorder.

Traumatic Dissociation: Neurobiology and Treatment

iatrogenesis in an erroneous classification of patients as DID. Obviously, if incorrect therapy is performed or correct treatments are not provided, misdiagnosis can have a profoundly damaging effect on the patient. This has been demonstrated in American psychiatry prior to the DSM-III era, when mood disorders were diagnosed less commonly than schizophrenia in the United States in comparison with Europe. However, American psychiatrists began to make the diagnosis of mood disorders more commonly due to the increasing availability of treatments for mood disorders such as lithium, better diagnostic systems to distinguish mood disorders from schizophrenia (Feighner et al. 1972; D.W. Goodwin and Guze 1989), and clinical studies that showed that the phenomenology of psychosis was similar across disorders (Pope and Lipinski 1978). Accordingly, many of these previously diagnosed schizophrenic patients were rediagnosed as having bipolar disorder, psychotic depression, or schizoaffective disorder. They often showed marked decreases in psychotic symptoms when the underlying affective disorder was treated. In some cases, patients were liberated from lengthy periods of institutionalization by treatment with medications for mood disorders. In addition, some patients diagnosed with personality disorders had remission in personality disorder symptoms when treated with antidepressants or lithium (Quitkin et al. 1979; Rifkin et al. 1972).

Would we really conclude that these incorrectly diagnosed patients had iatrogenic schizophrenia or iatrogenic personality disorders? Would we be more likely to call this situation iatrogenic if the patients accepted these diagnoses as accurate and made it the explanatory center of their lives? More likely, we would ascribe this situation to misdiagnosis, not iatrogenesis, although we might lament the iatrogenic complications of misdiagnosis: productive years wasted, secondary negative effects of long hospitalizations, disability, side effects from ineffective medications, loss of friends and family, and so on. All of these are factors among the many consequences of the (iatrogenic) failure to correctly diagnose and treat DID (see also Kluft 1989).

SUGGESTIBILITY

Suggestibility is also frequently invoked by sociocognitive model proponents as a putative central trait of DID patients. Like the use of the term *iatrogenesis, suggestibility* is used as though it were a clearly definable, well-accepted, well-understood, unitary construct. A brief tour of the literature on suggestibility provides a different perspective (Cardeña and Spiegel 1991; De Pascalis et al. 2000; Gheorghiu et al. 1989; Hilgard 1991;

Schumaker 1991b; D. Spiegel 1994). In fact, major reviews of the term *suggestibility* cite the multiple definitions and explanations that have been used both for the phenomenon of suggestion and the hypothesized trait of suggestibility (D.W. Brown et al. 1998; Eysenck 1991; Gheorghiu 2000; Gheorghiu and Kruse 1991; Gudjonsson 2003). These authors repeatedly cite the significant problems in defining either construct rigorously. They comment on the multiple ways in which these terms are used, based on the theoretical orientation of the researcher and the problems being studied.

In fact, the constructs of *suggestion* and *suggestibility* have been defined differently in terms of many research paradigms. These have included studies of hypnotic phenomena, unconsciously produced motor behaviors, possession states, false confessions, susceptibility to advertising, responses to psychotherapy, behavioral conditioning, and memory distortions, among many others (Cardeña and Spiegel 1991; Gheorghiu 2000; Gheorghiu and Kruse 1991; Groth-Marnat 1991; Hilgard 1991; Kaffman 1991; Rhue and Lynn 1991; Schumaker 1991a, 1991b; Ward and Kemp 1991). Reviews of the suggestibility literature have emphasized that there are many types of suggestions and different forms of suggestibility as well as a multitude of theoretical frameworks to account for various aspects of phenomena ascribed to suggestibility. In addition, research has shown that a type of suggestibility demonstrated in one research paradigm (e.g., hypnotic suggestibility) may not correlate with other types (e.g., interrogatory suggestibility) (Evans 2000; Gudjonsson 2003).

For example, clinical research on hypnotizability has repeatedly found that DID patients have the highest hypnotizability, defined on standardized hypnotizability protocols, of any clinical group (Frischholz et al. 1992). However, it is an important question whether DID subjects' capacity to readily enter into deep hypnotic states relates to any other kind of suggestibility or to some sort of general susceptibility to social influence, as implied by the sociocognitive model. Also, there are no studies that show whether suggestibility effects found in hypnosis research on nonclinical samples also will be found in samples of DID patients (e.g., increased confidence in a confabulated memory created during hypnosis). Recent studies demonstrated that there are different types of high hypnotizable people, with the dissociative disorder patients ("amnesia-prone" type) distinct from the "fantasy-prone" and the "positively set" (Barber 2000, p. 251). Despite these conceptual and research issues, Loftus (1993, 2000), for example, has made sweeping statements that her misinformation-suggestibility paradigm is a sufficient explanation for the development of iatrogenic DID and the construction of trauma memories during psychotherapy. Again, no research with clinical subjects (or for that matter, with research subjects) has been performed to demonstrate this contention. In fact, until recently, virtually no research on any type of suggestibility had been performed with DID subjects. Preliminary data from two series of DID subjects did not show elevated interrogatory suggestibility on the Gudjonsson Suggestibility Scale when compared with several clinical groups and Gudjonsson's nonclinical control sample (Gudjonsson 2003; Loewenstein et al. 2004; Williams et al. 2004).

BORDERLINE PERSONALITY DISORDER

The sociocognitive model argues that the substrate for DID is actually BPD (Benner and Joscelyne 1984; Brenneis 1996; Ganaway 1994; Lilienfeld et al. 1999). BPD patients are considered to have fluid subjective experience of self and identity and are hypothesized to be suggestible, presumably due to psychologically powerful needs for attention and validation from others (Kernberg 1975; Stone 1980). Lillienfeld et al. (1999) cited studies showing high rates of BPD in some DID samples. Ganaway (1994), among others, posited that the psychoanalytic construct of borderline personality organization is the actual substrate for DID, although Kernberg (quoted in Fink and Golinkoff 1990) stated that DID can occur at any level of personality organization, not just borderline organization.

Horevitz and Braun (1984) reported that 70% of 33 DID cases met DSM-III criteria for BPD. Ross (1997) reported on a series of studies in which up to about 60% of DID patients also met DSM-III criteria for BPD on the Dissociative Disorders Interview Schedule (DDIS; Ross et al. 1989; see also Chapter 13 in this volume, "Psychological Assessment of Posttraumatic Dissociation"). However, the DDIS is not validated to discriminate BPD from other disorders. The forced choice nature of the DDIS, with its yes-no format, may result in overendorsement of BPD items, leading to spurious overdiagnosis of BPD.

On the other hand, Ross (1997) viewed BPD as part of the trauma-dissociation spectrum of disorders, not as a separate condition. Based on data derived from the DDIS, Ross used comorbid BPD in DID patients as a kind of severity index. A DDIS diagnosis of BPD strongly correlated with more extensive trauma histories, higher scores on the Dissociative Experiences Scale (Bernstein and Putnam 1986), more Schneiderian/passive influence symptoms (Kluft 1987; Ross et al. 1990; Schneider 1959), more complex amnesia experiences, and other severe dissociative symptoms. To state it somewhat differently, the DDIS diagnostic section on BPD may be measuring generalized instability caused by posttraumatic and dissociative symptoms and not a comorbid personality disorder.

Several other studies using a variety of measures, including the Dissociative Experiences Scale, the DDIS, the Millon Clinical Multiaxial Inventory (Millon 1997), the Minnesota Multiphasic Personality Inventory–2 (Graham 1991), and the Trauma Symptom Inventory (Briere et al. 1995) found that some assessment tools, especially those designed to test for dissociation and trauma, discriminated the DID and BPD subjects (Dell 1998; Fink and Golinkoff 1990; Gleaves et al. 1995). The latter had lower dissociation scores and lower rates of traumatization. However, the Millon and Minnesota inventory profiles were similar in studies comparing DID and BPD patients (Dell 1998; Gleaves et al. 1995). On the other hand, these profiles were also similar to profiles of non-DID subjects with posttraumatic stress disorder (PTSD). As in the Ross studies, the latter findings were ascribed to general distress and traumatization in DID, BPD, and PTSD patients and not necessarily to DID being an epiphenomenon of BPD.

Boon and Draijer (1993; Draijer and Boon 1999) described a series of studies in which they used the Structured Clinical Interview for DSM-IV Dissociative Disorders—Revised (SCID-D-R) (Steinberg 1994) to differentiate patients with DID and dissociative disorders not otherwise specified (DDNOS) from those with DSM-IV (American Psychiatric Association 1994) Cluster B personality disorders, primarily BPD and histrionic personality disorder. In the first study, they showed that personality disorder patients and DID patients did not differ significantly on the depersonalization and derealization scales of the SCID-D-R. However, DID patients were significantly higher on the amnesia, identity alteration, and identity confusion scales. Both groups had trauma histories, but the DID group had a significantly higher rate of traumatic experiences and traumas at earlier ages.

Draijer and Boon (1999) described patients who did not meet DSM-IV diagnostic criteria for DID but had assumed the identity of a DID patient, encouraged by therapists who had misdiagnosed them or by their significant others. The DID identity had become the central organizing construct of these patients' lives. However, they did not present with typical DID phenomenology on clinical examination and did not show typical DID profiles on the SCID-D-R. Typically, these patients showed the pattern of SCID-D-R scores described for the Cluster B personality disorder patients in the prior study as well as having predominant clinical features of DSM-IV Cluster B personality disorders. These patients, as well as their concerned others, often resisted the SCID-D-R findings and insisted on the authenticity of the DID. Draijer and Boon conceptualized these patients as having a kind of factitious disorder, although they did not think that most of them were consciously feigning DID.

Thus, the patients might be conceptualized as having factitious disorder not otherwise specified, as based on the DSM-IV system (see Armstrong 1999, D.W. Brown and Scheflin 1999, High 1999, and Marmer 1999 for discussions of the relationship of factitious disorder, trauma disorders, and conscious feigning).

In terms of borderline personality organization, Armstrong and Loewenstein (1990) reported on a series of 100 patients with DID or DDNOS who were evaluated with the Exner Rorschach. In the original data set, dissociative patients were compared with Exner's samples of schizophrenic, depressed, and nonpsychiatric control subjects. Those with DID demonstrated a unique personality organization that significantly differentiated them from other groups.

DID patients had frequent, severe trauma intrusions throughout the testing, necessitating development of a Trauma Content score. On the other hand, they had a response style characterized by emotional restraint and complexity of responses. Although they gave some thought-disordered responses, these were primarily related to seeing features of multiplicity in the blots or being overwhelmed by traumatic intrusions. Otherwise, reality testing was intact. The DID patients showed a significantly hyperdeveloped capacity to reflect on the self in an insightful, nonemotional, distanced fashion (elevated form dimension score). This heightened self-observing capacity is thought to correlate with the ability to use insight-oriented psychotherapy effectively. DID subjects were two standard deviations higher than nonpsychiatric control subjects on this variable.

In addition, the DID subjects tended to try to back away from emotional stimuli and looked to their "inner world" for gratification rather than the outside world. They also showed a more active coping style than the depressive or schizophrenic subjects. DID patients were thought to show a personality organization characterized by obsessional features, not a borderline personality organization.

In a recent reanalysis of these data, Brand et al. (2006) compared the data on dissociative patients (approximately 75% DID with the remainder diagnosed with DDNOS with features of DID) with new samples, including patients with schizophrenia, BPD, PTSD, and acute stress disorder. Dissociative subjects had significantly different profiles from BPD patients on the Exner Rorschach. Compared with BPD subjects, the dissociative group showed significantly better capacity to form a therapeutic alliance, greater expectation of collaboration with others, better modulation of affect, and a much better self-observing capacity (as in the prior analysis). In addition, the dissociative patients showed an intellectualized, reflective coping style characterized by an ability for nonemotional introspection. They also showed significantly fewer cognitive distortions and better perceptual accuracy and logical thinking as well as markedly greater cognitive complexity. Consistent with their high hypnotizability, dissociative disorder subjects tended to become enthralled in the blots, seeming to lose themselves in the visual forms.

On the other hand, when flooded with traumatic associations, the dissociative patients' reality testing and emotional modulation deteriorated, leading to more misunderstanding of others and more cognitive distortions. Some dissociative patients even went into a flashback during testing, treating the Rorschach blot as though it were a traumatizing object. In addition, dissociative patients and BPD patients were similar in having high levels of chronic distress and social isolation as well as a tendency to avoid emotions.

Overall, these data are interpreted as showing dissociation to be an ideational, distancing defense and also support Armstrong's (1995) notion that dissociation allows for preservation of important aspects of healthy development that are not seen in BPD. However, when dissociation fails, patients are flooded with intrusive traumatic material resulting in cognitive disorganization and disruption of these more developed cognitive resources, perhaps leading to a more BPD-like clinical presentation.

CONCLUSION

The debate between the proponents of the sociocognitive model and those of the trauma model is unique in contemporary psychiatry (D. Spiegel 1988). Putnam (1995a, 1995b) has stated that the study of DID appears to be held to a different standard than that of other disorders. Nowhere else would a body of research data be so entirely discounted. This empirical base includes clinical case series; series studied with structured interview data; studies of phenomenology, prevalence, memory, hypnotizability, neurobiology, imaging, and psychophysiology; and psychological assessment profiles, among others. These studies include samples of children and adolescents and cross-cultural samples from North America, Europe, Latin America, Turkey, and Asia (International Society for the Study of Dissociation 2005).

In support of the trauma model, high rates of early trauma, maltreatment, and neglect have been found in every study of DID patients that has examined this question. Furthermore, documentation has been found for trauma in all studies that have attempted to do so, such as child studies in which maltreatment was substantiated in over 95% of dissociative disorders cases (Hornstein and Putnam 1992). In addition, a large body of

data has been acquired on dissociation as a dimensional construct studied in many populations, including samples with PTSD and acute stress
disorder (Bremner and Marmar 1998; Cardeña and Spiegel 1993; Classen
et al. 1998; Koopman et al. 1996). Virtually all of these studies have found
a robust relationship between dissociation and traumatic experiences.

Even more surprising is the lack of data presented by sociocognitive
model proponents to support their case. Articles that critique the DID/
trauma construct almost uniformly ignore the large research literature on
DID and the rigorous reviews and critiques of the data that are cited to support the sociocognitive model. With few exceptions, sociocognitive model
articles are mostly opinion pieces that rely on anecdotes and blanket dis-
missals of the literature on dissociation and DID (e.g., McHugh 1992,
1995a, 1995c; Merskey 1994). In general, these reports do not even cite the
small number of studies—primarily a few hypnotic demonstrations from
the 1940s with elicitation of phenomena having little relationship to clinical
DID (Harriman 1942a, 1942b, 1942c; Kampmann 1976; Leavitt 1947)—that
have purported to show that DID can be produced by hypnotic suggestions (D.W. Brown et al. 1999). To be sure, if there were a disorder that demonstrated the phenomena of deep trance naturalistically, characterized by
spontaneously occurring dissociative states, it would undermine considerably the underlying precepts of the sociocognitive model for hypnosis.

At best, as in the Lillienfeld et al. (1999) review, there is some attempt
to review a part of the DID literature and critique it in terms of data supporting the sociocognitive model for hypnosis. Nonetheless, broad gen-
eralizations are made about DID patients (suggestible, fantasy-prone)
for which data have been nonexistent until the recent studies cited earlier, studies that tend to disconfirm tenets of the sociocognitive model. It
is unlikely that refereed journals would publish articles like these about
any other psychiatric disorder.

It is hardly news that sociocognitive factors are likely to play a role in
shaping aspects of DID phenomenology, just as they may shape the presentation of other DSM-IV-TR (American Psychiatric Association 2000)
Axis I disorders (Ross 1997). Indeed, Richard Kluft (1984b), a major propo-
nent of the trauma model for DID, in his Four-Factor Model of DID explicitly cites a variety of developmental, intrapsychic, and social factors that
may influence the structuring and personification of the outward presentational characteristics of the DID self states. These can include a variety of
social and cultural substrates such as "imaginative involvement" with
characters in books, movies, or television; social role demands by the patient's family and/or significant others; and the effect of psychotherapy.

It is generally recognized that the content of psychotic delusions is
clearly shaped by cultural and social factors (e.g., persecution by the

Federal Bureau of Investigation or Central Intelligence Agency via elec-
tronic transmissions in twenty-first-century paranoid delusions or in-
corporation of a psychiatric hospital into a patient's delusions). Also,
somatoform presentations of mood disorders predominate in some
Asian cultures (Kirmayer 2001; Kleinman 1977). This may lead Western
psychiatrists to fail to correctly diagnose and treat depression appropriately in this population. However, these sociocultural factors are viewed
as only influencing the content or outward structure of the patient's
symptoms. They are not thought to nullify the basic diagnostic/phe-
nomenological constructs of delusions or of depression, respectively, or
to invalidate standard treatment paradigms for these disorders.

The idea that psychotic illness was a form of learned social role—a
lifestyle—validated by the "deviance management system" of modern
psychiatry was a major thrust of the anti-psychiatry movement in the
1960s–1970s (Scheff 1966; Sedgwick 1982). This idea has mostly been
discredited. However, in so doing, we have lost insights into the development of the social role of the "chronic mental patient" as distinct from
any particular diagnostic label. Adoption of this role may provide a
place in the world for mentally ill individuals. However, socialization as
a chronic psychiatric patient also may predict significant negative impact on clinical outcome, particularly in dissociative disorders (Fraser
and Raine 1992; Loewenstein 1994).

Sociocultural and sociocognitive factors have been hypothesized to influence the shared language and explanatory meaning and symbolic systems that develop between therapist and patient during psychotherapy.
Some theorists have conceptualized therapeutic interactions in terms of a
kind of mutually suggested ecology that develops in the shared perceptions, models, and metaphors that patients and their therapists come to
use in a highly dynamic interpersonal field (Fourie 2000). Similarly, some
modern psychoanalytic theorists have posited that psychotherapy occurs
in a kind of interpersonal, transference/countertransference "field" in
which both parties affect and influence the other during the course of therapy (Gill 1982; Peebles-Kleiger 1989). Research on demand characteristics
in cognitive-behavioral psychotherapy has shown that implicit demand
characteristics can shape patients' responses to and beliefs about that therapy (Kanter et al. 2002). Research on the process of hypnosis has shown
highly congruent motor behaviors in hypnotist and subject during hypnosis sessions. In another publication (Loewenstein 1993), I have discussed the potential impact of the DID patient's high dissociativity and
hypnotizability on the clinical field and the clinician during treatment.

Aspects of these complex matters are illustrated in the following an-
ecdote. Sheppard and Enoch Pratt Hospital was once home to Harry

Stack Sullivan (1953), who coined the term *interpersonal psychiatry* during his years of work there with schizophrenic patients. One night, a Sheppard Pratt resident admitted to the hospital an elderly, floridly schizophrenic man who was once a patient of Sullivan's. The patient's chief complaint: "I have an 'interpersonal problem'" (R. Chefetz, personal communication, November 1991).

Finally, since the study of hysteria began in the nineteenth century, it has been hard to separate conceptualization of these disorders from their social and cultural milieu. In our current world, dissociation and dissociative disorders touch on many complex and contentious aspects of our personal, political, philosophical, and even religious beliefs. These include the nature of memory, volition, and consciousness and the responsibility of individuals for their own behavior. Indeed, the debate touches on fundamental questions about the nature of the mind, the self, and the most intimate human behaviors.

When viewed within a larger sociopolitical perspective, dissociation theory intersects with many of the most controversial social issues of modern times. The role of trauma in our culture, particularly intergenerational violence and sexual abuse, crosses into historically taboo subjects such as rape, incest, child abuse, and domestic violence and their actual prevalence in our society. In addition, the study of trauma leads us into larger legal, social, and cultural questions related to peace and war, the meaning of violence in our society, the meaning of good and evil, and even varying religious views about the relationship between men, women, and children and the nature of the family.

In psychiatry and psychology, dissociative disorders are the focus of controversies well beyond the different theoretical schools at odds over the nature of hypnosis. These include the long-standing debates between mentalists and behaviorists, between psychodynamically oriented and biologically oriented clinicians, between various researchers in cognitive psychology, and among cognitive researchers, clinical researchers, and practitioners. Some fundamentalist Christian clinicians even have viewed demonic possession as part of the differential diagnosis of dissociative disorders. Furthermore, the existence of dissociative amnesias and delayed recall of traumatic events raises difficult questions about the reliability of traumatic memory. The latter controversy has led to a vociferous promulgation of the sociocognitive model, often in the context of highly contentious legal battles over false memories and the standard of care for patients diagnosed with DID and dissociative amnesia (D. W. Brown et al. 1998). This phenomenon led to a backlash in which the media, the public, and many professionals became far more skeptical of claims of childhood trauma and dissociative disorders. These false-memory cases have mostly subsided, and popular and professional culture has shifted back to a more receptive attitude to reports of trauma. Most probably, this shift is related to a more general awareness of the effects of trauma in the wake of the September 11, 2001, attacks; the Catholic Church priest abuse scandals; the events and devastation surrounding hurricanes Katrina and Rita; and the wars in Iraq and Afghanistan from which many combat veterans are returning with PTSD.

On the other hand, clinical interest in dissociative phenomena has reoccurred in every war since the beginning of the twentieth century, with the observation of amnesia, fugues, and conversion symptoms in traumatized soldiers (Archibald and Tuddenham 1965; W. Brown 1919; Henderson and Moore 1944; Sargent and Slater 1941). Unfortunately, the psychiatric and medical community then forgets these observations as the wars fade from memory. Similar oscillations have occurred for many of the more recent societal focuses in trauma, such as the concern for PTSD in the returning Vietnam veterans and the media interest in childhood sexual abuse. A cycle of concern and attention followed by backlash and forgetting, like the process of intrusion and numbing in PTSD, seems to characterize collective awareness of trauma and its spectrum of disorders.

Because of this, those who study and care for DID patients should be prepared to face criticism and skepticism in the long run. Wider social and cultural factors that also affect mental health professionals and researchers are likely to always make these disorders controversial. Because of the nature of these controversies, appeals to data, to reason, to intellectual integrity, and to the scientific method may not prevail, no matter how brilliantly presented. In addition, DID patients are often in an internal struggle over whether they believe themselves. This belief/disbelief split regarding the reality and implications of violence is mirrored in the countertransference brought to bear on DID patients from individual clinicians, psychiatric inpatient staff, and the culture at large.

REFERENCES

Archibald HC, Tuddenham RD: Persistent stress reaction after combat. Arch Gen Psychiatry 12:475–481, 1965

Armstrong JG: Reflections on multiple personality disorder as a developmentally complex adaptation. Psychoanal Study Child 50:349–364, 1995

Armstrong JG: False memories and true lies: the psychology of a recanter. J Psychiatry Law 27:519–547, 1999

Armstrong JG, Loewenstein R J: Characteristics of patients with multiple personality and dissociative disorders on psychological testing. J Nerv Ment Dis 178:448–454, 1990

American Psychiatric Association: Diagnostic and Statistical Manual of Mental Disorders, 2nd Edition. Washington, DC, American Psychiatric Association, 1968

American Psychiatric Association: Diagnostic and Statistical Manual of Mental Disorders, 3rd Edition. Washington, DC, American Psychiatric Association, 1980

American Psychiatric Association: Diagnostic and Statistical Manual of Mental Disorders, 4th Edition. Washington, DC, American Psychiatric Association, 1994

American Psychiatric Association: Diagnostic and Statistical Manual of Mental Disorders, 4th Edition, Text Revision. Washington, DC, American Psychiatric Association, 2000

Banyai EI: Toward a social-psychobiological model of hypnosis, in Theories of Hypnosis: Current Models and Perspectives. Edited by Lynn SJ, Rhue JW. New York, Guilford, 1991, pp 564–598

Barber TX: A deeper understanding of hypnosis: its secrets, its nature, its essence. Am J Clin Hypn 42:208–272, 2000

Becker-Blease KA, Freyd JJ: Beyond PTSD: an evolving relationship between trauma theory and family violence research. J Interpers Violence 20:403–411, 2005

Benner DG, Joscelyne B: Multiple personality as a borderline disorder. Psychiatr Clin North Am 7:89–99, 1984

Bernstein EM, Putnam FW: Development, reliability, and validity of a dissociation scale. J Nerv Ment Dis 174:727–735, 1986

Boon S, Draijer N: The differentiation of patients with MPD or DDNOS from patients with Cluster B personality disorder. Dissociation 6:126–135, 1993

Bowers KS: Hypnosis for the Seriously Curious. New York, WW Norton, 1976

Brand B, Armstrong JA, Loewenstein RJ: Psychological assessment of patients with dissociative identity disorder. Psychiatr Clin North Am 29:145–168, 2006

Bremner JD, Marmar CR (eds): Trauma, Memory, and Dissociation. Washington, DC, American Psychiatric Press, 1998

Brennan TA, Leape LL, Laird NM, et al: Incidence of adverse events and negligence in hospitalized patients: results of the Harvard Medical Practice Study I. N Engl J Med 324:370–376, 1991

Brenneis CB: Multiple personality: fantasy proneness, demand characteristics, and indirect communication. Psychoanalytic Psychology 13:367–387, 1996

Breuer J, Freud S: On the psychical mechanism of hysterical phenomena (1893), in The Standard Edition of the Complete Psychological Works of Sigmund Freud, Vol 2. Translated and edited by Strachey J, Strachey A. London, Hogarth Press, 2001, pp 1–17

Briere J, Elliott DM, Harris K, et al: Trauma Symptom Inventory: psychometrics and association with childhood and adult trauma in clinical samples. J Interpers Violence 10:387–340, 1995

Briquet P: Traité Clinique et Thérapeutique de l'Hystérie. Paris, Baillière et Fils, 1859

Brown D, Fromm E: Hypnotherapy and Hypnoanalysis. Hillsdale, NJ, L. Erlbaum Associates, 1986

Brown DW, Scheflin AW: Factitious disorders and trauma-related diagnoses. J Psychiatry Law 27:373–422, 1999

Brown DW, Scheflin AW, Hammond DC: Memory, Trauma, Treatment, and the Law. New York, WW Norton, 1998

Brown DW, Frischholz EJ, Scheflin AW: Iatrogenic dissociative identity disorder: an evaluation of the scientific evidence. J Psychiatry Law 27:549–638, 1999

Brown W: The treatment of cases of shell shock in an advanced neurological centre. Lancet August 17:197–200, 1919

Cardeña E, Spiegel D: Suggestibility, absorption, and dissociation: an integrative model of hypnosis, in Human Suggestibility: Advances in Theory, Research, and Application. Edited by Schumaker JF. New York, Routledge, 1991, pp 93–107

Cardeña E, Spiegel D: Dissociative reactions to the San Francisco Bay area earthquake of 1989. Am J Psychiatry 150:474–478, 1993

Chesler P: Women and Madness, 2nd Edition, Revised and Updated. New York, Doubleday, 1972

Classen C, Koopman C, Hales RE, et al: Acute stress disorder as a predictor of posttraumatic stress symptoms. Am J Psychiatry 155:620–624, 1998

Courtois CA: Complex trauma, complex reactions: assessment and treatment. Psychotherapy Theory, Research, Practice, Training 41:412–425, 2004

Dell P: Axis II pathology in outpatients with dissociative identity disorder. J Nerv Ment Dis 186:352–356, 1998

De Pascalis V, Gheorghiu VA, Sheehan PW, et al: Suggestion and Suggestibility: Theory and Research (Hypnosis International Monographs No 4). Munich, MEG-Stifung, 2000

Draijer N, Boon S: The imitation of dissociative identity disorder: patients at risk, therapists at risk. J Psychiatry Law 27:423–458, 1999

Ellenberger HF: The Discovery of the Unconscious. New York, Basic Books, 1970

Evans FJ: The domain of hypnosis. Am J Clin Hypn 43:1–16, 2000

Eysenck HJ: Is suggestibility? In Human Suggestibility: Advances in Theory, Research, and Application. Edited by Schumaker JF. New York, Routledge, 1991, pp 76–90

Feighner JP, Robins E, Guze SB, et al: Diagnostic criteria for use in psychiatric research. Arch Gen Psychiatry 26:57–63, 1972

Fink D, Golinkoff M: Multiple personality disorder, borderline personality disorder, and schizophrenia: a comparative study of clinical features. Dissociation 3:127–134, 1990

Fleming ST: Complications, adverse events, and iatrogenesis: classifications and quality of care measurement issues. Clin Perform Qual Health Care 4:137–147, 1996

Fourie DP: Friendliness and suggestibility: an ecosytemic perspective, in Suggestion and Suggestibility: Theory and Research (Hypnosis International Monographs No 4). Edited by De Pascalis V, Gheorghiu VA, Sheehan PW, et al. Munich, MEG-Stifung, 2000, pp 91–101

Fraser GA, Raine D: Cost analysis of the treatment of MPD, in Ninth Annual International Conference on Multiple Personality/Dissociative States. Edited by Braun BG. Chicago, IL, Department of Psychiatry, Rush Presbyterian-St. Luke's Medical Center, 1992, p 10

Freyd JJ: Betrayal Trauma: The Logic of Forgetting Childhood Abuse. Cambridge, MA, Harvard University Press, 1996

Freyd JJ, Putnam FW, Lyon TD, et al: The science of child sexual abuse. Science 308:501, 2005

Frischholz EJ, Lipman LS, Braun BG, et al: Psychopathology, hypnotizability, and dissociation. Am J Psychiatry 149:1521–1525, 1992

Ganaway G: Transference and countertransference: shaping influences on dissociative syndromes, in Dissociation: Clinical and Theoretical Perspectives Edited by Lynn SJ, Rhue JW. New York, Guilford, 1994, pp 317–337

Gheorghiu V: The domain of suggestibility: attempt to conceptualize suggestional phenomena, 1—particularities of suggestion, in Suggestion and Suggestibility: Theory and Research (Hypnosis International Monographs No 4). Edited by De Pascalis V, Gheorghiu VA, Sheehan PW, et al. Munich, MEG-Stifung, 2000, pp 1–15

Gheorghiu V, Kruse P: The psychology of suggestion: an integrative perspective, in Human Suggestibility: Advances in Theory, Research, and Application. Edited by Schumaker JF. New York, Routledge, 1991, pp 59–75

Gheorghiu V, Netter P, Eysenck HJ, et al: Suggestion and Suggestibility: Theory and Research. New York, Springer-Verlag, 1989

Gill MM: Analysis of Transference, Vol 1: Theory and Technique. New York, International Universities Press, 1982

Gleaves DH: The sociocognitive model of dissociative identity disorder: a reexamination of the evidence. Psychol Bull 120:42–59, 1996

Gleaves DH, May MC, Eberenz KP: Discriminating dissociative and borderline symptomatology among women with eating disorders. Dissociation 4:110–117, 1995

Gleaves DH, May MC, Cardeña E: An examination of the diagnostic validity of dissociative identity disorder. Clin Psychol Rev 21:577–608, 2001

Goodwin DW, Guze SB: Psychiatric Diagnosis, 4th Edition. New York, Oxford University Press, 1989

Goodwin J: Sexual Abuse: Incest Victims and Their Families, 2nd Edition. Chicago, IL, Year Book Medical Publishers, 1989

Graham JR: MMPI-2: Assessing Personality and Psychopathology, 3rd Edition. New York, Oxford University Press, 1991

Groth-Marnat G: Hypnotizability, suggestibility, and psychopathology, in Human Suggestibility: Advances in Theory, Research, and Application. Edited by Schumaker JF. New York, Routledge, 1991, pp 219–231

Gudjonsson GH: The Psychology of Interrogations and Confessions: A Handbook (Wiley Series in Psychology of Crime, Policing, and Law). West Sussex, England, Wiley, 2003

Guillain G: J.M. Charcot: His Life, His Work. London, Pitman, 1959

Harriman PL: The experimental induction of multiple personality. Psychiatry 5:179–186, 1942a

Harriman PL: The experimental production of some phenomena related to multiple personality. J Abnorm Soc Psychol 37:244–255, 1942b

Harriman PL: A new approach to multiple personality. Am J Orthopsychiatry 13:638–643, 1942c

Henderson JL, Moore M: The psychoneuroses of war. N Engl J Med 230:273–279, 1944

Herman JL: Father-Daughter Incest. Cambridge, MA, Harvard University Press, 1981

High JR: Deception through factitious identity. J Psychiatry Law 27:483–518, 1999

Hilgard ER: Divided Consciousness: Multiple Controls in Human Thought and Action, Expanded Edition. New York, Wiley, 1986

Hilgard ER: Suggestibility and suggestions as related to hypnosis, in Human Suggestibility: Advances in Theory, Research, and Application. Edited by Schumaker JF. New York, Routledge, 1991, pp 37–57

Horevitz RP, Braun BG: Are multiple personalities borderline? An analysis of 33 cases. Psychiatr Clin North Am 7:69–87, 1984

Hornstein N, Putnam FW: Clinical phenomenology of child and adolescent dissociative disorders. J Am Acad Child Adolesc Psychiatry 31:1077–1085, 1992

International Society for the Study of Dissociation: Guidelines for the treatment of dissociative identity disorder in adults. J Trauma Dissociation 6:69–149, 2005

Janet P: L'Automatisme Psychologique: Essai de Psychologie Expérimentale Sur les Formes Inférieures de l'Activité Humaine. Paris, Félix Alcan, 1889

Kaffman M: Monoideistic disorders and the process of suggestion, in Human Suggestibility: Advances in Theory, Research, and Application. Edited by Schumaker JF. New York, Routledge, 1991, pp 289–307

Kampmann R: Hypnotically induced multiple personality: an experimental study. Int J Clin Exp Hypn 24:215–227, 1976

Kanter JW, Kohlenberg RJ, Loftus EF: Demand characteristics, treatment rationales, and cognitive therapy for depression. Prevention and Treatment 5:Article 41, 2002

Kempe CH, Silverman FN, Steele BF, et al: The battered-child syndrome. JAMA 181:17–24, 1962

Kernberg O: Borderline Conditions and Pathological Narcissism. New York, Jason Aronson, 1975

Kirmayer LJ: Cultural variations in the clinical presentation of depression and anxiety: implications for diagnosis and treatment. J Clin Psychiatry 62(suppl):22–28, 2001

Kleinman AM: Depression, somatization and the "new cross-cultural psychiatry." Soc Sci Med 11:3–10, 1977

Kluft RP: An introduction to multiple personality disorder. Psychiatr Ann 14:19–24, 1984a

Kluft RP: Treatment of multiple personality disorder: a study of 33 cases. Psychiatr Clin North Am 7:9–29, 1984b

Kluft RP: Childhood multiple personality disorder: predictors, clinical findings, and treatment results, in Childhood Antecedents of Multiple Personality. Edited by Kluft RP. Washington, DC, American Psychiatric Press, 1985, pp 167–196

Kluft RP: First rank symptoms as a diagnostic clue to multiple personality disorder. Am J Psychiatry 144:293–298, 1987

Kluft RP: The dissociative disorders, in The American Psychiatric Press Textbook of Psychiatry. Edited by Talbot JA, Hales RE, Yudofsky SC. Washington, DC, American Psychiatric Press, 1988a, pp 557–584

Kluft RP: The phenomenology and treatment of extremely complex multiple personality disorder. Dissociation 1:47–58, 1988b

Kluft RP: The David Caul Memorial Symposium papers: iatrogenesis and MPD. Dissociation 2:66–104, 1989

Kluft RP: Multiple personality disorder, in American Psychiatric Press Review of Psychiatry, Vol 10. Edited by Tasman A, Goldfinger S. Washington, DC, American Psychiatric Press, 1991, pp 161–188

Kluft RP: Diagnosing dissociative identity disorder. Psychiatr Ann 35:633–643, 2005

Leape LL, Brennan TA, Laird N, et al: The nature of adverse events in hospitalized patients: results of the Harvard Medical Practice Study II. N Engl J Med 324:377–384, 1991

Leavitt MC: A case of hypnotically produced secondary and tertiary personalities. Psychoanal Rev 34:274–295, 1947

Lilienfeld SO, Kirsch I, Sarbin TR, et al: Dissociative identity disorder and the sociocognitive model: recalling the lessons of the past. Psychol Bull 125:507–523, 1999

Localio AR, Lawthers AG, Brennan TA, et al: Relation between malpractice claims and adverse events due to negligence: results of the Harvard Medical Practice Study III. N Engl J Med 325:245–251, 1991

Loewenstein RJ: Dissociation, development, and the psychobiology of trauma. J Am Acad Psychoanal 21:581–603, 1993

Loewenstein RJ: Diagnosis, epidemiology, clinical course, treatment, and cost effectiveness of treatment for dissociative disorders and multiple personality disorder: report submitted to the Clinton administration task force on health care financing reform. Dissociation 7:3–11, 1994

Loewenstein RJ, Putnam FW: The dissociative disorders, in Comprehensive Textbook of Psychiatry VIII, 8th Edition. Edited by Sadock BJ, Sadock VA. Baltimore, MD, Williams & Wilkins, 2004, pp 1844–1901

Loewenstein RJ, Vermetten E, Wilson K, et al: Suggestibility in dissociative identity disorder: relationship to factitious and "iatrogenic" DID, in Proceedings of the 19th International Fall Conference of the International Society for the Study of Dissociation. The Complexities of Dissociation: Trauma, Adaptation and Creativity. Edited by Steele K, Loewenstein RJ. Baltimore, MD, International Society for the Study of Dissociation, 2004, pp 50

Loftus EF: The reality of repressed memories. Am Psychol 48:518–537, 1993

Loftus EF: The most dangerous book. Psychology Today 33:126, 2000

Lyons-Ruth K, Dutra L, Schuder MR, et al: From infant attachment disorganization to adult dissociation: relational adaptations or traumatic experiences? Psychiatr Clin North Am 29:63–86, 2006

Mai FM, Merskey H: Briquet's treatise on hysteria: a synopsis and commentary. Arch Gen Psychiatry 37:1401–1405, 1980

Marmer SS: Variations on a factitious theme. J Psychiatry Law 27:459–481, 1999

McHugh PR: Psychiatric misadventures. The American Scholar 62:497–510, 1992

McHugh PR: Resolved: multiple personality disorder is an individually and socially created artifact. Affirmative. J Am Acad Child Adolesc Psychiatry 34:957–959, 1995a

McHugh PR: Resolved: multiple personality disorder is an individually and socially created artifact. Affirmative rebuttal. J Am Acad Child Adolesc Psychiatry 34:962–963, 1995b

McHugh PR: Witches, multiple personalities, and other psychiatric artifacts. Nat Med 1:110–114, 1995c

Merskey H: The artifactual nature of multiple personality disorder: comments on Charles Barton's "Backstage in psychiatry: the multiple personality controversy." Dissociation 7:173–175, 1994

Millon T: The Millon Inventories: Clinical and Personality Assessment. New York, Guilford, 1997

Orne MT: The nature of hypnosis: artifact and essence. J Abnorm Soc Psychol 58:277–299, 1959

Peebles-Kleiger MJ: Using countertransference in the hypnosis of trauma victims: a model for turning hazard into healing. Am J Psychother 43:518–530, 1989

Piper A: Multiple personality disorder. Br J Psychiatry 164:600–612, 1994

Piper A, Merskey H: The persistence of folly: a critical examination of dissociative identity disorder, part I. The excesses of an improbable concept. Can J Psychiatry 49:592–600, 2004a

Piper A, Merskey H: The persistence of folly: a critical examination of dissociative identity disorder, part II. The defence and decline of multiple personality or dissociative identity disorder. Can J Psychiatry 49:678–683, 2004b

Pope HG, Lipinski JF: Diagnosis in schizophrenia and manic-depressive illness: a reassessment of the specificity of "schizophrenic" symptoms in the light of current research. Arch Gen Psychiatry 35:811–828, 1978

Putnam FW: Diagnosis and Treatment of Multiple Personality Disorder. New York, Guilford, 1989

Putnam FW: Resolved: multiple personality disorder is an individually and socially created artifact. J Am Acad Child Adolesc Psychiatry 34:960–962, 1995a

Putnam FW: Resolved: multiple personality disorder is an individually and socially created artifact. Negative rebuttal. J Am Acad Child Adolesc Psychiatry 34:963, 1995b

Putnam FW: Dissociation in Children and Adolescents: A Developmental Model. New York, Guilford, 1997

Quitkin F, Rifkin A, Klein DF: Monoamine oxidase inhibitors: a review of anti-depressant effectiveness. Arch Gen Psychiatry 36:749–760, 1979

Rhue JW, Lynn SJ: Fantasy proneness, hypnotizability, and multiple personality, in Human Suggestibility: Advances in Theory, Research, and Application. Edited by Schumaker JF. New York, Routledge, 1991, pp 200–218

Rifkin A, Quitkin F, Carillo C, et al: Lithium carbonate in emotionally unstable character disorder. Arch Gen Psychiatry 27:519–523, 1972

Ross CA: Dissociative Identity Disorder: Diagnosis, Clinical Features, and Treatment of Multiple Personality. New York, Wiley, 1997

Ross CA, Heber S, Norton GR, et al: The Dissociative Disorders Interview Schedule: a structural interview. Dissociation 3:169–189, 1989

Ross CA, Miller SD, Reagor P, et al: Schneiderian symptoms in multiple personality disorder and schizophrenia. Compr Psychiatry 31:111–118, 1990

Roy A: Hysterical seizures. Arch Neurol 36:447, 1979

Sargent W, Slater E: Amnesic syndromes in war. Proc R Soc Med 34:757–764, 1941

Scheff TJ: Being Mentally Ill: A Sociological Theory. Chicago, IL, Aldine Atherton, 1966

Schneider K: Clinical Psychopathology, Fifth Edition. Translated by Hamilton MW, Anderson EW. New York, Grune and Stratton, 1959

Schreiber FR: Sybil. Chicago, IL, Regnery, 1976

Schumaker JF: The adaptive value of suggestibility and dissociation, in Human Suggestibility: Advances in Theory, Research, and Application. Edited by Schumaker JF. New York, Routledge, 1991a, pp 108–131

Schumaker JF (ed): Human Suggestibility: Advances in Theory, Research, and Application. New York, Routledge, 1991b

Sedgwick P: Psychopolitics. New York, Harper & Row, 1982

Soukhanov A: Iatrogenic. 1999. Available at: http://encarta.msn.com/dictionary_/iatrogenic.html. Accessed March 13, 2006.

Spanos NP: Multiple Identities and False Memories: A Sociocognitive Perspective. Washington, DC, American Psychological Association, 1996

Spanos NP, Burgess C: Hypnosis and multiple personality: a sociocognitive perspective, in Dissociation: Clinical and Theoretical Perspectives. Edited by Lynn SJ, Rhue JW. New York, Guilford, 1994

Spiegel D: Multiple personality as a post-traumatic stress disorder. Psychiatr Clin North Am 7:101–110, 1984

Spiegel D: Dissociation, double binds, and posttraumatic stress, in The Treatment of Multiple Personality Disorder. Edited by Braun BG. Washington, DC, American Psychiatric Press, 1986, pp 61–77

Spiegel D: Commentary: the treatment accorded those who treat patients with multiple personality disorder. J Nerv Ment Dis 176:535–536, 1988

Spiegel D: Dissociation and Trauma, in American Psychiatric Press Review of Psychiatry, Vol 10. Edited by Tasman A, Goldfinger SM. Washington, DC, American Psychiatric Press, 1991, pp 261–275

Spiegel D: Hypnosis and suggestion, in Memory Distortion. Edited by Schacter DL, Coyle JT, Fischback G, et al. Cambridge, MA, Harvard University Press, 1994

Spiegel D, Cardeña E: Disintegrated experience: the dissociative disorders revisited. J Abnorm Psychol 100:366–378, 1991

Spiegel D, Hunt T, Dondershine H: Dissociation and hypnotizability in posttraumatic stress disorder. Am J Psychiatry 145:301–305, 1988

Spiegel D, Koopman C, Classen C: Acute stress disorder and dissociation. Australian Journal of Clinical and Experimental Hypnosis 22:11–23, 1994

Spiegel H, Spiegel D: Trance and Treatment, 2nd Edition. Washington, DC, American Psychiatric Publishing, 2004

Steinberg M: The Structured Clinical Interview for DSM-IV Dissociative Disorders–Revised (SCID-D-R). Washington, DC, American Psychiatric Press, 1994

Stone MH: The Borderline Syndromes: Constitution, Personality, and Adaptation. New York, McGraw-Hill, 1980

Sullivan HS: The Interpersonal Theory of Psychiatry. New York, Norton, 1953

Ward C, Kemp S: Religious experiences, altered states of consciousness, and suggestibility: cross-cultural and historical perspectives, in Human Suggestibility: Advances in Theory, Research, and Application. Edited by Schumaker JF. New York, Routledge, 1991, pp 159–182

Williams TL, Loewenstein RJ, Gleaves DH: Exploring assumptions about DID: an investigation of suggestibility, hypnotizability, fantasy proneness, and personality variables, in Proceedings of the 19th International Fall Conference of the International Society for the Study of Dissociation. The Complexities of Dissociation: Trauma, Adaptation and Creativity. Edited by Steele K, Loewenstein RJ. Baltimore, MD, International Society for the Study of Dissociation, 2004, pp 12–13

Yapko MD: Suggestibility and repressed memories of abuse: a survey of psychotherapists' beliefs. Am J Clin Hypn 36:172–187, 1994

C H A P T E R   1 5

APPLICATIONS OF INNATE AFFECT THEORY TO THE UNDERSTANDING AND TREATMENT OF DISSOCIATIVE IDENTITY DISORDER

RICHARD P. KLUFT, M.D.

Despite the importance of affect in the trauma response and the dissociative disorders, there have been few efforts (e.g., Stone 1996) to apply contemporary affect theories to the understanding of these phenomena. In this chapter I attempt to build a bridge between the innate affect theory of Sylvan Tomkins (1962, 1963, 1991) and its exposition and clinical application by Donald Nathanson (1992) to the study of dissociative identity disorder (DID) and certain aspects of its treatment. I begin with the raw data of a brief clinical encounter and then use the analysis of its dissociative and affective infrastructures to illustrate the parallels and connections between the two and their potential to inform clinical interventions. With an emphasis on shame, I offer a preliminary exploration of how an awareness of innate affect theory can facilitate a more thorough understanding of traumatized dissociative patients, inform certain approaches to their treatment, and provide some new perspectives on well-known clinical phenomena.

Case Example: Lois

Lois, a bright and talented professional woman in her mid-30s, sits in my office, calm and composed. She expresses herself eloquently. She appears to be working very well in her therapy as she talks thoughtfully about a very embarrassing incident of a sort that frequently befalls her.

She is so smooth and insightful, and moving so far so fast, that the discrepancy between the mortification inherent in what she is discussing and the seamless untroubled facility of her self-expression is jarring.

I am moved to ask, "Lois, what are you feeling as you tell me this?" Her eyebrows arch up, and she blinks. "What did you say?" she asks. I repeat my question. She smiles very engagingly, and says, "Great!" "What does 'Great!' mean?" I persist. "Well, I feel nothing," She responds. "Nothing is bothering me. Everything is really the way it should be."

I remain silent. Lois's expression becomes frozen and pale. "What's going on?" I ask. Lois's face reddens, her jaw clenches, and she gives me a disapproving frown. She complains that I am never content when she feels well. "You can't leave well enough alone. You are only happy when I am suffering. This therapy is going nowhere." She picks up her purse, pushes her already well-styled hair into perfect order, and starts to get up.

I said, "Do you think it is possible that you have been trying to convince yourself that you can bypass how upset you were feeling, avoiding the painful emotions as best you could, and then got really angry at me when I tried to call your attention to your evasion?"

Lois' shoulders slump, she fixes her gaze on the floor, and turns her face away to hide her blush. "You didn't say it, but I knew you knew I blew it again. I feel like such a failure. I wish I could disappear into the wall. I hate it when you see me like this. Why do you waste your time with me?"

Lois is a severely traumatized DID patient with enough intelligence and strength to hide her disorder effectively and hold a prestigious executive position. She is a paradigm of the "high-functioning DID patient" I first described in 1986 (Kluft 1986). She serves as both our introduction to, and text for, a brief and necessarily incomplete discussion of how Sylvan Tomkins's innate affect theory, as applied to clinical phenomena by Donald Nathanson and others, can be useful in approaching the traumatized and dissociative patient.

Lois is a veritable encyclopedia of shame scripts, which are strategies for coping with the dysphoric affect of shame. In a few moments of conversation she enacted all four poles of the compass of shame (Nathanson 1992) as studied in innate affect theory: she initiated efforts to withdraw, to attack herself, to attack another, and to distract in order to avoid distressing embarrassment.

Strong affect and defense against strong affect are crucial components of both the experience of trauma and the development of the psychiatric conditions that follow in its wake. Affect regulation and affect tolerance are basic aspects of ego strength and are disrupted in most posttraumatic conditions. Problems dealing with affect abound in the treatment of the traumatized, whether one is studying the impact of flashbacks, traumatic nightmares (Lansky 1995), autonomic hyperreactivity, abreaction, incomplete responses to psychopharmacology, or the vicissitudes of exposure-based psychotherapies, among others. Furthermore, biological studies have demonstrated that although the prefrontal cortex may be "shut down" or hypoperfused in traumatized and dissociative patients, other brain structures, such as the amygdala, that are more closely linked to affect assume a more dominant role in their mental activity (Rauch et al. 1998).

INNATE AFFECT THEORY

My introduction to Tomkins's innate affect theory began in the 1980s in conversations with Donald Nathanson, M.D., my colleague at The Institute of Pennsylvania Hospital. However, my interest accelerated when I learned about Nathanson's "Compass of Shame" and typology of shame scripts. My initial exposure to his work dramatically improved the quality of the therapy I could deliver, especially to patients with dissociative disorders.

Sylvan Tomkins was a productive experimental psychologist who took off a sabbatical year to be at home with his firstborn child. Not only a dedicated father but also a keen observer, Tomkins rapidly appreciated that his son's expressions of distress, surprise, and joy in the first weeks and months of life were identical to those he observed in adults. He appreciated that these modes of expression were completely in place before his infant son could have had the slightest idea of what was sad, new, or delightful in terms of cognition and comparison with remembered experience. He inferred that these affects were programs that were genetically transmitted and hard-wired and that they amplified the stimuli that set them in motion. No matter whether the stimulus had come from something perceived or remembered, the stimulus would now become important in the way typical of that affect. Affect, Tomkins said, makes us care about things in different ways. Emotion becomes important to thinking because it controls or acts on the way we use thought, just as it takes over or influences bodily actions at the sites specific for it. When we are motivated, it is an affect that has made us so, and the direction and form of the motivation are determined by the affect. Affect conveys importance. Affect is the engine that drives us.

Although it was generally conceded that Tomkins was a genius, it was also generally acknowledged that his prose was dauntingly difficult to decipher. Furthermore, he took approximately 30 years to complete his masterful three-volume opus, *Affect/Imagery/Consciousness*. Few who began to read his work either completed the task or emerged with a useful understanding. Thus, his work languished. Nathanson, a

Philadelphia endocrinologist turned psychiatrist, became consumed with a passion to understand emotions, both biologically and psychologically. Nathanson studied Tomkins's work and received his blessing to make the work more accessible. The summaries of Tomkins's ideas cited in this chapter are drawn from Nathanson's efforts to make those ideas more accessible and to expand them from the developmental and phenomenological into the clinical realm.

Tomkins described nine innate affects. The affects and the facial expressions associated with them are listed in Table 15–1. Furthermore, Tomkins observed that affective experiences themselves can be linked into structures held in the mind and remembered as scenes. A stimulus triggers a whole set of responses, sequences of which become linked together to form a scene. Sequences or reiterations of the stimulus-response patterns create what Stern (1985) described as "representations of interactions that have been generalized," or RIGS. An affect script is "a sequence of RIGS connected by rules worked out through experience; it connects past and present to suggest, define, or determine a particular future" (Nathanson 1992, p. 246).

With this introduction to innate affect theory and affect scripts, it becomes possible to discuss some aspects of DID and to explore the relationship between script theory and dissociative identities in an effort to build a preliminary and tentative bridge between these classes of phenomena. The ideas shared are not represented as definitive formulations but as modest bridge-building heuristics. I hope they provide a sufficient basis for describing how I use concepts derived from innate affect theory to inform my therapeutic efforts with DID and allied dissociative conditions.

The dissociative identities in DID can be understood as personified adaptive strategies, each designed to enact a particular approach to general classes of dysphoric situations or to anticipate, prepare for, and/or avert such situations. Each personality also constitutes an ego state. Jack and Helen Watkins, the founders of ego state therapy, define ego states in the following way:

> We define an ego state as an organized system of behavior and experience whose elements are bound together by some common principle but that is separated from other such states by boundaries that are more or less permeable. Such a definition includes both true cases of multiple personalities and those less rigidly separated personality segments that lie in the middle of the differentiation-dissociation continuum and that may be more "integrated" and hence more adaptive. (Watkins and Watkins 1993, p. 278)

Clearly, what are called *scripts* or *script encyclopedias* (repertoires of scripts) in affect theory fall under the aegis of the ego state description

TABLE 15–1. The innate affects

Positive
1. Interest-Excitement: eyebrows down, track, look, listen
2. Enjoyment-Joy: smiles, lips widened and out

Neutral
3. Surprise-Startle: eyebrows up, eyes blink

Negative
4. Fear-Terror: frozen stare, face pale, cold, sweaty, hair erect
5. Distress-Anguish: cry, rhythmic sobbing, arched eyebrows, mouth down
6. Anger-Rage: frown, clenched jaw, red face
7. Shame-Humiliation: eyes down, head down and averted, blush
8. Dissmell: upper lip raised, head pulled back
9. Disgust: lower lip lowered and protruded, head forward and down

Source. Adapted from Tomkins 1962, 1991.

and paradigm without necessarily being alters able to assert executive control. That is, a person who can enjoy the healthy pride of competence or success but who also enacts a shame script under the influence of mortification is in different ego states when experiencing and coping with these different affects. I will return to this observation later, because it is important to appreciate that when one studies arrays of affect, behavior, cognition, and one's experience of self and others, one is studying mental processes and structures with much in common with dissociative identities. The ego states of DID (i.e., dissociative identities) can be understood as (among other things) personified and embodied scripts.

To illustrate the concept of an affect script in a more tangible way, I focus on what I consider Nathanson's most important clinical contribution to date: the Compass of Shame. Affect theorists are in the process of working out the compass model for all of the innate affects; for example, Grindlinger ("A Compass for the Affect Disgust," unpublished manuscript, 2001) has produced a masterful compass of disgust. However, shame is the compass that has been studied first and best. (For alternative perspectives on shame, see Lansky and Morrison 1997.)

Shame is considered the most uncomfortable affect, one that makes us feel different in a negative way, unlinked from others, alone and needing to be alone, and incapable of positive emotion. Shame severs interpersonal connections. When we experience the affect shame, we are rapidly forced to endure its cognitive sequelae. In the cognitive phase of shame we search our memories for previous similar experiences and generate layered associations to matters of prowess, potency,

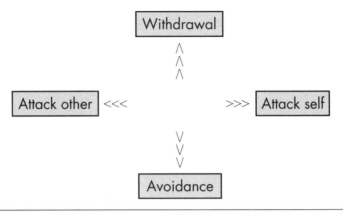

FIGURE 15–1.   The compass of shame.

Source.   Adapted from Nathanson 1992.

independence, competitiveness, sense of self, attractiveness, sexuality, personal visibility, and closeness. In each instance we are confronted by memories and cognitions that inform us that we are unique only to the extent that we are defective and unlovable. We feel like losers, helpless oafs, incompetents, and persons who are profoundly unattractive. We doubt the strength and genuineness of our sexuality, we want to escape from the sight of those who have witnessed or learned of our humiliation, and we both wish to be alone and fear we may have to be alone forever.

Not unexpectedly, this state of affairs is intolerable. We move to manage our shame affect. In his Compass of Shame model (Figure 15–1), Nathanson (1992) proposed that there are four major scripts with which we manage shame: withdrawal, avoidance, attack self, and attack other. We may withdraw to minimize our experience and risk of shame. We may, by avoidance, decline to acknowledge the shameful experience as shameful; disavow the experience and affect of shame as well; or try to minimize, shake off, or limit our shame exposure by changing our state with chemical substances, engaging in hedonistic or frantic activities, or making energetic efforts to distract ourselves and others from appreciating what might bring us shame.

Those who find the helplessness and isolation of shame predominant tend to take over the experience and place it under their control by attacking themselves. They tolerate shame by doing so voluntarily and in the service of maintaining rather than severing relatedness. Those who are unable to tolerate the cognitive aspect of shame that discloses information about their inferiority feel a profound need to make some-

TABLE 15–2.   Coping strategies and alter formation of Lois

Cognitive coping strategy	Alter created
This did not happen	A Lois who knows and a Lois who does not
I must have deserved it	Bad Lois, whose behavior would explain trauma as punishment
I must have wanted it	A sexual alter, Sherrie
I can control it better if I take charge	An aggressively sexual alter, Vickie
I would be safe if I were a boy	Louis, Lois's male "twin"
I wish I were a big man who could prevent this	Big Jack, based on some person of power
I wish I were the one who could hurt someone and not be hurt	Uncle Ben, or a more disguised identification with the aggressor
I wish I could feel nothing	Jessie, who endures all yet feels nothing
I wish someone could replace me	"The Girls" who encapsulate specific experiences of trauma unknown to Lois
I wish someone would comfort me	Angel, with whom Lois imagines herself to be while the body is being exploited and "The Girls" are experiencing the trauma

Source.   Adapted from Kluft 1998.

one lower than themselves, so they attack another person(s). Each of the four poles is a library for these crucial affect management strategies.

Now, if we study the personality system in Lois (see Table 15–2), with whose tactics of shame management this chapter began, we appreciate that Lois has developed an array of adaptations, all of which can be understood as scripts to avoid being overwhelmed and helpless with the intolerable affect of shame. Reviewing her personality system in terms of the Compass of Shame offers a useful perspective that does not fully explain Lois's system of personalities (i.e., her alters) but offers a heuristic for further deepening and broadening our understanding of DID.

From this perspective, Lois (as unaware of her alters) and her alters, such as the anesthetic Jessie and Louis, the boy (see Table 15–2), may be understood as enacting withdrawal scripts. They remove the self from the traumatic experience and the humiliation associated with being treated badly, being made to feel terrible, and enduring the helpless lot of a victimized female. Bad Lois, who blames the trauma on her own behavior, embodies an attack-self script, as does Sherrie, who represents herself as wanting sex and thus deserving her fate. Uncle Ben, the identification with the aggressor identity, is an attack-other script. However, I would argue that Big Jack, who is designed to counterattack against aggressors, is a latent attack-other adaptation, and that Vickie, who is prepared to seduce in order to dominate, is a combination of avoidance and attack other. Vickie uses counterphobic sexuality to distract herself (avoidance) and to disarm and defeat others (attack other). The remaining alters do not lend themselves to conceptualization within this model.

I note in passing that many therapists who violate boundaries by sexually exploiting DID patients have encountered an alter like Vickie, ostensibly seductive and willing but actually maneuvering to minimize damage from the anticipated reenactment of an attack, deemed to be inevitable, by influencing and directing aspects of what takes place. Such therapists have no idea what they are dealing with. Hopefully, the observations just discussed will begin to build some conceptual bridges between affect theory and dissociation theory and will make the language, dynamics, and topics of affect theory somewhat less foreign to students of dissociation.

Continuing the bridge-building, we must look to definitions of both dissociative identities (alters) and scripts in order to study their similarities and differences. In 1988 I wrote,

> I have tended to define a personality, alter, or disaggregate self state [i.e., dissociative identities] in a manner that stresses what such an entity does and how it functions….A disaggregate self state…is the mental address of a relatively stable and enduring particular pattern of selective mobilization of mental contents and functions, which may be behaviorally enacted with noteworthy role-taking and role-playing dimensions and sensitive to intrapsychic, interpersonal, and environmental stimuli. It is organized in and associated with a relatively stable…pattern of neuropsychophysiological activation, and has crucial psychodynamic contents. It functions both as a recipient, processor, and storage center for perceptions, experiences, and the processing of such in connection with past events and thoughts, and/or present and anticipated ones as well. It has a sense of its own identity and ideation, and a capacity for initiating thought processes and actions. (Kluft 1988, p. 51)

To define a *script*, I use an array of paraphrased observations and quotes from the work of Nathanson (1992). The process of growth and development, Nathanson wrote, creates *software scripts*, sequences of lived moments characterized by a variety of needs, affects, and responses. Similar situations are grouped and stored as a bundle, and a current experience of affect is compared with the bundles themselves. The existence of such bundles, which Tomkins calls scripts, allows us to bypass the full review that would be required in their absence. A script involves both a compression and condensation of all previous experiences with that affect, summated as an experiential pattern. "Stored along with our reminiscences of shame are our recollections of all of the ways we have made ourselves feel better when we are hurt...each of us has accumulated a library of defenses against painful experiences.... Intimately associated with the affect is our history of reaction to it" (p. 307). "So complex and pervasive are the habits and skills of script formation that we adults come to live more within these personal scripts for the modulation and detoxification of affect than in a world of innate affect" (p. 310). "When an event occurs, we analyze it to see if it fits into a script and we try to interpret it as one of a series of events that has been analyzed before" (p. 311).

Daniel Stern's (1985) concept of RIGS relates neatly to the scripts of affect theory and the dissociative identities of dissociation theory. Stern observed that infants have the ability to collect their experiences in the form of remembered scenes. Through RIGS, the infant derives highly personal rules about how life works. Stern defined RIGS not as memory, per se, but as the sum total of myriad experiences—the observations from which humans make assumptions about experiences that are novel but that resemble prior experiences.

In comparing and contrasting alters and scripts as two forms of RIGS and ego states, we can appreciate clearly that both are well-learned structures and processes for dealing with affect that is dysphoric in quality and/or quantity. Both are dedicated to the protection of self from awareness of that affect or disruption by it. Scripts are constructed of myriad interactions, and alters may be derived from a family of related experiences or from single incidents, but both are based on the conversion of experiences into mental structure. Both are related to biologically based response patterns.

A major difference between scripts and alters is related to the four cardinal points that distinguish an alter from the normal range of ego state phenomena (Kluft 1991). Alters differ from the wider range of ego state phenomena in having 1) their own identities, 2) self-representations, 3) memories, and 4) senses of ownership of various components and aspects of autobiographical memory. From this perspective, scripts are ego states (i.e., they do not have their own identities). Furthermore, although our self-representations are certainly different when different scripts are operative, this is not to the exclusion of our basic sense of self—that is, when we feel shame, we may feel diminished in size and strength and potency and feel unique only to the extent that we are faulty, but we do not become different people, changing in age or gender or race. Also, when we use or enact a script, we do not forfeit our autobiographical memory for our actions under the influence of other scripts; thus there is no differential amnesia, as is found at least across some alters in each person who qualifies for the DID diagnosis. Finally, although one alter may not have a sense of ownership of the experience of another alter, the use of a script per se does not encompass denial or disavowal of one's participation in the event that stimulated the script or the behaviors associated with enacting the script. Hence, it is the enactment of a pattern by an embodied personification that may distinguish dissociative identities and scripts, both of which are enacted rules or strategies for coping with actual or anticipated discomfort.

My initial description of Lois's behavior made no reference to her having DID and did not identify the alters associated with the manifested affects and scripts in that particular vignette. Yet her material can be studied in terms of the alters and the scripts involved. It is my experience that engaging the various dissociative identities (alters) about their major shame scripts is a very rich and rewarding approach to understanding and treating DID. Furthermore, and unexpectedly, it proves to be a frequently effective strategy for accessing as yet inaccessible memories without utilizing inquiries of the sort that may raise issues of suggestion and the risk of eliciting pseudomemories. In the following paragraphs I can only begin to review some of the concepts that I have found useful.

When engaging alters' shame scripts, it is important to bear in mind that at each pole of the Compass of Shame we encounter different assemblies of auxiliary affects that shore up defenses (Nathanson 1992). Withdrawal is often accompanied by distress and fear. Avoidance is usually joined by excitement, fear, and/or enjoyment. Attack other is commonly accompanied by anger. Attack self is associated with self-directed dissmell and disgust (often called self-dissmell and self-disgust).

Alters with attack-self scripts contribute major challenges to the treatment of DID, and attack-self scripts are common in chronically traumatized patients regardless of their psychiatric diagnosis. Alters embodying this script often are responsible for acting out and regression in the course of trauma work, leading many to believe such work is contraindicated. However, when work with auxiliary affects is incorporated as a preliminary to the trauma work, acting out often can be prevented or minimized. Grindlinger has offered a plan for approaching such work. *Disgust* involves rejection after sampling (an analogue of rejection after tasting something aversive) or rejection after having become acquainted ("A Compass for the Affect Disgust," unpublished manuscript, 2001). *Dissmell* (a term created by Tomkins as an analogue of rejection after smelling something aversive) involves rejection before sampling, rejection at a distance. Hence, disgust has similarities to suppression and dissmell to disavowal and dissociation. Clearly, an alter oriented to attack self with disgust and dissmell auxiliaries is very difficult to approach therapeutically because, in addition to the various forms of resistance and reluctance associated with shame per se, it will rebuff and reject therapeutic efforts that induce the slightest unacceptable dysphoria (disgust) and will evade anything that might expose the alter to something upsetting (dissmell). The affect scripts are reinforcing the pressures toward avoidance and dissociation associated with the traumatic material itself. These are often the parts that buttress their self-attack with avoidance scripts such as self-mutilation (an avoidance as well as an attack-self script), eating disorders, and addictions. The task of approaching such alters and bringing them into the psychotherapy can be arduous, because if all aspects are not somehow addressed, there is profound pressure to re-dissociate whatever is the occasion of distress in the treatment.

THERAPEUTIC APPLICATIONS

One of the most basic realizations apparent from innate affect theory with a focus on shame and its auxiliaries (those other basic affects that have become linked with it) is that since successful trauma treatment involves exposure to and mastery of what is upsetting and its impact on us, the successful operation of any shame script evades such material and renders deconditioning, exposure, or abreaction impotent. This freezes the patient in a posttraumatic or dissociative adaptation. The often-unnoticed component in failures to process trauma successfully is that processing trauma without addressing relevant affective scripts and auxiliary affects/scripts may increase rather than diminish distress and thus cause either decompensation or the erroneous determination that the patient cannot tolerate more than supportive psychotherapy. Not only do the shame scripts and the auxiliary affects and scripts discourage dealing with traumatic material, they encourage the rejection of alters who embody any perception of the affects being avoided. Disgust becomes an analogue of suppression: alters known to be a particular way are scorned, avoided, and disregarded. Dissmell becomes an analogue of dissociation or disavowal: alters suspected of being that particular way are not even acknowledged or, if acknowledged, are considered of no account or are pushed out of the treatment whenever possible.

An important related topic has a significant bearing on the management of painful memories. I have always tried to interest colleagues in the difference between resistance and reluctance (e.g., Kluft 1995). *Resistance* is an unconscious opposition to the goals and process of therapy, whereas *reluctance* is a conscious opposition. Resistances yield to confrontation, clarification, interpretation, and working through (Greenson 1967), whereas reluctances yield to reassurance, explanation, and persuasion. The alters' memories are often regarded as unconscious to the host, and their being accessed for recollection is often considered an exercise in memory retrieval subject to distortions of recall and the creation of pseudomemories. However, if the alters carrying traumatic memories have been ongoing since the time of the trauma, or even before the time of the trauma, then these memories have always been conscious in those alters and should not be considered either recovered memories or more unreliable than normal recall, which, admittedly, is far from perfect. From this perspective, the alters' memories are not so much repressed material as part of "elsewhere thought known" material in mental structures involved in parallel processing activities (Kluft 1995).

If this is so, then one of the simplest ways to access currently unavailable material would be to help the alters with those memories, or the alters fearing recovery of those memories, to alleviate the intensity of the activation of their shame scripts so that they will see the revelation of their memories as a constructive step toward competence and mastery rather than as an opportunity for demonstrating again how weak, bad, and shameful they are. Shame's capacity to sever interpersonal connections (Nathanson 1987, 1992) occurs among alters as well as among people. The reduction of shame relieves emotional isolation, decreases the desperation of dissociative reluctance, and lowers many forms of dissociative barriers by eliminating major aspects of their reasons for being. This occurs both within the alter system, promoting integration, and within the intersubjective field of the treatment, reducing the shame barriers that impede the therapeutic alliance and fostering the expression rather than the enactment of transference paradigms.

Skilled therapists may work on the reduction of shame through a variety of theoretical and technical perspectives, but they must, in their work, help patients toward self-efficacy and mastery. In Nathanson's words, the antidote to shame is competence. As early as 1990, I advocated systematic efforts toward the alleviation of shame responses as an aspect of the phase of safety in the stage-oriented treatment of trauma, assigning it to the phase of preliminary interventions (the second subphase of the stage of safety in specific DID treatment).

If one accepts the idea that alters are associated with "elsewhere thought known" material rather than repressed material, then when alters are helped to replace the enactment of shame scripts with the pride of mastery, the effort to actively pursue hidden material in many DID patients is reduced to asking the alters to tell their stories and to share their perspectives. Furthermore, when abreaction is managed competently under the aegis of pride and mastery as opposed to shame and guilt, regressive decompensation is very infrequent, and hospitalization in connection with the processing of trauma is very rare. In more than a dozen years of clinical work with DID, I have yet to encounter either a decompensation or need for hospital care when trauma work goes forward in this manner. Conversely, when abreaction takes place in an atmosphere of shame, self-disgust, and self-dissmell, no matter how competent the management of the affect, the pain of the traumatic experience is amplified by those affects and proves to be a more formidable challenge to the therapeutic process.

CLINICAL APPLICATIONS OF AFFECT THEORY TO THE TREATMENT OF DISSOCIATIVE IDENTITY DISORDER

Some mysteries are hidden in deep and byzantine labyrinths. Others are obscured in plain sight, as was the "missing" letter in Edgar Allan Poe's *The Purloined Letter.*

In the early 1990s a profoundly suicidal DID patient was referred to me for an inpatient evaluation. Her case follows.

Case Example: Ginger

Ginger was a brilliant medical student with a straight A average. She was seen as such an extreme risk for suicide that she had already been hospitalized for several months; she was on a leave of absence because she was not progressing in treatment. At the core of her plight was a particularly impulsive and violent alter named Asha (pronounced Ah-shah). Asha appeared determined to end Ginger's life and to fend off therapeutic efforts to enter Ginger's inner world in order to provide meaningful treatment and relief. Asha's labile and dangerous behaviors were keeping Ginger confined. Her skilled and dedicated psychiatrist was in a constant state of agitation not only about the risk of Ginger's suicide but also about her own personal safety when Asha would emerge and assume control.

Upon her arrival at the Dissociative Disorders Program at The Institute of Pennsylvania Hospital, Ginger was in the grips of profound gloom, and Asha threatened to attack anyone who tried to intervene to prevent Ginger's suicide. I noted that Ginger was several inches taller than I and easily outweighed me by 50 pounds. She also lifted weights. Anticipating that I (like my predecessors) might have to contend with physical confrontations, I took note that however physically imposing Ginger appeared, she was slow and clumsy and without training in the martial arts.

On her second hospital day, I asked to speak to Asha in order to see if I could begin to build a therapeutic alliance with her. Asha emerged, im-

mediately aggressive and threatening to attack me. After the usual pleas-
antries, I reviewed the history of the treatment to date. I asked Asha about
her history of violence toward herself and others and inquired about her
frequent attempts to withdraw from treatment. I asked her why she opposed therapy with such tenacity. She turned purple and clenched her
fists, so I changed the subject. "You have a curious name. Can you tell me
about it?" The patient ducked her head and tried to run from the room. I
blocked her, and we went down in a heap, fortunately with me on top.
"What are you bothering me for? My name is Asha and I am a medical
student. That's all I have to say." While keeping a firm grip on her, I began
to put her name and self-description together, and keeping in mind Poe's
"hidden in plain sight" letter and noting the shame signifier of the downward duck of her head, I said, "I guess I need to ask you the same question
in a different way. What are you Asha med about?" The patient thrashed
around for several minutes, throwing us both all over the room in a series
of efforts that resembled a crocodile's death roll. Finally, Asha withdrew
and Ginger returned and began to laugh. "Asha med? What are you talking about?" Still not relaxing my grip, I reviewed her behavior, talked to
her about the Compass of Shame, and told her that she seemed very adept
at attack-self, attack-other, and withdrawal scripts. I told her if we were
able to understand her mortification (Asha med = ashamed), we might be
able to break the cycle of her problem behavior. She found this formulation thought provoking and agreed to explore it in treatment.

We spent 2 very difficult years dealing with Asha's toxic shame scripts.
Asha held Ginger's mortification over father–daughter incest and dramatically enacted her wishes to deny it and make it unreal, and to reinsti-
tute an idealized picture of her father, or die. The attempt to resuscitate a
destroyed idealization and to kill one's self before one is disillusioned
once again is an exceptionally common precursor to successful suicides in
DID (Kluft 1995). In Ginger's case, this required a psychotic level of denial,
because her idealized father was in jail for the incest rape of her sister, who
herself was a witness to some episodes of Ginger's abuse, which Ginger
(through Asha) tried to disavow with ferocious dedication. The treatment
was tumultuous, but Ginger went on to complete medical school and res-
idency at her customary level of academic achievement. She is currently
an academic physician at a prestigious medical school.

CONCLUSION

The affect shame severs connections, which is analogous to the impact of
dissociation. The negative cognitions about one's self that are associated
with shame have much in common with those encountered in trauma
victims and DID patients. It is often helpful to approach the alter system
and its rules of operation in terms of what shame scripts are in play and

what auxiliary affects are reinforcing the intransigency of those shame scripts. Skilled therapists have often accomplished this without knowing or relying on affect theory, especially when they reframe alters' apparent motivations and roles into terms that address their defensive and self-protective dimensions. Because shame scripts are also ego states and RIGS that can be inferred from the careful study of the clinical material, affect theory can enrich therapists' understanding of what they are working with and the insights of affect theory are very easily translated into the language of dissociative disorder therapy. For the neophyte, affect theory provides some of the same constructs that experienced hands have had to learn by trial and error in the school of hard knocks and at considerable emotional expense to themselves and their patients.

The treatment of DID is arduous and demanding for therapist and patient alike. Any advance in understanding that holds the potential to make that treatment less painful and more empathic deserves the most thoughtful consideration by those who endeavor to identify, understand, and treat dissociative disorders.

REFERENCES

Greenson RR: The Technique and Practice of Psychoanalysis. New York, International Universities Press, 1967

Kluft RP: High-functioning multiple personality patients: three cases. J Nerv Ment Dis 174:722–726, 1986

Kluft RP: The phenomenology and treatment of extremely complex multiple personality disorder. Dissociation 1:47–58, 1988

Kluft RP: Multiple personality disorder, in The American Psychiatric Press Annual Review of Psychiatry, Vol 10. Edited by Tasman A, Goldfinger SM. Washington, DC, American Psychiatric Press, 1991, pp 161–168

Kluft RP: Psychodynamic psychotherapy of multiple personality disorder and allied forms of dissociative disorder not otherwise specified, in Dynamic Therapies for Psychiatric Disorders (Axis I). Edited by Barber JP, Crits-Cristoph P. New York, Basic Books, 1995, pp 332–385

Lansky M: Posttraumatic Nightmares. Hillsdale, NJ, Analytic Press, 1995

Lansky M, Morrison A (eds): The Widening Scope of Shame. Hillsdale, NJ, Analytic Press, 1997

Nathanson DL (ed): The Many Faces of Shame. New York, Guilford, 1987

Nathanson DL: Shame and Pride: Affect, Sex, and the Birth of the Self. New York, WW Norton, 1992

Rauch SL, Shin LM, Pitman RK: Evaluating the effects of psychological trauma using neuroimaging techniques, in Psychological Trauma. Edited by Yehuda R. Washington, DC, American Psychiatric Press, 1998, pp 67–96

Stern DN: The Interpersonal World of the Infant: A View From Psychoanalysis and Developmental Psychology. New York, Basic Books, 1985

Stone AM: Trauma and affect: applying the language of affect theory to the phenomena of traumatic stress, in Knowing Feeling: Affect, Script, and Psychotherapy. Edited by Nathanson DL. New York, WW Norton, 1996, pp 288–302

Tomkins SS: Affect/Imagery/Consciousness, Vol 1: The Positive Affects. New York, Springer, 1962

Tomkins SS: Affect/Imagery/Consciousness, Vol 2: The Negative Affects. New York, Springer, 1963

Tomkins SS: Affect/Imagery/Consciousness, Vol 3: The Negative Affects: Anger and Fear. New York, Springer, 1991

Watkins HH, Watkins JG: Ego state therapy in the treatment of dissociative disorders, in Clinical Perspectives on Multiple Personality Disorder. Edited by Kluft RP, Fine CC. Washington, DC, American Psychiatric Press, 1993, pp 277–299

C H A P T E R   1 6

TRAUMA, DISSOCIATION, AND IMPULSE DYSCONTROL

Lessons From the Eating Disorders Field

JOHAN VANDERLINDEN, PH.D.
WALTER VANDEREYCKEN, M.D., PH.D.
LAURENCE CLAES, PH.D.

The field of eating disorders (EDs) has been strongly influenced by the assumption that a history of physical and/or sexual abuse might play a crucial etiological role in the development of anorexia and bulimia nervosa. The fact that the vast majority of ED patients are female probably reinforced this idea, on account of the higher rates of sexual abuse in girls. The association between child abuse and EDs was also central to feminist thinking, which had a great influence on the sociocultural reconceptualization of EDs in the last decades of the twentieth century. In the same period, interest was growing in the dissociative experiences reported by ED patients, who were saying things like, "When bingeing, I am not myself anymore"; "It is as if someone else has taken over"; and "In my head there's something switching off or on, and then I seem to become someone else" (Pettinati et al. 1985). As a consequence, many publications appeared on the significance of dissociation and childhood trauma in EDs. Soon the field became divided between believers and nonbelievers in the link between child abuse, dissociation, and EDs (Vanderlinden and Vandereycken 1997). This was fueled by the fact that one of the infamous cases of recovered memory concerned a woman with an ED history (Pope and Hudson 1996).

Controversial issues may obscure critical thinking, but they can also stimulate creative research. Since the beginning of this century clinicians and researchers have abandoned narrow causal thinking and broadened their interest in moderating and mediating factors in the association between traumatic experiences, dissociative features, and EDs. In contrast with other fields, ED specialists have only rarely focused exclusively on the presence and treatment of dissociative symptoms in EDs. Hence dissociation has always been studied in relationship with other topics, such as the presence of trauma, impulse dyscontrol, and other comorbid behaviors. Following a short overview of the most important clinical and nonclinical findings in this area, we propose some general guidelines for the psychotherapeutic management of ED patients with a history of trauma, dissociative symptoms, or impulse dyscontrol problems. The clinical case of Laura is used to provide an example of the history of childhood abuse and the manifestation of dissociation sometimes present in EDs.

Case Example: Laura

Laura, a 28-year-old married woman, was referred for treatment of bulimia nervosa (purging type) following an increase in physical complaints such as headaches, sleep disturbances, and gastrointestinal problems. When asked about her eating pattern, Laura explained that she avoided eating during the day but totally lost control over her eating behavior in the evening. In her experience it was as though somebody else took control and forced her to eat huge portions of food and then purge it. "Some strange inner power is forcing me to binge and purge every evening. It frightens me a lot, because I really do not want to binge at all, but I just can't stop it." Dissociative experiences, suggestive in her description of bingeing, were confirmed by her high level of dissociation on the Dissociation Questionnaire (Vanderlinden et al. 1993a). Laura avoided her parents, especially her father whom she feared, and gradually during psychotherapy her familial history of physical violence and severe emotional abuse (especially humiliation) was revealed. Much later she also disclosed a history of sexual abuse by her father and grandfather.

RESEARCH

Studies in Clinical Samples

Prevalence of Abuse and Type of Eating Disorder

A growing number of studies have focused on the prevalence of sexual abuse and other traumatic experiences in ED patients. The figures range from 25% to 50%. In a meta-analysis of 53 studies, Smolak and Murnen (2002) found a small, significant positive relationship between reports of childhood sexual abuse (CSA) and ED. The authors emphasized the need to study what aspects of eating pathology are most influenced by CSA. Waller (1991) found in a sample of 100 ED women that the reporting of abuse (in 50% of the sample) was clearly associated with a diagnostic subcategory; women with bulimic disorders reported significantly higher rates of unwanted sexual experiences than restricting anorexic women. Another study of 100 women with anorexia nervosa (Waller 1993b) revealed a strong association between unwanted sexual experiences (in 37% of the total sample) and purging behavior (vomiting and abuse of laxatives). Overall, these studies support a strong association between CSA and a specific type of ED characterized by bingeing and purging behaviors.

Comparison of Abuse in Eating Disorders and Other Samples

Welch and Fairburn (1994) investigated four individually matched groups: 50 community cases of bulimia nervosa, 50 community control subjects without an ED, 50 community control subjects with other psychiatric disorders (mostly depression), and 50 inpatients with bulimia nervosa. Assessment of sexual abuse histories before the onset of an ED was established by means of an interview in the subjects' own homes. Significantly more community patients with bulimia nervosa reported a history of sexual abuse before the onset of the ED (26%) compared with community control subjects (10%). However, there was no difference between the rates of sexual abuse in the community cases of bulimia nervosa and the psychiatric control subjects (24%). A surprising result was the smaller number of inpatient patients with bulimia nervosa who had sexual abuse histories (16%). Welch and Fairburn concluded that an abuse history does increase the risk of developing a psychiatric disorder but that this higher risk is not specific to bulimia nervosa.

Whereas many studies have focused on the incidence of sexual abuse, some researchers have highlighted the importance of examining the full range of possible abusive experiences (Schmidt et al. 1993). For example, Rorty et al. (1994) compared 80 women with a lifetime history of bulimia nervosa and 40 women who had never had an ED or related difficulties. The bulimic women reported higher levels of childhood physical abuse, psychological abuse, and multiple abuse. In a case-control design study of anorexia nervosa patients and discordant twin sisters (Karwautz et al. 2000), the anorexic subjects differed from their healthy sisters in terms of personal vulnerability traits and exposure to high parental expectations and sexual abuse. Clearly these studies show no direct or specific link between traumatic experiences and the development of ED. However, they do seem to point to an increased risk or vulnerability for developing an ED following childhood interpersonal trauma. Whether and why such an outcome is to be expected also depends on other risk and protective factors.

Abuse, Eating Disorders, and Dissociation

ED patients with a history of trauma report significantly higher levels of dissociation compared with nonabused subjects (Vanderlinden and Vandereycken 1997). In one early study (Vanderlinden et al. 1993b), approximately 13% of the ED sample (*n*=98; mostly bingeing and purging patients) reported severe dissociative symptoms such as identity confusion and fragmentation, loss of control, and amnesia. Most of these patients received a diagnosis of dissociative disorder not otherwise specified; a diagnosis of dissociative identity disorder was very rare in this group. Dissociative symptoms appear more prevalent in those ED patients with bingeing and purging behaviors (Dalle Grave et al. 1997). However, Hartt and Waller (2002) found that only neglect and sexual abuse were correlated with dissociation in a group of bulimic patients. In another study, Waller et al. (2003) reported robust associations between the presence of somatoform dissociative symptoms and the specific bulimic behaviors of laxative abuse, diet pill abuse, diuretic abuse, and excessive exercise, as well as bulimic attitudes. The authors stressed the need for assessment of both psychological and somatoform dissociative symptoms in ED patients with bulimic features.

Abuse, Eating Disorders, and Comorbidity

If ED patients—especially those with bingeing and purging behaviors— report a history of abuse, they are at a higher risk of developing substance abuse (Deep et al. 1999; Wonderlich et al. 2001), self-injurious behavior (SIB; Favaro and Santonastaso 1998), dissociative symptoms, body dissatisfaction, depression, and low self-esteem (Grilo and Masheb 2001). In a more recent series of studies, self-injuring ED patients showed more clinical symptoms (anxiety, depression, suicidal ideation, and hostility) than ED patients without SIB (Claes et al. 2001, 2003). Furthermore, within the SIB group, the highest scores on clinical symptoms were found in those patients who showed more than one type of SIB. In addition the more SIBs, the greater the likelihood of self-reported traumatic experiences in the past, especially sexual abuse. Patients with SIB, especially those who did not feel any pain during the behavior, showed a greater tendency toward dissociative experiences. Perhaps the link with comorbidity explains the poorer prognosis in ED patients with a history of abuse (Anderson et al. 1997; Cachelin et al. 1999; Matsunaga et al. 1999).

Mediating Factors Between Abuse and Development of an Eating Disorder

Despite the extensive research on the adverse effects of reported sexual abuse, the process linking abuse and ED remains unclear. As suggested in other populations, a link has been found between the age at onset of abuse and development of ED: abusive experiences at a younger age seem to be associated with more severe problems (Waller 1993a, 1993b). This also applies to specific characteristics of the abuse; symptoms such as bingeing and vomiting are more marked when the abuse was intrafamilial and involved force (Waller 1993a, 1993b). The extent of psychopathology, particularly the frequency of vomiting and the presence of borderline personality disorder symptoms, may be associated with the nature of the perceived response to an attempted disclosure (Waller and Ruddock 1993): a perceived lack of response or a negative, hostile response is associated with greater levels of both borderline personality disorder and bulimia nervosa symptoms (particularly vomiting).

Another line of research focuses on the influence of a negative self-image, based on self-blame in combination with poor self-esteem, often present in trauma victims (Waller et al. 2001). More specifically, in ED it is assumed that self-esteem is strongly related to the way patients perceive their own body. In fact, negative perceptions and cognitions of one's own body were the best predictors of the presence of dissociative symptoms at follow-up after ED treatment (Vanderlinden et al. 1995). The negative body experiences seem to be strongly related to the severity of abuse history (especially sexual abuse), and it is assumed that these negative body experiences mediate between the trauma experience and the development of the ED and dissociative symptoms. This also implies that in traumatized ED patients, the disturbed body experience is probably not only related to a wish to be thin but also to a wish to make the body unattractive or to punish the body because of feelings of guilt. If this is indeed the case, the treatment should focus on this aspect. Another mediating factor between a trauma experience and the development of an ED may be the family environment. A retrospective study by Schmidt et al. (1993) suggested that negative life events, together with negative family experiences, may affect the course of an ED: bulimic patients reported more childhood adversity in their family environment than restricting anorexia nervosa patients. Hastings and Kern (1994) reported significant connections between bulimia, sexual abuse, and a chaotic family environment. According to Kinzl et al. (1994), the quality and amount of family support given to the child were more important in the link between abuse and ED than the abuse experience per se.

Studies in Nonclinical Samples

The previous studies have the major limitation of focusing on selected samples in clinical populations, except that of Welch and Fairburn (1994), who also used comparisons with a community sample. The selection bias due to the presence of psychopathology can be avoided by studying nonclinical populations, which can be very meaningful in putting the clinical studies into a broader perspective. For example, Kent et al. (1999) studied the full range of abusive experiences in a nonclinical sample and found that emotional abuse was the only form of childhood trauma that predicted unhealthy eating attitudes. Other studies in various population samples (urban, rural, and statewide) have shown that sexual victimization places girls at risk for various unhealthy eating behaviors, such as purging and dietary restriction, along with body dissatisfaction (Thompson et al. 2001; Wonderlich et al. 2001). Baldo et al. (1996) reported that female university students with histories of intrafamilial sexual assaults were more likely to have an ED than women with no history of CSA and women with experiences of extrafamilial assaults. In a large community sample, purging bulimic subjects were distinguishable from nonpurging subjects on the basis of several factors, including a history of sexual abuse (Garfinkel et al. 1996). A younger age of sexual abuse experience appears to be linked to a higher likelihood of developing an ED (Kenardy and Ball 1998). Moreover, the association between CSA and a chaotic family environment increases in an additive manner the probability of developing an ED, particularly bulimia (Hastings and Kern 1994). According to the findings of Perkins and Luster (1999), sexual abuse may be related to purging behavior, but the latter is more strongly influenced by physical abuse as well as familial (e.g., family support and communication) and extrafamilial factors (e.g., social support). Strong familial relationships may decrease the risk of developing ED behavior in young women reporting abuse experiences (Neumark-Sztainer et al. 2000). Finally, Ackard et al. (2001) underscored the importance of disclosure of the abuse experience: adolescents who did not discuss the abuse were more likely to develop bingeing and purging behaviors than those who did disclose their traumatic experience.

Summary of Research Findings

In general, abusive experiences increase the vulnerability in young women to develop an ED, in particular one with bingeing and purging characteristics. In addition, a history of trauma is associated with a greater likelihood of comorbidity, such as depression (including low self-esteem and negative self-talk), dissociative symptoms, and a series of other problems in which both impulsivity and dissociation seem to play a common role (e.g., substance abuse, suicidality, SIB, borderline personality disorder). This higher prevalence of comorbidity, and especially the presence of dissociative symptoms, probably explains the poorer outcome in ED patients with a history of abuse. The mediating factors in this developmental process are complex. The impact of a traumatic experience depends on several factors, including 1) the functioning of the subject prior to the trauma (e.g., age and vulnerability at the time of the abuse); 2) the nature, severity, and extent of traumatization (e.g., sexual abuse vs. physical abuse alone or a combination of both); 3) the initial coping response to the trauma (e.g., disclosure or nondisclosure); and 4) the general family environment and educational atmosphere. The research data especially underline the importance of the family context as a basic factor in increasing the vulnerability or enhancing the protective resources of the victim.

CLINICAL GUIDELINES

Clearly, the relationship between traumatic experiences and the development of an ED with dissociative symptoms is complex. Even without abusive experiences someone might develop anorexia nervosa or bulimia nervosa. In others a trauma history may be linked with totally different disorders. From a clinical viewpoint, we consider it more fruitful to try to understand the interplay between trauma, dissociative symptoms, and ED in a more functional—rather than causal—way (Vanderlinden and Vandereycken 1997). Perhaps the abusive experience has reshaped an already developing or existing ED into a more self-destructive way of life, or perhaps the victim "learned" to dissociate and to use bingeing and purging as an escape or avoidance strategy for feelings, memories, sensations, and cognitions linked to the trauma. The trauma history may have undermined the victim's self-esteem to such an extent that the ED is one way of expressing a basic dissatisfaction with oneself and one's body in particular. Alternatively, the opposite mechanism may be involved; the

ED patient over time developed such a negative self-image that past experiences are filtered through a negative self-perception. These are the types of hypotheses that guide our psychotherapeutic work, the basic principles of which are discussed in the following section.

Basic Principles

The fundamental goal of our clinical work in traumatized ED patients with dissociative symptoms can be summarized as "back to reality." Our approach can be best described as eclectic, integrating principles from cognitive-behavioral therapy and strategic systems therapy. First, we want to help patients cope with the reality of their present lives, and this means developing alternatives to dissociation. For many, coping with a present life implies ultimately turning their back on the past and heading toward the future. Yet it also means that therapists have to face the emotional reality of traumatic life histories.

Closely linked to this endeavor is the issue of control that lies at the heart of the ED, whether it is the almost-obsessional need for self-mastery in anorexic patients or the terrible sense of loss of control in bulimic patients. From this core perspective we are inclined to consider a great deal of comorbidity, such as dissociative symptoms in (traumatized) ED patients as an expression of disturbed or dysfunctional self-control. This is quite obvious for symptoms of impulse dyscontrol such as self-injury and substance abuse, but it also applies to dissociative phenomena that reflect a state of being (temporarily) "out of control." Impulsiveness should not only be considered a key feature in ED with a bulimic component. It also seems closely related to the lack of stability in borderline cases and to the maladaptive behavioral repertoire of victims of childhood trauma.

Whatever its theoretical interpretation, from learned helplessness to neurobiological dysfunction, a pragmatic approach to treatment goals for these patients is required that enhances self-control within a well-structured daily life. We continuously give the message that, from the moment the therapy starts, patients must accept responsibility for their behaviors, including dissociation. We stress that, notwithstanding their bad experiences in the past, they can now take control of their lives and make their own positive choices.

Screening of traumatic experiences has become a highly controversial issue. In our view, the first task of a clinician or therapist is accepting the patient's subjective experience and narrative truth within a relationship of growing mutual trust. Testing the factual truth is not the primary function (Vanderlinden and Vandereycken 1997). In some instances, however, we are forced to consider the implications of information revealed to us, especially when there is good reason to believe the patient or another person is still the victim of serious violations of their personal rights and integrity. Then the first step is to ensure protection of the (potential) victim against repetition of abuse. The patient's safety is always a primary concern and is a basic condition for therapy itself. If actions outside the therapeutic context are necessary, we should remain in the therapeutic role and leave it up to an otherwise uninvolved colleague who 1) evaluates the information on its factual reliability, 2) involves other parties when and where needed without violating the rights of the patient or significant others, and 3) discusses these actions and all their implications with the patient (informed consent).

Treating the Eating Disorder

Based on clinical experience with both in- and outpatient treatment of ED patients, we consider the following rules essential in creating the necessary conditions for therapeutic change in those ED patients with a history of trauma (Vanderlinden et al. 1992).

1. Therapy should be based on a biopsychological assessment. This multidimensional assessment includes an examination of the physical condition of the patient, a functional analysis of the disturbed eating pattern, and an assessment of the psychosocial functioning of the patient.
2. Therapy should interrupt the perpetuating influences and focus first on the factors that appear to perpetuate the disorder.
3. Therapy should give maximum responsibility to the patient. We elaborate this principle in a treatment contract in which patients are asked to make their own treatment plan.
4. Therapy should improve self-esteem and body experience. This treatment goal is of crucial importance in the case of ED patients with trauma and dissociation.
5. Therapy should include the family context. Often, distorted family interactions are part of the perpetuating influences of an ED. Therefore, as early as possible in the beginning of treatment, we try to establish a collaborative alliance with the patient's parents (or partner). The patient may decide him- or herself whether to attend the family sessions. In the case of ongoing abuse, the parents will be invited by another team member but without the presence of the patient. To guarantee as much security as possible, the patient's therapist will have no contact at all with the abusive family members.

6. Therapy should be well structured but transparent. This is done in a very concrete and clear way (transparency with written agreements) to avoid debate about when certain rules must be applied.
7. Therapy should be time limited, with regular evaluations. Therapeutic goals should be shaped accordingly, which includes the evaluation of whether it is worthwhile to continue (this form of) treatment.

Guidelines for Patients With a History of Dissociation

Compared with nontraumatized, nondissociative ED patients, ED patients with a history of trauma and dissociative symptoms present the therapist with a more complicated task. He or she will be forced not only to focus on the typical eating symptoms such as bingeing and purging behaviors but also often on a wide variety of impulse dyscontrol behaviors. Hence this group of patients requires additional therapeutic measures. Many have to find a way to regain control over the dissociative episodes frequently linked to impulsive and self-destructive behaviors. They often believe themselves to be out of control. Therefore, a basic treatment goal is to reach sufficient "internal control" over what they do, think, and feel (Vanderlinden and Vandereycken 1997). To reach this inner control, our approach has been largely influenced by Linehan's (1993) dialectical behavior therapy focusing on the emotional dysregulation of patients with borderline personality disorder. Basic strategies include the self-monitoring of situations that may trigger dissociative reactions and learning alternative and more efficient coping behaviors when confronted with these triggers.

Coping With Dissociative Experiences

Our principle of back to reality is inseparably connected to the basic idea of self-responsibility. In patients with dissociative reactions, a basic element of their back-to-reality script is learning strategies to reorient themselves in the here-and-now situation. While in a dissociative state, patients find it difficult to realize where they are, what time it is, what they are actually doing, and so on. Moreover, they may be overwhelmed with all kinds of negative emotions and thoughts they cannot understand or explain. The ability to realistically evaluate the actual situation is often also decreased at moments of impulse dyscontrol, including binges. Nevertheless, patients can learn to acquire a better sense of self-mastery, first of all through self-observation by means of a self-monitoring form. Throughout treatment, patients continue this self-observation by writing down thoughts, images, feelings, and circumstances that (might) lead to a loss of control over their behavior. This self-monitoring includes all kinds of possible "triggers" connected to dissociative reactions and impulse dyscontrol, such as 1) situations (cues) that refer directly or indirectly to the trauma, 2) certain emotional states, 3) certain physiological states and bodily sensations, 4) certain foods that may be closely associated with the original trauma situation, and 5) revictimization experiences. This way the therapist may discover, for example, that the traumatized ED patient's avoidance of certain foods (e.g., not wanting to eat sweets) has a different meaning compared with ED patients without a trauma history.

Once the patient has identified the most important triggers, alternative and more efficient coping behaviors must be tested and learned. Both behavioral (e.g., jogging, writing, singing, asking for help) and emotional strategies (e.g., self-hypnosis relaxation, listening to music, taking a bath, touching a safe object) can be practiced. However, after their long-lasting experience of being out of control, patients often find it hard to believe that they can learn to take better control over themselves. They have to be convinced, first, that triggers do not provoke immediate and sudden uncontrollable changes in their behavior, thoughts, and feelings; in short, it is not just a matter of on/off switching. In many cases careful self-monitoring reveals that the experienced loss of control was preceded by a predictable chain of events in an important number of situations or conditions. Once these triggers have been identified, patients have to take responsibility over their actions in these situations: Where and how can I stop this chain? Dealing with dissociation can be broken down into the following principles:

- *Self-monitoring:* Patients keep a diary of environmental and psychological cues that trigger dissociative episodes.
- *Stimulus control:* Strategies are developed to stop the chain of reaction from trigger to dissociation.
- *Response prevention:* If patients are faced with triggers, the alternatives to dissociation can be utilized. Such alternatives may include physical exercises (such as running, cycling, fitness training) designed to reduce tension. The guiding principles in the selection of these exercises are that they should 1) be easily available, 2) be harmless (for both the patient and other people), and 3) quickly "discharge" emotional energy by reducing rather than increasing the likelihood of dissociation.

Case Example: Laura's Control Over Dissociation

Laura's diary shows that she was at risking of losing control when

- She was confronted with her body
- Her body was touched
- She received specific messages from her father
- She had to eat specific food, such as bread and pudding
- It got dark
- She heard people screaming

A list of alternative behavioral, emotional, and cognitive strategies to be executed when she was at risk of losing control, was developed with Laura. She chose the following strategy: "When I am confronted with difficult situations and fear dissociating and losing control, I will stay in the living room with the other patients and start painting while listening to some relaxing music. Other alternatives may be to listen to my self-hypnosis audiotape in order to imagine a safe and secure situation or firmly touch my little bear who symbolizes 'safety and security,' while I remain in the presence of others."

CONCLUSION

The research data suggest a close association between dissociative symptoms and negative body experiences that trigger these symptoms in ED. Perhaps body dissatisfaction may function as a specific mediating factor between the traumatic experience and the development of an ED. Overall, research findings as well as our clinical experience underline the importance of a therapeutic approach focusing on positively changing or influencing the way patients experience and evaluate their bodies, thus reducing triggers of dissociation. However, it still remains a great challenge to help ED patients with a history of trauma to positively change their body experience. A person's body image often reflects in a concrete way that person's self-image, especially in Western societies where bodily appearance is assumed to "mirror" a person's inner and social life as well as their past history and present circumstances. Further research is needed to support our clinical conviction that a therapeutic approach aimed at positively changing the body experience of a (traumatized) ED patient with dissociative symptoms is the cornerstone for long-lasting change. Meanwhile, the therapeutic work with ED patients who dissociate remains a great challenge for every therapeutic approach.

REFERENCES

Ackard DM, Neumark-Sztainer D, Hannan PJ, et al: Binge and purge behavior among adolescents: associations with sexual and physical abuse in a nationally representative sample: the Commonwealth Fund survey. Child Abuse Negl 25:771–785, 2001

Anderson KP, LaPorte DJ, Brandt H, et al: Sexual abuse and bulimia: response to inpatient treatment and preliminary outcome. J Psychiatr Res 31:621–633, 1997

Baldo TD, Wallace SD, O'Halloran MS: Effects of intrafamilial sexual assault on eating behaviors. Psychol Rep 79:531–536, 1996

Cachelin FM, Striegel-Moore RH, Elder KA, et al: Natural course of a community sample of women with binge eating disorder. Int J Eat Disord 25:45–54, 1999

Claes L, Vandereycken W, Vertommen H: Self-injurious behaviors in eating-disordered patients. Eat Behav 2:263–272, 2001

Claes L, Vandereycken W, Vertommen H: Eating disordered patients with and without self-injurious behaviors: a comparison of psychopathological features. European Eating Disorders Review 11:379–396, 2003

Dalle Grave R, Oliosi M, Todisco P, et al: Self-reported traumatic experiences and dissociative symptoms with and without binge-eating disorder. Eat Disord 5:105–109, 1997

Deep AL, Lilenfeld LR, Plotnicov KH, et al: Sexual abuse in eating disorder subtypes and control women: the role of comorbid substance dependence in bulimia nervosa. Int J Eat Disord 25:1–10, 1999

Favaro A, Santonastaso P: Impulsive and compulsive self-injurious behavior in bulimia nervosa: prevalence and psychological correlates. J Nerv Ment Dis 6:157–65, 1998

Garfinkel PE, Lin E, Goering P, et al: Purging and nonpurging forms of bulimia nervosa in a community sample. Int J Eat Disord 20:231–238, 1996

Grilo CM, Masheb RM: Childhood psychological, physical, and sexual maltreatment in outpatients with binge eating disorder: frequency and associations with gender, obesity, and eating-related psychopathology. Obes Res 9:320–325, 2001

Hartt J, Waller G: Child abuse, dissociation and core beliefs in bulimic disorders. Child Abuse Negl 26:923–938, 2002

Hastings T, Kern JM: Relationship between bulimia, childhood sexual abuse, and family environment. Int J Eat Disord 15:103–111, 1994

Karwautz A, Rabe-Hesketh S, Hu X, et al: Individual-specific risk factors for anorexia nervosa: a pilot study using a discordant sister pair design. Psychol Med 31:317–329, 2000

Kenardy J, Ball K: Disordered eating, weight dissatisfaction and dieting in relation to unwanted childhood sexual experiences in a community sample. J Psychosom Res 44:327–337, 1998

Kent A, Waller G, Dagnan DA: A greater role of emotional than physical or sexual abuse in predicting disordered eating attitudes: the role of mediating variables. Int J Eat Disord 25:159–167, 1999

Kinzl JF, Traweger Ch, Guenther V, et al: Family background and sexual abuse associated with eating disorders. Am J Psychiatry 151:1127–1131, 1994

Linehan MM: Cognitive-Behavioral Treatment of Borderline Personality Disorder. New York, Guilford, 1993

Matsunaga H, Kaye W, McConaha C, et al: Psychopathological characteristics of recovered bulimics who have a history of physical or sexual abuse. J Nerv Ment Dis 187:472–477, 1999

Neumark-Sztainer D, Story M, Hannan PJ, et al: Disordered eating among adolescents: associations with sexual/physical abuse and other familial/psychosocial factors. Int J Eat Disord 28:249–258, 2000

Perkins DF, Luster T: The relationship between sexual abuse and purging: findings from community-wide surveys of female adolescents. Child Abus Negl 23:371–382, 1999

Pettinati HM, Horne RL, Slaats JM: Hypnotizability in patients with anorexia nervosa and bulimia. Arch Gen Psychiatry 42:1014–1016, 1985

Pope HG, Hudson JI: "Recovered memory" therapy for eating disorders: implications of the Ramona verdict. Int J Eat Disord 19:139–146, 1996

Rorty M, Yager J, Rossotto E: Childhood sexual, physical, and psychological abuse in bulimia nervosa. Am J Psychiatry 151:1122–1126, 1994

Schmidt U, Tiller J, Treasure J: Setting the scene for eating disorders: childhood care, classification and course of illness. Psychol Med 23:663–672, 1993

Smolak L, Murnen SK: A meta-analytic examination of the relationship between child sexual abuse and eating disorders. Int J Eat Disord 31:136–150, 2002

Thompson KM, Wonderlich SA, Crosby RD, et al: Sexual victimization and adolescent weight regulation practices: a test across three community based samples. Child Abuse Negl 25:291–305, 2001

Vanderlinden J, Vandereycken W: Trauma, Dissociation, and Impulse Dyscontrol in Eating Disorders. New York, Taylor & Francis, 1997

Vanderlinden J, Norré J, Vandereycken W: A Practical Guide to the Treatment of Bulimia Nervosa. New York, Brunner Mazel, 1992

Vanderlinden J, Van Dyck R, Vandereycken W, et al: The Dissociation Questionnaire: development and characteristics of a new self-reporting questionnaire. Clin Psychol Psychother 1:21–27, 1993a

Vanderlinden J, Vandereycken W, Van Dyck R, et al: Dissociative experiences and trauma in eating disorders. Int J Eat Disord 13:187–194, 1993b

Vanderlinden J, Vandereycken W, Probst M: Dissociative symptoms in eating disorders: a follow-up study. European Eating Disorders Review 3:174–184, 1995

Waller G: Sexual abuse as a factor in eating disorders. Br J Psychiatry 159:664–671, 1991

Waller G: Sexual abuse and eating disorders: borderline personality disorder as a mediating factor? Br J Psychiatry 162:771–775, 1993a

Waller G: Sexual abuse as a factor in anorexia nervosa: evidence from two separate case series. J Psychosom Res 37:1–7, 1993b

Waller G, Ruddock A: Experiences of disclosure of childhood sexual abuse and psychopathology. Child Abuse Rev 2:185–195, 1993

Waller G, Meyer C, Ohanian V, et al: The psychopathology of bulimic women who report childhood sexual abuse: the mediating role of core beliefs. J Nerv Ment Dis 10:700–708, 2001

Waller G, Babbs M, Wright F, et al: Somatoform dissociation in eating-disordered patients. Behav Res Ther 41:619–627, 2003

Welch SL, Fairburn CG: Sexual abuse and bulimia nervosa: three integrated case control comparisons. Am J Psychiatry 151:402–407, 1994

Wonderlich S, Crosby R, Mitchell J, et al: Pathways mediating sexual abuse and eating disturbance in children. Int Eat Disord 29:270–279, 2001

C H A P T E R   1 7

TREATMENT OF TRAUMATIC DISSOCIATION

JAMES A. CHU, M.D.

Traumatic dissociation is an essential feature of many of the dissociative disorders (including dissociative amnesia, dissociative fugue, and dissociative identity disorder [DID]) and posttraumatic stress disorder (PTSD). In discussing the treatment of traumatic dissociation, this chapter addresses the principles and modalities used in clinical work with PTSD and trauma-related dissociative disorders. Although the basic fundamentals of treatment apply across these diagnostic categories, there are significant differences in practice depending on the severity and chronicity of the clinical syndromes. In addition, there are specific techniques that must be incorporated when working with dissociative disorders for which there are elaborations of different identity states.

Patients with PTSD often have traumatic experiences that are *dissociative*—that is, the memories are fragmented and poorly integrated into patients' overall mental schemas. In their review, van der Kolk et al. (2001) concluded, "[f]or over 100 years clinicians have observed and described the unusual nature of traumatic memories. It has been repeatedly and consistently observed that these memories are characterized by fragmentary and intense sensations and affects, often with little or no verbal narrative content" (p. 9). Confronting and integrating traumatic experiences are core elements of trauma treatment. It is generally accepted among experienced clinicians that this work with traumatic experiences diminishes acute posttraumatic and dissociative symptoms and allows patients to develop new perspectives about themselves and the world. Working through traumatic memories involves tolerating the associated overwhelming affect and bodily sensations, finding words to describe them, and integrating them into the context of normal experiences and existing mental schemas. The process of confronting and working through traumatic memories has been termed *abreaction* and *working through* by psychodynamic clinicians and *desensitization, exposure,* and *deconditioning* by cognitive-behavioral practitioners. However, regardless of the terms and theoretical orientation used, the essential principles remain the same.

In general clinical practice, most individuals with PTSD are treated with an eclectic mix of approaches, often including psychodynamic and interpersonal therapy perspectives along with cognitive-behavioral therapy (CBT) and sometimes hypnosis or guided imagery. All of these approaches may provide important elements to the overall treatment. A psychodynamic formulation helps patients with PTSD understand the impact of the trauma on their current lives as well as the contributions of pretrauma experiences. (However, it is not useful to utilize classic psychodynamic assumptions that trauma creates conflict because of fulfillment of unconscious fears and wishes rather than acknowledging helplessness in the face of trauma.) Interpersonal support and interaction are essential in helping patients tolerate memories of overwhelming events so that they feel their experiences have been witnessed and shared rather than judged. Interpersonal interactions also provide outside perspectives with which to reframe and change the way the experiences are understood. CBT approaches may be used for controlling symptoms; learning skills for coping with anxiety, such as guided visualization, breathing retraining, or biofeedback; managing negative thoughts through cognitive restructuring techniques; learning anger management; and using social skills training to enhance patients' ability to communicate effectively and to engage in supportive relationships. Closely related to guided imagery, hypnotherapy can be used to help control anxiety, access memories and emotions, and fractionate exposure to traumatic material.

Although few clinicians practice using a single approach, some specialized treatments have been developed that demonstrate efficacy for certain populations of PTSD patients. Three approaches—exposure therapy, stress inoculation training (SIT), and eye movement desensitization and reprocessing (EMDR)—have been deemed "probably effective" for PTSD by the American Psychological Association's Division 12 (Society of Clinical Psychology) (Chambless et al. 1998). Exposure therapy, a specific type of CBT, was initially shown to be effective with combat veterans (Foa and Kozak 1986; Foa et al. 1989; Keane et al. 1989) and subsequently with traumatized civilians, such as rape victims (Foa et al. 1993). Exposure therapy is used to detoxify and desensitize the traumatic experience, often using detailed mental imagery to help survivors confront the trauma in a controlled environment with high levels of social support.

SIT is a combination of CBT interventions used to teach a set of skills for managing anxiety and stress in order to "inoculate" people with PTSD from heightened stress responses (Meichenbaum 1996). SIT typically consists of education and training in coping skills, including emotional self-regulation, self-soothing and acceptance, deep muscle relaxation, breathing retraining, assertiveness training, role playing, cognitive restructuring, problem solving, and interpersonal communication skills training. SIT is instituted as a three-phase intervention in which clients learn about the nature and impact of stress, acquire and practice coping skills, and apply their newly learned coping skills to situations with increasingly higher levels of stress.

EMDR is a therapeutic technique developed by Francine Shapiro (2001). The essential part of the therapy involves alternating sensory stimulation of the right and left brain hemispheres (through eye movements, audio signals, or tapping on parts of the body) while mentally focusing on the traumatic experience. In theory, the treatment helps integrate and process verbal and nonverbal components of the trauma. The use and efficacy of EMDR remains controversial. Proponents claim widespread efficacy and point to controlled studies demonstrating its effectiveness. Detractors suggest that positive results may be due to placebo effects and the general positive but nonspecific effects of education and psychotherapy. Some authors and investigators have suggested that EMDR works primarily through relaxation and fractionated exposure and that the eye movements or alternating stimulation of different sides of the body is not necessary for symptom reduction (Perkins and Rouanzoin 2002).

TREATMENT OF COMPLEX POSTTRAUMATIC STRESS DISORDER

Judith Herman (1992a, 1992b) originally formulated the concept of complex PTSD to describe many features commonly seen in individuals subjected to severe and persistent traumatization. Persons with complex PTSD not only have classic posttraumatic symptoms but also have profound alterations in the way they view themselves and the world and in the way they function and interact with others. In Herman's conceptualization of complex PTSD, the individual is harmed by being held under the control of a perpetrator of abuse and unable to escape. Although such conditions can be found in situations such as prisons, chronic traumatization occurs much more frequently in ongoing domestic violence and most commonly in the form of severe and chronic childhood abuse.

Herman described changes in certain core domains in complex PTSD: alterations in emotional regulation, such as persistent sadness, suicidal thoughts, or explosive or inhibited anger; alterations in consciousness, such as forgetting or reliving traumatic events or having episodes in which one feels detached from one's mental processes or body; alterations in self-perceptions, such as helplessness, shame, guilt, stigma, and a sense of being completely different from others; alterations in perception of the perpetrator, such as attributing total power to the perpetrator or becoming preoccupied with the relationship to the perpetrator, including revenge fantasies; alterations in relations with others, such as isolation, distrust, or repeated searches for a rescuer; and alterations in one's system of meanings, such as a loss of sustaining faith or a sense of hopelessness and despair.

The deficits in ego functioning and relational capacity found in complex PTSD can grossly interfere with the ability of patients to do active work with traumatic memory. Such work can be complicated and stressful. It requires that patients be able to reexperience traumatic events with powerful associated affects—such as terror, fear, horror, rage, helplessness, despair, and shame—and to tolerate these feelings and remain functional. Patients must also have the ability to forge and sustain strong and trusting relationships with their therapists in order to feel heard, understood, and supported and to avail themselves of the perspectives of others. Their history of abuse profoundly affects transference feelings and expectations of therapists, whose examination of traumatic memories may be experienced as a deliberate reinflicting of harm. Finally, they must be able to remain grounded in their current reality rather than feeling consumed by the traumatic experience. In short, before attempting to process traumatic experiences, patients must have good ego functioning in terms of affect tolerance and impulse control. They must be able to maintain stable, supportive relationships, and they must have established both an ability to maintain their functioning and some positive sense of their lives and themselves.

STAGE-ORIENTED TREATMENT

Stage-oriented treatment consists of a hierarchy of treatment interventions designed to address specific symptomatology, beginning with an initial (often lengthy) period of developing fundamental skills prior to embarking on any significant exploration of childhood trauma. Stage-oriented or phase-oriented approaches were extensively developed in the 1990s and are now considered the standard of care in working with patients who have an extensive history of traumatization (Chu 1992b, 1998; Courtois 1999; Herman 1992b; van der Kolk et al. 1996a). The best outcomes for patients grappling with complex posttraumatic and dissociative symptoms occur with those who attempt to gain control of themselves and their lives and persist in efforts to attain some semblance of a "normal" life. The initial gains from these efforts often feel fragile and superficial. However, eventual gains in functioning may result in 1) a positive sense of self, 2) an ability to manage feelings and control impulses, 3) the capacity to interact with the external environment and develop a stable daily structure, and 4) the ability to cultivate and maintain a network of social supports. These gains are made slowly over time through the interventions (described in the following section) in the early or stabilization stage of treatment. They may be a part of a solid foundation that provides some grounding in current reality and permits eventual exploration of early abuse.

Virtually all stage-oriented treatment models include an initial stage of stabilization that is followed by active work with traumatic memories and ends with further personal growth and connection with the external world. The current description of a stage-oriented treatment model divides the treatment course into early, middle, and late stages (see Chu 1992b, 1998). The early stage consists of building the fundamentals of good ego functioning, including basic relational skills, coping strategies, and a positive self-identity. The middle stage involves the exploration, working through, and integration of traumatic experiences. The late stage consists of stabilization of gains and increased personal growth, particularly in relation to the external world.

Early-Stage Treatment

The mnemonic SAFER—Self-care and Symptom control, Acknowledgment, Functioning, Expression, and Relationships—outlines the major areas of focus of early-stage treatment (Chu 1992b, 1998).

Self-Care

Survivors of long-standing physical or sexual abuse have little inherent understanding of self-care. They often have a sense of detachment from their own bodies, perhaps related to chronic depersonalization experiences and a dissociated sense of self-identity. Furthermore, they have been exposed to a paradigm in which their bodies were exploited by others for tension relief. As adults, they may employ the same paradigm, using their bodies to relieve their own intolerable feelings and impulses. Many persons with complex PTSD engage in clandestine, nonlethal repetitive self-harming—usually in the form of cutting (Brodsky et al. 1995; Connors 1996; De Yong 1982; Himber 1994; Santa Mina and Gallop 1998; S. Shapiro 1987; Wise 1989). Dissociative anesthesia appears to mask the pain; the primary experience is of almost instant anxiety relief. Given the level of mistrust that derives from early abuse, persons with complex PTSD may habitually engage in self-harming behaviors as a means of relieving tension that is "safer" than asking for support from others. Alternatively, painful self-cutting may also be used to end dysphoric numbing or depersonalization and derealization.

Persons with complex PTSD often develop other self-destructive and dysfunctional behaviors. Substance abuse may serve as a way of numbing dysphoria related to traumatization and dissociation (Najavits et al. 1997; Stewart 1996; Triffleman 1998). Other dysfunctional behaviors are common in traumatized persons, including eating disorders (Hastings and Kern 1994; Miller and McCluskey-Fawcett 1993; Zlotnick et al. 1996; see Chapter 16 in this volume, "Trauma, Dissociation, and Impulse Dyscontrol," for review), somatization (North 2002; van der Kolk et al. 1996b), and risk-taking behaviors (N. L. Brown et al. 2003; Paul et al. 2001).

Major issues concerning personal safety must be addressed as a first-order priority in treatment. Traumatized persons need to learn that they can trust others to provide support rather than relying on self-harming behaviors that repeat the victimization and are associated with shame and isolation. However, abuse survivors are often ambivalent about abandoning self-destructive patterns of coping, reasoning that relying on others may lead them to feel extremely vulnerable. Functional ways of coping with stress are prerequisites to any exploration of traumatic experiences, because such work requires support from others.

Symptom Control

Although early-stage treatment does not emphasize exploration of traumatic events, patients with complex PTSD are likely to have trauma-related symptoms such as intrusive reexperiencing of traumatic memories and emotions, flashbacks, chronic anxiety, and high autonomic arousal. Rather than exploring the etiological events at this early stage, these symptoms need to be modulated and controlled in order to bring some stability into patients' lives. It is indeed possible for patients to achieve control of intrusive symptoms without having to explore the related traumatic experiences, but only if the patient is in alliance with efforts to reduce the rate and intensity of such symptoms.

Many of the techniques to control posttraumatic symptomatology fall into the category of "grounding techniques" that reinforce the current reality, enabling patients to avoid being drawn into consuming re-experiences of traumatic events. These techniques are most effective when patients are *beginning* to experience symptoms and not when they are completely overwhelmed. A well-lit environment can be very helpful for grounding; too often, traumatized individuals feel drawn to darkened bedrooms or even closets, which only increases the likelihood of losing grounding in current reality. Eye contact—particularly in therapy—is enormously effective and conveys two important therapeutic messages: 1) control of symptoms is possible and 2) other people can be helpful and safe. Looking around the room, naming objects, or looking at photographs or picture books may also be helpful. Using the sense of smell can help ground patients, and carrying a small container of a strong-smelling item such as potpourri, coffee beans, or orange peel may be very useful. Often touch can be a valuable grounding mechanism, using familiar and soothing objects or substances, such as ice, that induce a strong sensation. Finally, using hearing can be helpful, with music, singing, or even listening to the therapist's voice-mail messages. Patients are often the most successful in devising ingenious grounding techniques that are particularly effective for their personal needs.

Patients with complex PTSD should formulate a crisis plan to be implemented when they *begin* to feel overwhelmed. The crisis plan should consist of a list of grounding techniques, cognitive strategies, and activities that have proven to be effective in controlling symptoms. Calling one's therapist or going to an emergency department should be at the end of the list—not only to spare the clinician but also to reinforce that patients themselves can achieve control over their symptoms.

Acknowledgment

Although intensive exploration of past traumatic experiences is not appropriate in the early stage of treatment, it is important to acknowledge the central role of the early trauma in patients' lives. Victims of childhood abuse tend to believe that they were somehow to blame for their abuse. These beliefs seem to derive from the child's need to find personal meaning in their abusive experience and to have some sense of control over them—in effect, the abuse must be happening because they were "bad" and would stop if only they could learn to be "good." It results from a child's inability to comprehend independent causation (pre-formal operations in Piaget's sense). Therapists should simply reiterate how patients have used normal adaptive responses to cope with extraordinarily overwhelming events, thus beginning the process of helping survivors to understand many of their current difficulties. This means facing their essential helplessness and working against their tendency to assume control by identifying with the aggressor.

Patients have strong ambivalence about acknowledging the role of past trauma. Often they will continue to believe in their own defectiveness as their only ongoing sense of self and as a way of avoiding feeling helpless. Denial concerning the meaning and impact of the abuse may also serve a need to maintain a bond with idealized caretakers who in reality were abusive. It may be well into the therapy before patients are able to let go of an entrenched sense of defectiveness and to establish some positive sense of self.

Functioning

The reexperiencing of traumatic memories can intrude into every aspect of patients' lives, interfering with vocational and social functioning and even personal care and daily activities. These traumatic memories often are experienced as all-consuming, and feelings of victimization, hopelessness, powerlessness, and isolation become superimposed on current realities. If patients are poorly prepared to tolerate such memories and lack the basic skills to manage their symptoms and accept support, they may rapidly decompensate and regress, often becoming unable to function in virtually all aspects of their lives.

Therapists must educate patients about maintaining functioning as an antidote to regression. Maintaining regular employment, a volunteer job, educational programs, or recreational activities can provide a sense of mastery, positive self-identity, and grounding in current reality. Maintaining a social network and interacting with others also can dilute the dysphoric dependency on their therapists that patients often experience. If patients are unable to meet the challenges of regular work or educational activities, therapeutic programs such as groups, partial hospital programs, or Alcoholics Anonymous or Narcotics Anonymous–related activities can be important as areas of functioning.

Expression

Traumatic memories are often experienced as literally unspeakable. Even those patients who are otherwise highly articulate often have difficulty describing the feelings related to their maltreatment, instead experiencing them as dysphoric, wordless, and overwhelming sensations. This kind of experience is supported by research that suggests that traumatic experiences are linked to predominantly nonverbal right brain activity (Schiffer et al. 1995).

Over time, part of the therapeutic process is to help patients translate their "unspeakable" feelings into words, allowing them to communicate their experience to others and to use cognitive processes to gain a sense of control over them. However, in the early stages of treatment, verbalization of very intense feelings can only gradually be acquired. Nonetheless, patients must learn to express these feelings in nondestructive and therapeutic ways. Even when patients are encouraged to limit exploration of traumatic experiences in the early stage of treatment, they still often have some overwhelming negative affects such as intense depression and anxiety, hopelessness and despair, panic and terror, and rage and sadism. Therapy must help patients find healthy expressions, avoiding ingrained and destructive coping mechanisms.

Expressive therapy can permit and facilitate appropriate expression, first in nonverbal ways and ultimately in words. In the early stage of therapy, expressive therapy should be directed primarily at therapeutic expression (e.g., venting tension) rather than exploration of traumatic experiences. As such, it can be a powerful force in helping patients to find both relief from tension and words for their unspeakable feelings. Patients also can be trained to use relaxation techniques, guided imagery or autohypnosis, and regular physical exercise to combat both dysphoric feelings and the bodily overactivation that occurs in posttraumatic conditions.

Relationships

Many patients with complex PTSD are survivors of chronic childhood trauma, and they bring the abuse-related interpersonal assumptions of their childhood relationships into all their adult relationships, including the therapeutic one. Because relationships are seen only through the lenses of abuse and control, vulnerability, betrayal, and abandonment, patients tend to reenact relational dynamics in which they and others take abuse-related roles—most often victim or abuser, but sometimes rescuer or indifferent bystander (Davies and Frawley 1994). The recapitulation and reenactment of early abusive paradigms within the therapeutic relationship often seems to make collaborative work on resolving past traumatic experiences impossible. However, it is a core part of the treatment to help patients broaden their understanding and experience of how relationships can be maintained, using the relationship with the therapist as a model.

It is a critical part of the early stage of therapy for the patient and therapist to repeatedly renegotiate the therapeutic alliance. Because the patient is unconsciously compelled to precipitate abusive reenactments that disrupt the treatment relationship, the therapist must help the patient to develop a sense of collaboration and mutuality. This process of disconnection and reconnection must occur repeatedly, with endless variations, before even a minimal sense of basic trust is formed. This is the therapeutic dance (Chu 1998), a seemingly endless cycle of disconnection and reconnection—sometimes in the course of even a single therapy session, and certainly over the weeks, months, and sometimes years early in treatment.

In order to actually experience a sense of collaboration and mutuality, patients permit themselves to connect and trust others, a process that makes them feel enormously vulnerable. However, this process provides a new model of relating that is in sharp contrast to the abusive style of relatedness that the patient has experienced and expects. Establishing and providing this transforming interpersonal process is the corrective emotional experience, providing patients with mechanisms to obtain support, resolve conflict, and feel a powerful sense of connection with others.

Middle-Stage Treatment

Experts in the trauma field agree that effective abreaction (or exposure and restructuring in cognitive terms)—remembering, tolerating, reframing, and integrating overwhelming events—will allow individuals to gain a sense of control over the experiences, to understand their reactions to the experiences, and to build a better understanding of their own personal history and sense of self. When traumatized patients have mastered the tasks of early-stage therapy, they may then cautiously proceed to the explorative, abreactive, and restructuring work of the middle stage of treatment. However, it is important to understand that patients vary considerably in their ability to move beyond early-stage treatment, with stabilization, symptom management, and the other early-stage interventions remaining the long-term goals of treatment for some severely distressed individuals. (In addition to this overview, more in-depth discussions of working with traumatic memories can be found elsewhere [see D. Brown et al. 1997; Courtois 1988, 1999; Davies and Frawley 1994; Herman 1992b; van der Kolk et al. 1996a].)

Active work with traumatic memories should not involve crisis and almost always takes place in an outpatient setting. Achieving full understanding of the past and integrating traumatic experience is often very painful, but with the work of early-stage therapy, patients should tolerate the dysphoria and not act on dysfunctional impulses. Abreaction only very rarely takes the form of a single cataclysmic catharsis. Instead, although there may be breakthroughs of understanding and instances of intense emotional release, working through trauma is a progressive process that is accomplished over time. As early abreactive work is successfully completed, patients feel empowered by new understandings about their lives. They may feel progressively freed from internal conflict, intrusive memories, and self-hate. This new strength allows them to go on to work on the resolution of other conflictual areas or even to return to and rework areas already broached.

Patterns and timing of effective abreaction differ according to the individual characteristics of patients. However, some common phases often occur: 1) increased symptomatology, particularly more intrusive reexperiencing, resulting in 2) intense internal conflict, followed by 3) acceptance and mourning, which is transformed into 4) mobilization and empowerment.

An increase in the reexperiencing of traumatic events in the form of memories, thoughts, and emotions often occurs early in the abreactive process. The early-stage work helps patients to tolerate and control the intense memories and feelings associated with reexperiencing traumatic events. In addition, patients are better able to enlist and utilize support from others. Using these new skills, patients begin to endure and acknowledge the reality of past events and begin to attempt to reframe these experiences. Maintaining interpersonal connections is crucial in this process, enabling the patient to utilize the adult perspectives of others—perspectives that often cannot be gained by the patient alone. Patients come to view the events from a more adult vantage point rather than reexperiencing them from the perspective of a helpless abused child.

New perspectives about past abusive experiences produce intense internal conflict. For example, patients have difficulty letting go of deeply held feelings of self-blame at the same time that they understand that they were not responsible for their abuse. Patients may retain a sense of identification with the perpetrators of abuse and may still feel intensely protective of them while also feeling enraged at them. Patients should be helped to understand and have compassion for their adaptations to traumatic events. Somewhat paradoxically, accepting and integrating these "old" feelings and beliefs, as opposed to rejecting and disavowing them, leads to the resolution of these internal conflicts.

When survivors understand the full extent of their victimization and what it has meant in terms of their life course, patients begin to mourn what did and did not occur and the consequences of the abuse. This is often a slow and painful process as patients examine all the significant aspects of their lives and reframe how they understand them. This process of confronting past helplessness and disempowerment paradoxically leads to feeling a sense of current control and empowerment as they surrender the role of victim and replace it with a sense of self as a survivor of abuse.

Effective working through and integration of past traumatic experiences frees traumatized patients from the anxiety that they will be overwhelmed by dissociated memories. Perpetrators of abuse that seemed huge and malevolent become smaller and less powerful, and even horrific events become memories of the past rather than being relived in the present. Often, having understood and overcome painful past events, abuse survivors feel a new sense of control, including the sense that they can protect themselves from future victimization. Sometimes, having been able to acknowledge their own victimization and come to terms with human failings such as selfishness, aggression, and malevolence, abuse survivors grow in character in terms of self-understanding and true empathy toward others. Abreaction (i.e., exposure and restructuring) becomes the process through which survivors of trauma begin to build a credible personal narrative that helps them truly understand how they have become who they are, why they feel what they feel, why they do what they do, and how they can go on with their lives.

Late-Stage Treatment

The resolution and integration of past traumatic experiences enables trauma survivors to proceed with their lives with much less dysfunction and disability. Late-stage therapy consists of consolidating gains and increasing healthy interactions with the external world. The reduction of survivors' symptoms and dysphoria lessens the need for internal preoccupation concerning their distress, allowing them to become involved with outside activities and others. In addition, a new sense of personal empowerment enables patients to have increased confidence in their ability to engage in interpersonal relationships and other activities in ways that previously eluded them. Work with patients in the late stage of trauma-related treatment is similar to patients who enter therapy with good ego strength but who are experiencing impediments in their ability to function.

CONSIDERATIONS IN THE STAGE-ORIENTED TREATMENT OF COMPLEX DISSOCIATIVE DISORDERS

This discussion briefly outlines several pertinent considerations when moving from the stage-oriented treatment of complex PTSD to that of complex dissociative disorders such as DID. More comprehensive papers and texts on this subject can be readily found in the psychiatric literature (International Society for the Study of Dissociation 2005; Kluft 1999, 2001; Nijenhuis 1999; Putnam 1989; Putnam and Loewenstein 2000; Ross 1997).

Treating the Dissociative Identity Disorder System

The DID system must be seen as a whole. The alternate identities or personalities are *not* independent entities but representations of components of the patient's experience, affects, somatic sensations, and personal identities. From a psychodynamic perspective, the dramatic and somewhat bewildering presentations of identities may be understood as representing split-off manifestations of intolerable events, affects, or characteristics in the face of overwhelming trauma. At any given time in the therapy of DID patients, the therapist should be working with a relatively small number of identities who represent the current issues to be resolved. The particular identities active in the therapy will change as issues are resolved and the therapeutic process progresses. For example, if persistent self-injury is a major issue, the identities that contain anger, sadism, and self-hate should be part of the current treatment in addition to those who have overall executive control of the person's body and consciousness.

The conceptual model of family/systems theory is useful in understanding and negotiating difficult interpersonality dilemmas. In family/systems theory, the family itself is the patient rather than any particular family member. The family as a whole takes on the responsibility of understanding, resolving, and containing the behaviors of each family member. In DID patients, family/systems theory is applicable to the *internal* family of identities (Kluft 1999; Putman 1989). Using this theoretical framework, there are no bad personalities, only personalities that are compelled to behave in a particular way because of past events and because other identities have disowned certain intolerable experiences, affects, or beliefs.

Despite the tendency for therapists to most strongly identify with the functional host identity, many interpersonality dilemmas can be resolved through gentle confrontation of the host identity's need not to know or not to feel. For example, rather than attempting to induce an angry persecutor personality to behave, the therapist should point out to the host that the persecutor has served a very useful function in holding the anger and aggression that the host has not been able to tolerate, praising assertiveness while restraining aggression. The host identity can then be urged to gradually own more of the disavowed affects as a way of resolving the conflict. In this process, the host identity must actively participate. The therapist cannot be primarily responsible for communication between identities, because this allows the dissociative barriers to be maintained.

It is not always necessary to have important underlying identities immediately emerge to take executive control of the patient's body and consciousness in the therapy. The technique of "talking through" to underlying identities can be very useful in allowing the patient to control the timing of when to expose previously hidden parts. All that is usually required is for the therapist to make it clear that he or she is addressing all parts that are relevant to the situation, for example, "It is very important that all parts involved in the current problem listen to what I have to say."

Therapists working with the personality system as a whole must keep in mind that their role is as facilitator, not peacemaker. No therapeutic efforts can bring about internal agreements within the conflicted personality system unless there is a clear motivation on the part of the patient as a whole to do so. Thus, the primary impetus for internal cooperation must come from the patient, particularly from the host personality. In the psychopathological process, the host personality disowns and dissociates overwhelming or unacceptable events, affects, impulses, and behaviors. To the extent that these experiences remain disavowed, they increasingly take on autonomous functioning in the form of separate personalities. Somewhat paradoxically, if the host personality is able to begin to acknowledge and accept disavowed experiences, they can be more controlled and integrated into the self as a whole.

A particular problem with DID is that the personality system also allows the patient to maintain ambivalent feelings. The inevitable ambivalence of childhood abuse survivors about important issues, such as wanting to live/wanting to die, wanting to trust/fearing relationships, remembering the past/blocking out the past, and so on may be apportioned to the various identities in DID patients, with dissociated parts holding radically different views and feelings. It is common for therapists to lose the perspective that they are dealing with only a part of the patient at any given time, resulting in so-called negative therapeutic reactions. For example, a therapist might feel as though the patient is making good progress in trusting and fostering a therapeutic alliance, only to discover that other identities are feeling vulnerable and angry. Therapists should be constantly aware—particularly early in treatment—that they are being presented with a very limited perspective about the patient and must consider the full range of the patient's thoughts and feelings.

In the treatment of DID patients, increasing internal communication with the goal of co-consciousness is a crucial task. The amnesic and dissociative barriers are significant liabilities, limiting both therapists' and patients' understanding of their needs as a whole. Thus, even from the beginning of treatment, the therapy must encourage the various identities to understand that they are part of the personality system as a whole and to seek awareness of other parts. The identities must see themselves as a kind of family system (albeit dysfunctional) that must find a way to act in concert without exploiting, scapegoating, or attempting to destroy any other member of the family.

PSYCHOPHARMACOLOGY FOR TRAUMATIC DISSOCIATION

Psychotropic medications are generally considered adjunctive treatments for traumatic dissociation. There is a considerable literature concerning the use of medications in PTSD (e.g., Davidson 1997; Friedman 1998; Marshall et al. 1996), mostly for intrusive symptoms and hyperreactivity. However, it is unclear whether various medications are treating the dissociative processes in PTSD or decreasing autonomic overactivation, thus reducing the potential for patients to be triggered to remember traumatic events. The literature for the use of medications in dissociative disorders is much sparser (e.g., Loewenstein 1991).

The use of psychotropic medications in PTSD and dissociative disorders is remarkably common, with virtually all classes of psychotropic medications having being utilized. The newer antidepressant medications are commonly used to treat depressive and anxiety symptoms. There have been well-controlled studies that show effectiveness in treating relatively uncomplicated PTSD with fluoxetine (van der Kolk et al. 1994), sertraline (Brady et al. 2000; Davidson et al. 2001), and paroxetine (Marshall et al. 2001); the latter two medications are approved by the U.S. Food and Drug Administration for use in PTSD.

Anxiolytics have been widely used to treat the anxiety associated with PTSD and dissociative disorders. However, the commonly used benzodiazepine medications (lorazepam, clonazepam, diazepam, chlordiazepoxide and others) have the potential to result in habituation and psychological and physiological addiction, particularly in patients who are vulnerable to substance abuse.

Neuroleptic or antipsychotic medications, particularly the newer atypical agents (e.g., risperidone, quetiapine), have been used to treat the autonomic overactivation and intrusive symptoms of PTSD as well as the chronic anxiety, insomnia, and irritability experienced by many PTSD and dissociative disorder patients. There is a burgeoning body of research that supports the use of these medications for PTSD patients (Reich et al. 2004).

Mood stabilizers have also been used to treat dysphoria in PTSD and dissociative disorder patients. Some patients describe a decrease in PTSD symptoms and mood instability in response to these agents. The use of these mood stabilizers is largely empirical, although there have been open-label studies of valproate (e.g., Clark et al. 1999).

Other medications used to treat PTSD and dissociative disorder patients include naltrexone, which may (at least in theory) counteract endogenous opioids that might be produced by self-harmful and self-destructive behaviors, although there is little evidence of efficacy. So-called β-blockers such as propranolol have been used to treat the subjective experience of hyperactivation and panic. α-Agonists such as clonidine, whose primary indication is as an antihypertensive medication, have been used to treat intrusive PTSD symptoms, including nightmares.

There is clearly a need for more systematic research concerning pharmacotherapy for dissociative disorder patients and for PTSD patients who have survived chronic childhood maltreatment. Until such investigations are done, the pharmacological treatment for traumatic dissociation remains largely based on clinical experience.

CONCLUSION

In summary, the successful treatment of patients with traumatic dissociation depends on a thoughtful and rational approach. Because many such patients have experienced severe traumatization, they must be encouraged to build solid coping skills before attempting to explore and work through their experiences. Until patients can control dysfunctional behavior, tolerate intense affect, control symptoms, maintain functioning, and sustain good collaborative relationships, they cannot work through traumatic events, and premature abreaction (exposure) is largely retraumatizing. Many patients with traumatic dissociation have intense interpersonal vulnerability, and therapists should use good clinical judgment to guide the therapeutic process.

The rational treatment of patients with complex dissociative disorders such as DID must always primarily focus on the treatment of the *patient* and not on the separate identities or on dissociative phenomenology. The goals of treatment should be to increase communication, cooperation, and integration. Therapists should keep in mind that excessive fascination or preoccupation with dissociative phenomenology may interfere with patients' treatment or even encourage the development of further fragmentation.

The treatment of traumatic dissociation—particularly for patients with complex dissociative disorders—sometimes does require therapists to make thoughtful modifications of certain psychotherapeutic stances. However, therapists should adhere to the basic principles of sound psychotherapy that have been established and tested over generations of patient–therapist interactions. Traditional principles concerning interpersonal interactions, boundaries and limits, the therapeutic alliance, and treatment pacing must be respected. Not doing so can and does result in potential therapeutic impasses and negative therapeutic outcomes.

The late David Caul, M.D., was an important teacher in the 1970s and 1980s. He observed that "[t]herapists should always remember that good basic psychotherapy is the first order of treatment regardless of any specific diagnosis" (Chu 1992a, p. 101). This wise advice should be heeded by all therapists treating patients with traumatic dissociation. Many of these patients who have survived profound childhood maltreatment provide challenges for even experienced therapists, and their difficulties have the potential to lead to serious pitfalls and impasses. However, good clinical judgment and the use of sound psychotherapeutic practices permit rational and productive treatment for even the most challenging patients.

REFERENCES

Brady K, Pearlstein T, Asnis GM, et al: Efficacy and safety of sertraline treatment of posttraumatic stress disorder: a randomized controlled trial. JAMA 283:1837–1844, 2000

Brodsky BS, Cloitre M, Dulit RA: Relationship of dissociation to self-mutilation and childhood abuse in borderline personality disorder. Am J Psychiatry 152:1788–1792, 1995

Brown D, Scheflin AW, Hammond DC: Memory, Trauma Treatment and the Law. New York, WW Norton, 1997

Brown NL, Wilson SR, Kao Y-M, et al: Correlates of sexual abuse and subsequent risk taking. Hisp J Behav Sci 25:331–351, 2003

Chambless DL, Baker MJ, Baucom DH, et al: Update on empirically validated therapies, II. Clin Psychol 51:3–16, 1998

Chu JA: Empathic confrontation in the treatment of childhood abuse survivors, including a tribute to the legacy of Dr. David Caul. Dissociation 5:98–103, 1992a

Chu JA: The therapeutic roller coaster: dilemmas in the treatment of childhood abuse survivors. J Psychother Pract Res 1:351–370, 1992b

Chu JA: Rebuilding Shattered Lives: The Responsible Treatment of Complex Posttraumatic and Dissociative Disorders. New York, Wiley, 1998

Clark RD, Canive JM, Calais LA, et al: Divalproex in posttraumatic stress disorder: an open-label clinical trial. J Trauma Stress 12:395–401, 1999

Connors R: Self-injury in trauma survivors: functions and meanings. Am J Orthopsychiatry 66:197–206, 1996

Courtois CA: Healing the Incest Wound: Adult Survivors in Therapy. New York, WW Norton, 1988

Courtois CA: Recollections of Sexual Abuse: Treatment Principles and Guidelines. New York, WW Norton, 1999

Davidson JRT: Biological therapies for post-traumatic stress disorder: an overview. J Clin Psychiatry 58:29–32, 1997

Davidson JRT, Rothbaum BO, van der Kolk BA, et al: Multi-center, double-blind comparison of sertraline and placebo in the treatment of posttraumatic stress disorder. Arch Gen Psychiatry 58:485–492, 2001

Davies JM, Frawley MG: Treating the Adult Survivor of Childhood Sexual Abuse: A Psychoanalytic Perspective. New York, Basic Books, 1994

De Yong M: Self-injurious behavior in incest victims: a research note. Child Welfare 61:577–584, 1982

Foa EB, Kozak MJ: Emotional processing of fear: exposure to corrective information. Psychol Bull 99:20–35, 1986

Foa EB, Steketee G, Rothbaum BO: Behavioral/cognitive conceptualizations of post-traumatic stress disorder. Behav Ther 20:155–176, 1989

Foa EB, Rothbaum BO, Steketee GS: Treatment of rape victims. J Interpers Violence 8:256–276, 1993

Friedman MJ: Current and future drug treatment for PTSD. Psychiatr Ann 8:461–468, 1998

Hastings T, Kern JM: Relationship between bulimia, childhood sexual abuse, and family environment. Int J Eat Disord 15:103–111, 1994

Herman JL: Complex PTSD: a syndrome in survivors of prolonged and repeated trauma. J Trauma Stress 5:377–391, 1992a

Herman JL: Trauma and Recovery. New York, Basic Books, 1992b

Himber J: Blood rituals: self-cutting in female psychiatric patients. Psychother 31:620–631, 1994

International Society for the Study of Dissociation: Guidelines for the treatment of dissociative identity disorder in adults. J Trauma Dissociation 6:69–149, 2005

Keane TM, Fairbank JA, Caddell JM, et al: Implosive (flooding) therapy reduces symptoms of PTSD in Vietnam combat veterans. Behav Ther 20:245–260, 1989

Kluft RP: An overview of the psychotherapy of dissociative identity disorder. Am J Psychother 53:289–319, 1999

Kluft RP: Dissociative identity disorder, in Treatment of Psychiatric Disorders, Vol 2. Edited by Gabbard GO. Washington, DC, American Psychiatric Publishing, 2001, pp 1653–1693

Loewenstein RJ: Rational psychopharmacology in the treatment of multiple personality disorder. Psychiatr Clin North Am 14:721–740. 1991

Marshall RD, Stein DJ, Liebowitz MR, et al: A pharmacotherapy algorithm in the treatment of post-traumatic stress disorder. Psychiatr Ann 26:217–226, 1996

Marshall RD, Beebe KL, Oldham M, et al: Efficacy and safety of paroxetine treatment for chronic PTSD: a fixed-dose, placebo-controlled study. Am J Psychiatry 158:1982–1988, 2001

Meichenbaum D: Stress inoculation training for coping with stressors. Clin Psychol 4:4–7, 1996

Miller DAF, McCluskey-Fawcett K: The relationship between childhood sexual abuse and subsequent onset of bulimia nervosa. Child Abuse Negl 17:305–314, 1993

Najavits LM, Weiss RD, Shaw SR: The link between substance abuse and posttraumatic stress disorder in women: a research review. Am J Addict 6:273–283, 1997

Nijenhuis ERS: Somatoform Dissociation: Phenomena, Measurement, and Theoretical Issues. Assen, The Netherlands, Van Gorcum, 1999

North CS: Somatization in survivors of catastrophic trauma: a methodological review. Environ Health Perspect 110:637–640, 2002

Paul JP, Catania J, Pollack L, et al: Understanding childhood sexual abuse as a predictor of sexual risk-taking among men who have sex with men: the urban men's health study. Child Abuse Negl 25:557–584, 2001

Perkins BR, Rouanzoin CC. A critical evaluation of current views regarding eye movement desensitization and reprocessing (EMDR): clarifying points of confusion. J Clin Psychol 58:77–97, 2002

Putnam FW: Diagnosis and Treatment of Multiple Personality Disorder. New York, Guilford, 1989

Putnam FW, Loewenstein RJ: Dissociative identity disorder, in Comprehensive Textbook of Psychiatry, Vol 7. Edited by Kaplan HI, Sadock BJ. Baltimore, MD, Williams & Wilkins 2000, pp 1552–1564

Reich DB, Winternitz S, Hennen J, et al: A preliminary study of risperidone in the treatment of posttraumatic stress disorder related to childhood abuse in women. J Clin Psychiatry 65:1601–1606, 2004

Ross CA: Dissociative Identity Disorder: Diagnosis, Clinical Features, and Treatment of Multiple Personality. New York, Wiley, 1997

Santa Mina EE, Gallop RM: Childhood sexual and physical abuse and adult self-harm and suicidal behaviour: a literature review. Can J Psychiatry 43:793–800, 1998

Schiffer F, Teicher MH, Papanicolaou AC: Evoked potential evidence for right brain activity during the recall of traumatic memories. J Neuropsychiatry Clin Neurosci 7:169–175, 1995

Shapiro F: Eye Movement Desensitization and Reprocessing: Basic Principles, Protocols, and Procedures, 2nd Edition. New York, Guilford, 2001

Shapiro S: Self-mutilation and self-blame in incest victims. Am J Psychother 41:46–54, 1987

Stewart SH: Alcohol abuse in individuals exposed to trauma: a critical review. Psychol Bull 120:83–112, 1996

Triffleman E: An overview of trauma exposure, posttraumatic stress disorder, and addictions, in Dual Diagnosis and Treatment: Substance Abuse and Comorbid Medical and Psychiatric Disorders. Edited by Kranzler HR, Rounsaville BJ. New York, Marcel Dekker, 1998, pp 263–316

van der Kolk BA, Dreyfuss D, Michaels M, et al: Fluoxetine in post-traumatic stress disorder. J Clin Psychiatry 55:517–522, 1994

van der Kolk BA, McFarlane AC, Weisaeth L (eds): Traumatic Stress: The Effects of Overwhelming Experience on Mind, Body, and Society. New York, Guilford, 1996a

van der Kolk BA, Pelcovitz D, Roth S, et al: Dissociation, somatization, and affect dysregulation: the complexity of adaptation to trauma. Am J Psychiatry 153: 83–93, 1996b

van der Kolk BA, Hopper JW, Osterman JE: Exploring the nature of traumatic memory: combining clinical knowledge with laboratory methods. Journal of Aggressoin, Maltreatment and Trauma 4:9–31, 2001

Wise ML: Adult self-injury as a survival response in victim-survivors of childhood abuse. Journal of Chemical Dependency and Treatment 3:185–201, 1989

Zlotnick C, Hohlstein LA, Shea MT, et al: Relationship between sexual abuse and eating pathology. Int J Eat Disord 20:129–134, 1996

AFTERWORD

Traumatic dissociation is neither an oxymoron nor a redundancy. As the chapters in this book indicate, trauma commonly but not inevitably triggers dissociation, and those with dissociative symptoms or disorders often but not always have histories of traumatic stressors. Traumatic stress is a sudden discontinuity of experience, substituting threat for safety; overwhelming fear, pain, and uncertainty for predictability of the environment and internal state; and autonomic and hypothalamic-pituitary-adrenal (HPA) axis arousal for internal homeostasis. There is accumulating evidence that dissociative responses during and immediately after trauma are common and often adaptive, allowing for potentially life-saving control in the face of overwhelming threat. It is often better not to get the big picture at a time of extreme danger but rather to focus attention on control of responses that might elicit more harm or to find safe means of exiting the threatening situation. There seems to be a poststress time period of days to weeks in which most individuals engage in processing of traumatic experiences, allowing them to acknowledge, bear, and put into perspective traumatic experiences and their implications. This can allow for a modulation of the emotional and physiological impact of the trauma, providing a gradual desensitization of traumatic stimuli.

However, persistent dissociation seems to set some individuals on a different path. Although dissociation may provide the appearance of emotional control over the arousing impact of life-threatening stress, it can have the paradoxical effect of transforming physical helplessness at the time of the trauma into psychological helplessness during the periodic incursions of traumatic memories and associations into consciousness. Such individuals often feel strangely in control of events at the time of the trauma, denying their fundamental helplessness at times of being physically overwhelmed, but then experience intrusive thoughts, flashbacks, nightmares, numbing, amnesia, and hyperarousal as a kind of retraumatization. Thus these symptoms seem to sensitize rather than produce habituation to traumatic experiences, perpetuating further acute stress disorder, posttraumatic stress disorder (PTSD), and dissociative symptoms.

As this book demonstrates, major advances have occurred in our understanding of traumatic dissociation. We have more systematic measures of the phenomena associated with it and more knowledge of comorbid risk factors, such as disorganized attachment in childhood, early physical and sexual abuse, and depression. We have a better understanding of the activation of stress response systems, such as sympathetic nervous system arousal, impaired parasympathetic soothing, and HPA dysregulation, including initial hyperactivation followed by low cortisol levels, loss of normal diurnal variation, and hyperresponsiveness to subsequent stressors. This HPA abnormality has been associated with a dysregulatory cascade either associated with or causing hippocampal damage. Smaller hippocampal volume has been found to be associated with PTSD and dissociative symptoms. Although debate continues regarding the possibility that the smaller volume is a genetically based vulnerability to PTSD and dissociation or a result of glucocorticoid abnormalities, the association has become clear.

Imaginative use of functional magnetic resonance imaging and other new brain imaging technologies has provided fascinating glimpses into the activity of brain regions involved in dissociative symptoms. The normal integration of systems that regulate emotion (dorsolateral prefrontal cortex, anterior cingulate, subgenual cingulate, and amygdala), autonomic nervous system activity (insula, thalamus), sensation (parietal and temporal lobes, occipital cortex, and cerebellum), attention (thalamus, anterior cingulate, frontal cortex), and memory (hippocampus) can be disrupted in specific ways that compromise integration of identity, memory, and consciousness. Traumatic dissociation is a special kind of body/mind problem in which psychosomatic threat and damage is reflected in dysfunction of the brain.

Moving beyond the neuropsychological and neurobiological understanding of traumatic dissociation, the clinical section of the book outlines a series of imperatives for treatment. In completion of psychiatric assessment, multidimensional psychometric assessment should be based on empirically validated instruments designed to help clarify not only *whether* patients dissociate but *how* they dissociate. The clinical chapters argued that treatment of patients with dissociative disorders related to traumatic experiences includes working through cognitive, affective, and social components of the traumatic experiences to provide methods for ongoing integration of the traumatic experience and a restructured framework of meaning. A phase-oriented approach is essential in treatment. Patients must be encouraged to build solid coping skills before exploring and working through their experiences. It should be borne in mind that until patients can control dysfunctional thoughts and behavior, tolerate intense affect, maintain functioning, and sustain good collaborative relationships, they should not work through traumatic events. Therapists should always be aware how compromised and vulnerable patients with dissociative disorders based on traumatic experiences can be in the face of interpersonal contact and even moderate levels of affect.

Therefore, we feel that key issues in the treatment of traumatic dissociation include developmental history, neurobiological function, interacting effects of traumatic experience, and specific vulnerabilities to dissociative processes that all contribute to the clinical phenotype of traumatic dissociation. It is hoped that the neurobiology and treatment as described in this book provided a firm empirical basis for further clinical and theoretical formulations of traumatic dissociation and its resolution.

INDEX

*Page numbers printed in **boldface** type refer to tables or figures.*

363